Young People in Forensic Mental Health Settings

Young People in Forensic Mental Health Settings

Psychological Thinking and Practice

Edited by

Andrew Rogers
Changing Minds Ltd, UK

Joel Harvey
King's College London, UK

Heather Law
Greater Manchester West Mental Health NHS Foundation Trust, UK

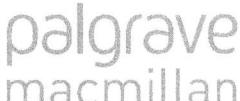

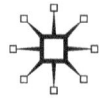

Selection, introduction and editorial matter © Andrew Rogers, Joel Harvey and Heather Law 2015
Individual chapters © Respective authors 2015
Foreword © James McGuire 2015

All rights reserved. No reproduction, copy or transmission of this publication may be made without written permission.

No portion of this publication may be reproduced, copied or transmitted save with written permission or in accordance with the provisions of the Copyright, Designs and Patents Act 1988, or under the terms of any licence permitting limited copying issued by the Copyright Licensing Agency, Saffron House, 6–10 Kirby Street, London EC1N 8TS.

Any person who does any unauthorized act in relation to this publication may be liable to criminal prosecution and civil claims for damages.

The authors have asserted their rights to be identified as the authors of this work in accordance with the Copyright, Designs and Patents Act 1988.

First published 2015 by
PALGRAVE MACMILLAN

Palgrave Macmillan in the UK is an imprint of Macmillan Publishers Limited, registered in England, company number 785998, of Houndmills, Basingstoke, Hampshire RG21 6XS.

Palgrave Macmillan in the US is a division of St Martin's Press LLC, 175 Fifth Avenue, New York, NY 10010.

Palgrave Macmillan is the global academic imprint of the above companies and has companies and representatives throughout the world.

Palgrave® and Macmillan® are registered trademarks in the United States, the United Kingdom, Europe and other countries.

ISBN 978–1–137–35978–0 hardback
ISBN 978–1–137–35979–7 paperback

This book is printed on paper suitable for recycling and made from fully managed and sustained forest sources. Logging, pulping and manufacturing processes are expected to conform to the environmental regulations of the country of origin.

A catalogue record for this book is available from the British Library.

Library of Congress Cataloging-in-Publication Data
Young people in forensic mental health settings : psychological thinking and
   practice / [edited by] Andrew Rogers, Changing Minds Ltd, Joel Harvey,
   King's College London, UK, Heather Law, Greater Manchester West Health
   NHS Foundation Trust, UK.
     pages   cm
   ISBN 978–1–137–35978–0 (hardback)
   1. Forensic psychology.   2. Mentally ill offenders.   3. Behavioral
assessment of children.   4. Behavioral assessment of teenagers.
   I. Rogers, Andrew, 1975–   II. Harvey, Joel.   III. Law, Heather, 1984–
RA1148.Y69 2015
614'.15—dc23   2015013462

Contents

List of Illustrations vii

Foreword ix

Acknowledgements xi

Notes on Contributors xii

List of Abbreviations xx

1 Introduction 1
   Andrew Rogers, Joel Harvey, Heather Law and Jenny Taylor

2 'Through My Eyes': A Young Person's Experience of Forensic
   Mental Health Settings 20
   Lola-Rose Morris, Emma Jamieson and Rebecca Marshall

3 Psychological Practice in Community Settings 44
   Simone Fox and Berit Ritchie

4 Psychological Practice in Secure Settings 64
   Clare Snodgrass and Jackie Preston

5 Youth Violence Risk Assessment: A Framework for Practice 96
   Lorraine Johnstone and Leanne Gregory

6 Whole Systems Approaches 123
   Brigitte Squire, Tom Jefford and Cindy Cupit Swenson

7 Violence among Young People: A Framework for Assessment and
   Intervention 143
   Wendy Morgan

8 Sexually Harmful Behaviour 167
   Trudy Potter and Sarah Reeves

9 Fire-Setting in Adolescence 204
   Abigail Willis

10 Self-Harming Behaviour 226
   Joel Harvey, Alison Sillence and Kirsty Smedley

11 Substance Misuse 253
   Lisa Shostak and Ben Harper

12	Intellectual Disabilities *Charlotte Staniforth and Yve Griffin*	286
13	Autism Spectrum Disorder *Yve Griffin and Charlotte Staniforth*	316
14	Young People's Self-Disclosure in Secure Forensic Settings *Joel Harvey and Luke Endersby*	344
15	Developing Safe and Strong Foundations: The DART Framework *Andrew Rogers and Miranda Budd*	356

Index 390

Illustrations

Figures

1.1	Overview of services	5
3.1	'Fit' for aggression	54
4.1	A model of psychological provision	74
5.1	Formulation of risk of violence	107
5.2	The process of risk formulation	108
7.1	Framework for the assessment and intervention with violence (FAIV)	145
7.2	Social-ecological model of youth violence	151
8.1	'Fit' for problem sexual behaviour	190
8.2	'Fit' for social isolation	191
9.1	Triage assessment pathways	211
9.2	Developmental formulation	214
9.3	Formulating Jake	215
11.1	Eoin's individual psychologically informed formulation	277
11.2	Example of Eoin's maintenance cycles for use of cannabis	279
11.3	Example of Eoin's maintenance cycles for use of cocaine	279
12.1	Psychological formulation	309
15.1	The DART house of parenting	371
15.2	Feeling safe	377
15.3	Comfort and co-regulation	380
15.4	Making relationships	381
15.5	Managing behaviour and risk	382

Tables

4.1	Overview of secure settings	65
5.1	Summary of risk factors for Eric	112
9.1	Areas of work for high-risk fire-setting, to be completed with individual and wider system	220
11.1	The classification of substances and maximum penalties for drug possession, supply (dealing) and production for adults in the UK	259
12.1	Table of impairments associated with ID	288
13.1	Difficulties associated with ASD	317
15.1	High-risk attachment behaviours	366

Boxes

4.1	Case example 1	77
4.2	Case example 2	79
4.3	Case example 3	80
4.4	Case example 4	84
4.5	Case example 5	85
4.6	Case example 6	86
11.1	Factors indicating high risk	265
12.1	Suggested adaptations of interventions for young people with an ID	302

Foreword

Adolescence has long been regarded in Western cultures as a period of transition, a time of protracted uncertainty and unease. Expectations are unclear and boundaries confused, as developing individuals 'experiment' with gradually maturing versions of themselves. One well-known manifestation of the turbulence that sometimes results is that the mid-teenage years represent the peak of the 'age-crime curve'. The social context within which all this occurs is itself constantly evolving, as large-scale cultural, economic and political forces bear down upon families and individuals. The changing structure of society is such that this period is now viewed as extending even later in life, as the concept of 'emerging adulthood' has been articulated and explored.

The majority of us come through this reasonably unscathed. But for a proportion, the sequence of events can be less favourable. Our awareness of the difficulties they face is compounded by recognising that what is at stake may be more than just their immediate needs. Whether or not the sometimes severely pressing problems are resolved can have profound implications for future years, even decades, of someone's life. We might think of the teenage years as a series of choice points where young people can travel in multiple directions with a risk at each stage of options closing off or difficulties worsening, with serious long-lasting consequences of some pathways.

To work with troubled young people in the course of such a journey would be challenging enough. It is often made all the more so by the somewhat disconnected nature of service provision for this age group. Such issues arise perhaps most sharply of all in forensic mental health. As the authors of the opening chapter of this book indicate, services are too often experienced as fragmented and chaotic, mirroring some of the conditions and influences in individuals' histories and backgrounds.

But it is also possible to talk ourselves needlessly into a state of gloom and despondency. Fortunately, there is help at hand for any such tendency. There are many texts on adolescence that offer useful outlines of major theories, and others that provide informative reviews of research. The present book departs from these familiar conventions and enters new territory by harnessing both theory and research to inform everyday practice. In seeking to achieve their aims in this respect, its editors and authors have produced a volume that offers us, as readers, some major advantages, and there are several reasons why the book is to be welcomed.

A first and perhaps most crucial one is the applied emphasis of the contents. The book has a strong practical focus, deriving from the choice of authors, who are highly experienced clinicians. If any book is intended, using contemporary terms, to be 'translational' in its approach then this is an excellent example. It is invaluable to hear at first hand, from those involved in this work, of the day-to-day challenges they face, to take just two examples, in providing services to looked after children, or on the implementation of functional and multisystemic approaches which have been among the most promising innovations of recent years.

Second, and allied to this, there is a key emphasis here on genuine systemic thinking, integrating different perspectives on a person's problems with contextual influences both from the immediate surroundings and from farther afield in society. Without that approach, broadly conceived, any attempt to address problems with the level of complexity and intricacy often encountered here is unlikely to succeed.

Third, this is enriched by the extensive use of case studies and vignettes. These not only bring material further to life, they also greatly facilitate the application of ideas to practice – we never feel as if what is being said is detached from the real demands of practice. It is refreshing to find the approach to the topic beginning from the perspective of an expert-by-experience service user.

A fourth element is the recurring emphasis on ethical aspects of practice. Although often seen as marginal or tangential, this is a dimension that arises repeatedly in applied work, far more often than its near-invisible place in most books would lead us to believe.

A final feature is the book's firm developmental emphasis. That might seem obvious and to be anticipated in a book concerned mainly with one phase of life, but it often eludes writers on adolescent and youth offending that growing individuals are in a dynamic state and are themselves looking forward. Yet, when writing about them, there is a risk of losing sight of the important connections with what went before and what may or may not come afterwards. That has not happened here and the perspective of developmental continuity has been maintained.

In terms of coverage, the book has a wide-ranging remit. Some chapters focus on fundamental process issues, including assessment, relationship building, and the seldom addressed one of disclosure and how to manage it. Others deal with substantive problem areas, including violence, sexual coercion, self-harm, fire-setting, substance misuse, intellectual disabilities, autism and other developmental problems. Within this diversity, chapters adopt a methodical template, comprising sections devoted to definition, assessment, formulation, practical implications, ethical aspects and case illustration. Overall, this book is an important addition to the literature in its field, and one which practitioners from many backgrounds will find to be an invaluable resource.

James McGuire
University of Liverpool
February 2015

Acknowledgements

We would firstly like to thank all of the authors for their hard work and willingness to join us in this venture, but also for their dedication to promoting psychological practice and supporting young people and families in need. Particular thanks to Lola-Rose Morris, a young person who has shown tremendous insight and courage in sharing her story and experiences with us.

We are grateful to the many people who have helped us develop some of the ideas and themes in the creation of this book, not least the young people and families that we have encountered during our respective careers to date. We are also grateful to the many colleagues who have offered support in various ways while we were editing this book. In particular, our thanks to Kim Golding for her wisdom and permission to use her ideas, including published and unpublished material.

Many thanks to Dominic Walker at Palgrave for his support and guidance, and blind faith that we would deliver the final product! Thanks also to Alex Franklin who took the time to proofread the full manuscript.

Finally, we are aware of the impact that working on such a project can have on those around us, particularly the long evenings of limited conversation and monotonous tapping away on a keyboard in front of the TV. Therefore, we are particularly grateful to our respective partners, families and friends for their tolerance, love and unstinting support.

Contributors

Miranda Budd is a clinical psychologist and works in both the NHS (National Health Service) and for an independent organisation known as Changing Minds. In the NHS, she is based in a medium secure unit for adolescents who have a forensic history and who are also experiencing mental health difficulties. As part of Changing Minds, she works in a variety of settings, providing teaching and consultation to foster carers and staff in residential children's homes. Prior to this she has worked in an inpatient adolescent unit and a young offender institution (YOI). The work centres on offering specialist psychological assessment and formulations, including risk assessments and psychological interventions. Additionally, she has worked in the complex needs unit in the YOI, providing consultation within an attachment and trauma framework. She holds a BSc in Psychology from the University of Liverpool, and then went onto study a doctorate at the University of Manchester. She has subsequently been involved with teaching and providing supervision for research projects for doctorate-level students.

Luke Endersby trained as a clinical psychologist at the University College London. He has worked in secure forensic settings for over 17 years. He has worked in prison and medium secure units. He has also been involved in the training of other professionals and has been a visiting lecturer at London Metropolitan University.

Simone Fox is a consultant clinical and forensic psychologist, and Multisystemic Therapy (MST) supervisor. She is employed by South West London and St George's Mental Health NHS Trust. She is also Deputy Clinical Director and Senior Lecturer on the Doctorate in Clinical Psychology Programme, Royal Holloway, University of London. She has previously worked with adult mentally disordered offenders in medium secure units and prison, and started working with young offenders in 2004 within a young offender institution. She also has significant experience in undertaking psycho-legal assessments for young people for criminal courts.

Leanne Gregory is a clinical psychologist at Dublin North City and County Child and Adolescent Mental Health Services (HSE), and an associate of the Centre for Youth and Criminal Justice at the University of Strathclyde. She has worked clinically in a range of health, prison and social work settings between Scotland and Ireland. Most of her experience to date has involved the assessment, formulation and treatment of individuals, especially young people who would be considered high risk in terms of vulnerability to harm and/or posing a risk of harm. She has spoken at national, European and international conferences in relation to high-risk youth. She is particularly interested in the impact of childhood trauma on development and offending behaviour.

Yve Griffin is a clinical psychologist working in the Adolescent Service at St Andrew's Northampton. For the past six years, Yve has been working with young people with intellectual and developmental disabilities, primarily autism, in a secure psychiatric hospital. Yve's specialist interests include relationships between risk and offending behaviour in young people with ASD (Autism Spectrum Disorder).

Ben Harper is a principal clinical psychologist working within academia and NHS clinical services for children and families. He works as a clinical tutor on the Lancaster DClinPsy course and the programme director for the Increasing Access to Psychological Therapies (IAPT) Cognitive Behaviour Therapy (CBT) training programme. He has completed postgraduate training in systemic psychotherapy and cognitive analytical therapy and is also an accredited cognitive behaviour psychotherapist, supervisor and trainer with the British Association for Behavioural & Cognitive Psychotherapies (BABCP). Over the past ten years, he has experience of working psychologically within adoption services, and has 'looked after children' teams and youth offending services (YOS) in Northern Ireland and England. He has previously worked as a clinical lead within a young person's substance misuse service and developed practice-based research with this population. He has a particular interest in relational models of working and applying psychological theory within complex systems.

Joel Harvey is Lecturer in Clinical Psychology at the Institute of Psychiatry, Psychology and Neuroscience, King's College London. He holds a PhD in Criminology from the Institute of Criminology, University of Cambridge, and then trained as a clinical psychologist at the University of Manchester. He has worked across various community and secure forensic services, with both adults and young people. He has previously published *Young Men in Prison: Surviving and Adapting to Life Inside* (2007/2012) and co-edited *Psychological Therapy in Prisons and Other Secure Settings* (2010).

Emma Jamieson has been a manager of a countywide service for the last seven years. In 2012, she completed an MSc in Criminology, Penology and Management. This involved completing a thesis that explored young people and their families' experiences of mental health services. In 2000, she completed a Diploma in Probation Studies and qualified with the first cohort of probation-trained probation officers. Since qualifying as a probation officer she has also worked for the National Probation Service and as a manager in a city youth offending service. She is particularly interested in youth justice and young people's emotional and mental health.

Tom Jefford is Head of Youth Support Services at Cambridgeshire County Council and has over 20 years of local government experience. He has a long-standing interest in evidence-based practice, and set up the first multi-systemic therapy (MST) team in England in 2000/1. He has supported the implementation of MST with other local authorities, and has introduced new clinical variants into the UK, including child abuse and neglect and substance abuse. He holds a Master's degree from the Tavistock Centre, and is studying for a professional doctorate at Anglia Ruskin University. He is a board member of the company delivering the first social impact bond in Essex, which utilises MST to prevent care entry.

Lorraine Johnstone is a consultant clinical and forensic psychologist and Head of Child and Family Clinical Psychology, NHS Forth Valley. She also holds a position at the Centre for Youth and Criminal Justice, University of Strathclyde, where she is a clinical lead for a project developed to manage high-risk youth – the IVY Project. Previously, she worked as an interim lead clinician at the Forensic Child and Adolescent Mental Health Service, NHS GG&C. Before that, she worked with mentally disordered offenders in adult settings and was employed in high, medium, low secure and forensic outpatient settings. Her research activities have included studies designed to examine a range of phenomena associated with violence and risk assessment. She has a long-standing interest in the development of psychopathy in youth. She has published on various topics in peer-reviewed journals, edited books, and has produced reports, monographs and a set of structured professional guidelines. She recently co-edited a textbook on risk assessment. She has also delivered papers in many national and international settings.

Heather Law is a research trial manager at the Psychosis Research Unit, Greater Manchester West Mental Health NHS Foundation Trust, and an honorary research fellow in the School of Psychological Sciences at the University of Manchester. In her role as a trial manager, she currently works on a variety of research trials funded by the National Institute for Health Research (NIHR). She holds a PhD in Clinical Psychology from the University of Manchester on the topic of recovery in psychosis. She has also worked with young people and adults in both community and secure settings in her previous roles as an assistant psychologist and research assistant. She is currently working on developing a series of research studies with young people in a variety of care settings.

Rebecca Marshall has been a clinical psychologist within the NHS for over 12 years. She started her career working with children with learning disabilities and within child and adolescent mental health services, where she specialised in working with families with children diagnosed with autistic spectrum disorders. In 2009, she became the supervisor for the Multisystemic Therapy team, working with young people and families at risk of out-of-home placement or custody due to a variety of antisocial behaviours. In 2014, she took up the role of UK MST consultant as part of the MST UK National Implementation Team, and now offers consultation and training to a number of MST teams around the UK.

Wendy Morgan has almost 20 years of experience of working within forensic psychology. During this time she has been employed by or worked as a consultant to HM Prison Service, the Parole Board of England and Wales, schools, charities and voluntary sector organisations. She has worked with offenders who have been convicted of sexual and violent offences, domestic abuse and homicide. She specialises in working a multidisciplinary manner which focuses on risk and protective factors within individuals. As such, she has written and spoken about the need for great integration of offender assessment and intervention work, with the focus on the individual and not the offence for which they have been convicted. In addition to acting as a consultant for a variety of organisations, she is a principal lecturer and course director of the MSc in Forensic Psychology at London Metropolitan University.

Lola-Rose Morris is working as a supervisor for a well-known toy store. She has worked in retail for the last two years and has held an assistant team manager role with another retail outlet. She went to school until the age of 16 and achieved 9 GCSEs grade A to C. She then went on to be a student at a well-regarded sixth form college and achieved a Diploma in Health, Social Care and Early Years, for which she gained a Merit. She is specialised in social care during her second year and is now keen to become a social worker or youth justice officer. She has recently applied and been accepted to be a Youth Offending Service volunteer and is just about to start her training to be a referral order panel member.

Trudy Potter is a registered social worker currently managing a specialist sexual behaviour service working for a local authority. She has previously worked in adolescent mental health, specialist residential placements and the Race Equality and Diversity Service with Travellers and Gypsies. She is an EMDR

(Eye movement, desensitisation and reprocessing) practitioner working with children and adolescents.

Jackie Preston is a consultant clinical psychologist at the Bluebird House, a secure mental health NHS hospital for young people near Southampton. Bluebird House is one of six units which form the national Secure Forensic Mental Health Service for Young People. She helped to develop standards for psychologically informed care across the national service. Her clinical area of specialism is working with young people with complex attachment and trauma histories and emerging personality disorder, particularly enhancing the skills, expertise and psychological thinking of staff working most closely with the young people.

Sarah Reeves is a consultant clinical psychologist, currently managing a multisystemic therapy (problem sexual behaviour) team. She has previously worked in both adult mental health services and child and adolescent mental health services.

Berit Ritchie is a principal clinical psychologist working as the supervisor and clinical lead for the Multisystemic Therapy for Problem Sexual Behaviour Service in Sheffield. This is a specialist service for young people between the ages of 10 to 17 who display problem sexual behaviour, and is only the third such team in the UK. In previous roles, she was a lead clinical psychologist for the Forensic Child and Adolescent Mental Health Service in Wakefield. This was a new service and much of her role was to develop the clinical psychology service provision within that team. She further provided clinical psychology input to the Rivendell Unit (HMP New Hall) and East Moor Secure Children's Home, as part of a multidisciplinary team. Prior to her work with young people and adolescent, she worked in adult medium secure services. She has worked for the NHS for 13 years and has specialist knowledge within the forensic field, both with adults and young people.

Andrew Rogers is a consultant clinical and forensic psychologist and has over 17 years' experience working in community, residential, prison and secure and open hospital settings with young people (and their families) who present with high-risk behaviour, including serious offending. He was a professional lead for Psychological Therapies in a nationally recognised NHS Adolescent Forensic Mental Health Service, until moving to work in independent practice in 2014. He is an associate fellow of the British Psychological Society and past-chair of the BPS Division of Clinical Psychology Faculty for Children, Young People and Families, the representative body for clinical psychologists working with children, young people and families across the UK. He is also a visiting associate for the Institute of Psychiatry, Psychology and Neuroscience at King's College London.

Lisa Shostak is a clinical psychologist who provides supervision and consultation to a range of third sector providers of mental health provision. Her practice focuses on supporting organisations in understanding and embedding psychological formulation and systemic thinking into all the work they do. Prior to this she spent four years with Hackney Multi-Systemic Therapy Team, initially as a therapist and then as the MST supervisor. The team offered MST as an alternative to custody for those young people at very high risk across four north-east London boroughs. She is also the policy officer for the Division of Clinical Psychology's Faculty for Children, Young People and their Families within the British Psychological Society.

Alison Sillence is a clinical psychologist in a Community Mental Health Team for Older People in South Cambridgeshire. She has previously worked with the Cambridgeshire Youth Offending Service and at a low secure hospital. She has also volunteered at HMP & YOI Chelmsford.

Kirsty Smedley is a consultant clinical psychologist who has worked in adolescent inpatient services for over 17 years. She is working as the psychology lead at the Young People's Services based at the Priory Hospital Cheadle Royal. Previously she worked in the Adolescent Forensic Service in Manchester for ten years, including developing and providing an in-reach clinical psychology service for young men at HMYOI Hindley. She was the clinical supervisor for a University of Manchester pilot study aimed at delivering CBT to young offenders in secure units and prisons. She also has a background in working with looked after young people in residential care and foster placements. She has a specialist interest in working psychologically with young people with psychosis. She is an honorary lecturer at the University of Manchester and was a member of the Guideline Development Group for the NICE guidance on psychosis and schizophrenia in children and young people.

Clare Snodgrass is a principal clinical psychologist for CAMHS (Child and Adolescent Mental Health Service) in secure settings in Leeds, and works in Wetherby Young Offender Institute and East Moor Secure Children's Unit. Wetherby Young Offender Institute currently looks after around two hundred 15–18-year-olds, and will shortly be the only young offenders' institute in the north of England. East Moor Secure Children's Unit looks after up to 24 young people on criminal justice or welfare grounds. Clare's clinical area of specialism is working with young people who present with high risk to themselves or others, and have complex attachment and trauma histories.

Brigitte Squire is a consultant clinical psychologist and systemic therapist, seconded to Cambridgeshire County Council as an MST programme director leading the MST services group. For the past 12 years, she has driven the commissioning and progression of MST (Multisystemic Therapy) within Cambridgeshire County Council. Having been an MST supervisor for eight years for an MST standard team, she is now leading on three MST adaptations for specialist client groups: serious adolescent substance abuse, child abuse and neglect, and adolescent sexual problem behaviour. She is also the programme manager of two new MST teams in Northamptonshire. For the past two years, she has been a sector advisor for the Department of Health, assisting in setting up new similar teams in the UK. In 2007, she received a Cambridge Justice Award for outstanding contribution to Cambridgeshire's Criminal Justice System, and in 2009 she was a finalist for a national NHS Leadership Award under the category NHS Innovator of the Year. In 2010, she was awarded an honorary MBE for her services to youth justice. She has an interest in research and service evaluation, and completed some research at the Institute of Psychiatry, the University of East London, and is now involved in the evaluation of the MST CAN (Child Abuse and Neglect) pilot scheme research project, in collaboration with the Medical University of South Carolina, USA.

Charlotte Staniforth is a principal clinical psychologist working in the Adolescent Service at St Andrew's Northampton. For the past six years, she has been working with young people with intellectual and developmental disabilities in a secure psychiatric hospital. Her special interests include transitions, developmental trauma and personality disorder. She is also a visiting research associate in the Department of Forensic and Neurodevelopmental Science at the Institute of Psychiatry, Psychology and Neuroscience, King's College London.

Cindy Cupit Swenson is Professor of Psychiatry and Behavioral Sciences at the Medical University of South Carolina. She holds a PhD in Clinical Psychology from Florida State University and a postdoctoral fellowship in Child Clinical and Pediatric Psychology at the Medical University of South Carolina. She is a principal investigator on a National Institute on Drug Abuse-funded randomised controlled trial evaluating the Multisystemic Therapy Building Stronger Families Model for co-occurring child maltreatment and parental substance abuse. In addition, she is conducting research on treatment for child abuse and neglect in multiple European countries, and is the co-founder of Project Okurase, a community development and health project in a rural village in Ghana, West Africa. She has published many journal articles, book chapters and three books.

Jenny Taylor holds a PhD in Clinical Psychology from the Institute of Psychiatry in London, after she had studied Human Sciences at the University of Sussex. She joined the committee of the BPS's Clinical Faculty for Children and Families shortly after qualifying, and went on to chair the Faculty, and then later to twice chair the Division of Clinical Psychology. Her key focus as chair was to increase understanding of clinical psychologists' role as applied scientists, in order to ultimately improve psychological science's contribution to our mental health. Her main clinical and research interests are in the application of psychology to the problems of socially excluded families. She managed a specialist CAMHS team in South London, working with looked after children and their families and carers for several years, was the Borough Psychology Lead for Hackney CAMHS and oversees the North East London Multi-Systemic Therapy Service for young people at risk of care or custody. She has recently been involved in the development of the NICE Guidelines for Conduct Disorder. Jenny is an associate fellow of the British Psychological Society.

Abigail Willis is a consultant clinical psychologist employed in the All Wales Forensic Adolescent Consultation and Treatment Service. She has worked in community, residential and custodial settings with young people presenting high-risk behaviour.

Abbreviations

ABAS-II	Adaptive Behaviour Assessment System: Version II
ACCT	Assessment, Care in Custody and Teamwork
ACT	Acceptance and Commitment Therapy
ADHD	Attention Deficit Hyperactivity Disorder
ADOS-2	Autism Diagnostic Observation Schedule: Version 2
AHRQ	Agency for Healthcare and Research Quality
AIM	Assessment, Intervention and Moving-On
AMBIT	Adolescent Mentalisation-Based Integrative Therapy
AMHS	Adult Mental Health Services
APA	American Psychiatric Association
ARA	Actuarial Risk Assessment
ARC	Attachment, Self-Regulation and Competency
ARMADILO	Assessment of Risk Manageability of Individuals with Developmental and Intellectual Limitations who Offend
ASB	Antisocial Behaviour Co-ordinators
ASBO	Antisocial Behaviour Order
ASD	Autism Spectrum Disorder
AUDIT	Alcohol Use Disorders Identification Test
BME	Black and Minority Ethnic
BPS	British Psychological Society
BYI-II	Beck Youth Inventories: Version 2
CAMHS	Child and Adolescent Mental Health Service
CAN	Child Abuse and Neglect
CASE	Child and Adolescent Self-Harm in Europe
CAT	Cognitive Analytic Therapy
CBT	Cognitive Behaviour Therapy
CFIR	Consolidated Framework for Implementation Research
CHAT	Comprehensive Health Assessment Tool
CJS	Criminal Justice System
CPA	Care Programme Approach
CYP IAPT	Children and Young People's Increasing Access to Psychological Therapies
CYT	Cannabis Youth Treatment Trial
DART	Developmentally Informed Attachment, Risk and Trauma
DBT	Dialectical Behavioural Therapy
DCP	Division of Clinical Psychology
DH	Department of Health

DICA-R	Diagnostic Interview for Children and Adolescents – Revised
DSM	*Diagnostic and Statistical Manual of Mental Disorders*
DTO	Detention and Training Order
EARL-20B	Early Assessment Risk List for Boys
EARL-20G	Early Assessment Risk List for Girls
ERASOR	Estimate of Risk of Adolescent Sexual Offence Recidivism
FACE-CARAS	FACE – Child and Adolescent Risk Assessment Suite
FAIV	Framework for the Assessment and Intervention with Violence
FASM	Functional Assessment of Self-Mutilation
FCAMHS	Forensic Child and Adolescent Mental Health Services
FFT	Functional Family Therapy
FGC	Family Group Conferencing
FIPS	Family Intervention Projects
FSE	Fire Safety Education
GLM	Good Lives Model
HCPC	Health and Care Professions Council
HCR-20 V2	Historical Clinical Risk-20, V2
HoNOS	Health of the Nation Outcome Scales
HoNOSCA	Health of the Nation Outcome Scales for Children and Adolescents
I-AIM	Internet-Assessment Intervention and Moving-On
ICD-10	*International Classification of Diseases*: Version 10
ID	Intellectual Disability
IEP	Incentives and Earned Privileges
IES	Impact of Events Scale
ITSO	Integrated Theory of Sexual Offending
JETS	Juvenile Enhanced Thinking Skills
J-SOAP-II	Juvenile Sex Offender Assessment Protocol
KEEP	*Key Elements of Effective Practice*
LAC	Looked After Child
LSCB	Local Safeguarding Children's Board
MACI	Millon Adolescent Clinical Inventory
MATCH	Modular Approach to Therapy for Children
MDT	Multidisciplinary Team
MEGA	Multiplex Empirically Guided Inventory of Ecological Aggregates for Assessing Abusive Children and Adolescents
MET	Motivational Enhancement Therapy
MST	Multi-Systemic Therapy
MST-CAN	Multi-Systemic Therapy – Child Abuse and Neglect
MST-CM	Multi-Systemic Therapy – Contingency Management

MST-PSB	Multi-Systemic Therapy – Problem Sexual Behaviour
MST-SA	Multi-Systemic Therapy – Substance Abuse
MTFC	Multidimensional Treatment Foster Care
NAS	National Autistic Society
NHS	National Health Service
NICE	National Institute for Health and Care Excellence
NIDA	National Institute on Drug Abuse
NSSI	Non-Suicidal Self-Injury
NTA	National Treatment Agency
OCD	Obsessive Compulsive Disorder
OFSTED	Office for Standards in Education, Children's Services and Skills
OHRN	Offender Health Research Network
OJJDP	Office of Juvenile Justice and Delinquency Prevention
PACE	Playfulness, Acceptance, Curiosity and Empathy
PARiHS	Promoting Action on Research Implementation in Health Services
PEERS	Programme for the Education and Enrichment of Relational Skills
PICU	Psychiatric Intensive Care Unit
PIE	Psychologically Informed Environment
PIPE	Psychologically Informed Planned Environment
PSB	Problem Sexual Behaviour
PTSD	Post-Traumatic Stress Disorder
RCP	Royal College of Physicians
RCT	Randomised Controlled Trial
RNR	Risk-Need-Responsivity
RSVP	Risk for Sexual Violence Protocol
SABER	Social and Behavioural Engagement Rating Scale
SAM	Stalking Assessment Manual
SARA	Spousal Assault Risk Assessment
SASII	Suicide Attempt Self-Injury Interview
SAVRY	Structured Assessment of Violence Risk in Youth
SCH	Secure Children's Home
SCIE	Social Care Institute of Excellence
SDQ	Strength and Difficulties Questionnaire
SHARP	Sexually Harmful Adolescent Risk Protocol
SM	Substance Misuse
SMART	Specific, Measurable, Attainable, Relevant and Time-Bound
SPELL	Structure, Positive, Empathy, Low Arousal, Links
SPJ	Structured Professional Judgement
SQIfA	Screening Questionnaire Interview for Adolescents

START: AV	Short-Term Assessment of Risk and Treatability: Adolescent Version
STC	Secure Training Centre
SVR-20	Sexual Violence Risk, 20
TASIT	The Awareness of Social Inference Test
TAU	Treatment as Usual
TEACHH	Treatment and Education of Autistic and Related Communication Handicapped Children
TSCC	Trauma Symptom Checklist for Children
UCJ	Unstructured Clinical Judgement
WAIS-IV	Wechsler Adult Intelligence Scale: 4th Edition
WISC-IV	Wechsler Intelligence Scale for Children: 4th Edition
YJB	Youth Justice Board
YJS	Youth Justice System
YLS-CMI	Youth Level of Service/Case Management Inventory
YOI	Young Offender Institution
YOS	Youth Offending Service
YOT	Youth Offending Team
YRO	Youth Rehabilitation Order

1
Introduction

Andrew Rogers, Joel Harvey, Heather Law and Jenny Taylor

This book examines the application of psychological thinking and practice with young people across a broad range of forensic settings across the UK. Whilst the book focuses on working with young people under the age of 18, we would hope that its developmental focus will have relevance to those working across the lifespan with individuals who present with high-risk and complex needs.

What exactly constitutes a forensic setting is also difficult to define. Settings included in the book span both community and secure environments and include: youth offending services (YOSs), secure inpatient settings, young offender institutions (YOIs), child and adolescent mental health services (CAMHS) and secure children's homes (SCHs). However, we would advocate that, in many ways, there is not a clear distinction between forensic and non-forensic settings; rather, a better description would be services and settings with whom young people who present with high-risk (to self and/or others) and complex needs come into contact.

This book draws upon the experience of practitioner psychologists and psychological therapists working within the field, and provides an up-to-date account of current thinking and practice, and the challenges of applying effective psychological approaches with young people who present in forensic settings. This collection of chapters serves as a platform for debate and as a forum for discussing the future delivery of psychologically informed services with young people who display high-risk behaviours.

The book has six key aims:

1. To examine the role of psychology and practitioner psychologists across a range of forensic settings for young people.
2. To examine psychologically informed approaches to addressing need across forensic settings for young people.
3. To explore psychological thinking and practice with young people who present with a range of complex needs and high-risk behaviours in the context of their care systems.

4. To examine the practical and ethical challenges surrounding the provision of psychological approaches to the care and treatment of young people within forensic settings.
5. To highlight the experience of young people and carers in receipt of psychologically informed assessment and intervention.
6. To encourage further debate and promote enhanced service delivery.

The book explores psychologically informed approaches with young people who display high-risk behaviour and who are experiencing psychological difficulties. We argue that young people are not 'mini-adults', and that it is vital that the psychological needs of young people (and their care systems) should not be separated from an understanding of their offending behaviour; the two are inextricably linked. Furthermore, in this book it is argued that interventions to meet these needs should be guided by a comprehensive psychologically informed formulation. Such a formulation should integrate a wide range of psychological, biological, social, systemic and cultural factors, and should aim to describe a young person's presenting difficulties and needs, how they developed and how they are being maintained, all framed within the context of their developmental trajectory. The formulation should also cover positive and protective aspects of the young person's presentation that may be helpful in ameliorating any difficulties. The book also explores the importance of providing psychologically informed systems of care and support in the treatment of young people within forensic settings, and the role of the practitioner psychologist in supporting this.

Highlighting psychological thinking and practice in this area is timely given the challenges faced by traditional mental health services for young people, the ongoing concern about the well-being and development of young people in 21st-century society, and the ongoing policy developments which aim to improve the emotional well-being and mental health of young people within the youth justice system (YJS) and beyond. Furthermore, the breadth of experience of the contributors is unique, for their practice is current and their experience stretches across a range of environments.

Whilst this book strives to emphasise a needs-led, formulation-based approach to thinking about and working with young people, we acknowledge that much of the research involving young people in forensic settings takes a more diagnostic and categorical approach to understanding their needs. With the dearth of research focusing on descriptive need and formulation, rather than diagnosis, it is inevitable that this book will, at times, engage with the diagnostically based literature. In this sense, we have tried hard not to arrange the chapters in terms of any presenting diagnosis, but rather focus on young people's presentations in a variety of contexts.

We are strongly of the view that a diagnostically led approach is too simplistic in understanding the complex needs of young people in forensic settings, and that a developmentally informed, multifactorial formulation-based approach should be paramount.

In particular, we want to challenge the often-dominant discourse of biomedical and diagnostically led explanations of high-risk and offending behaviour, which, in our experience, often lead to ineffective outcomes and reinforce the wider societal view that young people who display such behaviour are inherently 'mad or bad'. In line with Kinderman (2014a), we would support a system of understanding that is based on multifactorial and psychologically informed formulation and the notion that most behaviour is understandable (although not necessarily condonable), in the context of personal experience. This does not in any way discount genetic and biological influences, but does not put them front and centre as primary 'reasons', 'disorders' or 'illnesses' to be 'fixed'. Rather, the influence of our genetics and underlying biology are all viewed as being filtered through psychological processes – in effect, the processes by which our brain learns to makes sense of the world around us. Formulating and understanding in this way leads to interventions that are as much focused on the societal and environmental influences that the person is experiencing, as on the individual themselves. There is now a growing body of evidence to suggest that the most promising interventions for young people who display high-risk and offending behaviour (and, in fact, mental health difficulties in general) are multifactorial, systemic and largely psychologically and socially informed (Kinderman 2014a, 2014b).

Whilst there is not space in this book to debate the use of diagnostic and medically driven approaches in addressing mental health and high-risk behaviour, there has been increasing cross-professional debate and concern for a number of years (for a further debate see BPS 2000; Coppock and Hopton 2000; Boyle 2002; BPS 2003 (Division of Clinical Psychology (DCP) position statement on diagnosis); Bentall 2004; Barker 2011; BPS 2011; Bracken et al. 2012; Johnstone 2008; Moncrieff 2008; Kinderman 2014a, 2014b). Thankfully, we do seem finally to be moving away from the notion that the difficulties that young people present with are simply because they are 'ill', have a 'disorder', or that there is something inherently 'wrong' with them. We hope, therefore, that the following chapters highlight the need to look beyond any diagnostic label to really understand and address the complex origins of high-risk behaviour and psychological need in adolescent forensic populations.

The needs of young people in forensic settings

Research with young people involved with forensic services is expanding as the complex needs of this population become more apparent. There is a growing evidence base that the prevalence of mental health problems among detained young people is substantially higher than in adolescents in the general population (Lader, Singleton and Meltzer 2000). The potential health and mental health needs of young offenders has been highlighted in various reports (e.g. NACRO 1999; Farrant 2001).

High prevalence rates of mental health problems have been consistently highlighted in studies with adolescent offenders in both the UK (Kroll et al. 2002; Bailey 2003) and internationally (Lader, Singleton and Meltzer 2000; Teplin et al. 2002; Vermeiren 2003; Vreugdenhil et al. 2004). There is some evidence that detained young people have a higher percentage of mental health problems, although Chitsabesan and colleagues (2006) found no significant difference between the mental health needs of detained young offenders and those in the community.

Chitsabesan and colleagues (2006) highlight that almost one in five young people had significant depressive symptoms, one in ten reported anxiety or post-traumatic stress symptoms and almost one in ten young offenders reported self-harm within the past month. This study also suggested that young offenders in the community have significantly more needs than those who were detained in relation to education, relationships, risky behaviour, and alcohol and drug misuse. Stallard, Thomason and Churchyard (2003) also found that young people attending a community youth offending team (YOT) had high rates of emotional and behavioural problems; more than twice those expected in the general population.

In addition to a high incidence of mental health needs, young people in secure settings have high rates of learning difficulties and educational needs (Hall 2000; Anderson, Vostanis and Spencer 2004; Chitsabesan et al. 2006), and substance misuse (SM) among young offenders is a significant problem (Audit Commission 1996); 38 per cent of 'persistent and serious' offenders had drug and alcohol problems.

Research also indicates that young people in forensic settings have high levels of exposure to traumatic and stressful life events. For example, Lader and colleagues (2000) found that the majority of young male offenders (over 96 per cent) had experienced at least one stressful life event, and about two-thirds had experienced five or more. The most commonly reported stressful events were exclusion from school and running away from home, whilst 1 in 20 males had experienced sexual abuse (Lader et al. 2000). Similarly, Abram and colleagues (2004) found that 90 per cent of young offenders had experienced at least one traumatic event, and over half (56.8 per cent) had experienced six or more. The HM Inspectorate of 'Young Prisoners' reported that 17 per cent of young offenders had suffered abuse of a violent, sexual or emotional nature, with over two-thirds claiming not to have received any help (HMIP 1997).

Not surprisingly, Laub and Sampson (2003) found that the social consequences of family environment, especially deficient parental attachment, are strongly related to offending in young people. Kroll and colleagues (2002) found that the majority of young people in secure care (70 per cent of a sample of 97) had difficulties in social relationships. Dolan, Holloway and Bailey (1999) commented that the extent of homelessness among young offenders is of concern. Additionally, many young people who have offended have experienced local authority care at some point (Lader et al. 2000; Chitsabesan et al. 2006). The high prevalence of having experienced local authority care may also be an indicator of difficulties in early attachment relationships.

Imprisonment itself has been identified as having a significant negative impact on the mental health of young offenders (Mental Health Foundation 1999). Events that may occur whilst the young person is in custody can also have an impact. Over two-thirds of young offenders disclosed having come into contact with bullying whilst in prison (HMIP 1997), and Farrant (2001) also highlighted that bullying is frequently rife in YOI and is likely to affect the individual's mental health.

Overview of systems

As we have established, most of the young people who come into contact with forensic services have extremely chaotic histories and present with high levels of need and complexity. There is no one pathway for young people into forensic settings and, as such, there are a myriad of services that have evolved in an attempt to meet the extreme needs of this population. Figure 1.1 attempts

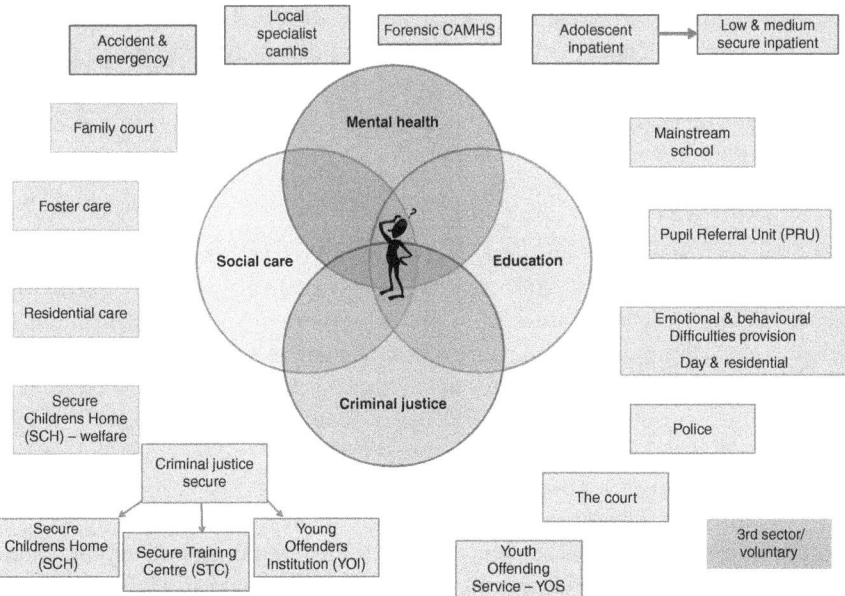

Figure 1.1 Overview of services

to show some of the statutory services that young people displaying high-risk behaviour may find themselves in contact with. In addition, there are a whole host of voluntary and third sector services that both complement, and at times overlap, with the statutory services, and have often developed organically as attempts to fill the gaps.

The services identified in Figure 1.1 are by no means an exhaustive list, and, certainly, young people may find themselves in contact with one or more of these systems at any one time. If we were to add arrows onto this diagram to represent all the connections, it would look so complicated as to be incomprehensible. Funding of these services adds an even more complex layer, and to add where the funding streams link in would be an almost impossible task.

Young people are supported across multiple systems such as criminal justice, mental health, education and social care. These systems all have different fundamental aims and approaches, which, whilst potentially complementary, can also, at times, be contradictory. For example, arguably the primary aim of mental health services is to improve well-being, whereas the main aim of the criminal justice system (CJS) is to protect the public and reduce reoffending.

To complicate matters further, legislation and service delivery varies across the United Kingdom, and across the different systems. Each system (criminal justice, education, social care and mental health) is underpinned by different funding streams, is governed by different legislation and report to different governmental departments, which makes any sense of co-ordination among services highly problematic. In summary, different systems, governed by different principles, funded differently and with different aims, are all trying to support young people in a co-ordinated manner. What is clear, from experience of working within and across these systems, is that there is often no overarching theoretical and therapeutic rationale, and that there is a lack of consistency and co-ordination of approach across services.

In practice, therefore, young people and families presenting with high-risk behaviours often become shunted between mental health services, social care, education and the CJS, or are, too often, left without any support, because they do not 'fit' into any one system in terms of their presentation. For example, education may view the difficulty as a learning problem, CAMHS view it as a mental health difficulty, and social care and criminal justice may view it as 'behavioural' – often because no one system has the 'answers' or intervention on their own to treat the presenting concerns.

What this often means is that the systems themselves may be experienced (both by young people and the practitioners within them) as fragmented, blaming, chaotic and inconsistent, with no one service having oversight or taking responsibility for the intervention plan. This process often mirrors the earlier care experiences of the young people. Recognising this mirroring of fragmented support is important in that it is not a 'neutral' intervention. Such corporate 'caregiving' can often, in our experience, serve to reinforce the very behaviours and emotional needs that they are trying to address.

The role of the practitioner psychologist

Practitioner psychologists might be employed across any or a mixture of the systems outlined in the section 'Overview of systems'. Practitioner psychologists have a core undergraduate degree covering a broad range of psychological knowledge and theory. In order to go on to train as a practitioner psychologist, the undergraduate qualification needs to be recognised by the British Psychological Society (BPS) as providing Graduate Basis for Chartered Membership (or equivalent for international students). This ensures that anyone pursuing a career as a practitioner psychologist has a good grounding in scientific method and psychological science. Practitioner psychologists are statutorily registered by the Health and Care Professions Council (HCPC), and there are seven protected titles: clinical, forensic, counselling, health, occupational, educational, and sport and exercise. The training route for all of these professions is different, with, currently, some requiring a Masters-level and others requiring a doctoral-level qualification to enable registration with the HCPC.

Practitioner psychologists are not only able to deliver psychological therapy. They are trained in a broad range of psychological knowledge, theory, scientific method, research and applied practice. As applied scientists, trained to determine, from considering the relevant (and ever-changing) scientific knowledge base, what type of psychological intervention would be most appropriate to address particular needs, they are able to draw on and integrate multiple models and theories to facilitate their understanding of the presenting needs, individual and their environment. Rather than being trained in a single paradigm or model (such as cognitive behavioural theory or psychodynamic theory), they are able to integrate different psychological models and deliver psychological therapies flexibly from a range of modalities, driven by a multifactorial psychological formulation that draws from a range of psychological knowledge.

The practitioner psychologist working with adolescents in forensic settings has a range of roles in supporting psychologically informed service delivery. These include:

- Psychological assessment – including risk assessment.
- Complex formulation drawing on a broad range of 'pure' and 'applied' psychological science.
- Psychological intervention – including, but not limited to, traditional 'psychological therapy'.
- Psychological consultation.

- Training and supporting others in the promotion of psychological thinking and practice.
- Evaluation, audit, research and service development.

Psychological assessment

A key role of the practitioner psychologist is to undertake a psychologically informed assessment of need. This may or may not include the use of scientifically validated psychometric tools and tests, which are designed to measure empirically derived psychological constructs such as impulsivity, attention, suggestibility, self-esteem, developing personality and so on. However, no assessment should be based on psychometric tools alone, and other assessment techniques such as observation, clinical interviews, gathering of collateral information (from families, professionals and clinical notes) are also used in any comprehensive assessment process.

To illustrate some of the ways in which psychological assessment may be undertaken, the following vignette will be used.

Case vignette

Ty is awaiting sentencing for his involvement in a robbery. He is 15 years old, and has two previous convictions for which he is currently serving a community sentence. He has been out of school for the last two years. He and his 12-year-old sister live with his grandmother, who says she has no control over him anymore. His grandmother has a history of depression and SM. The YOS are preparing to write a pre-sentence report to inform the court decision-making process.

An assessment at this stage has the potential to impact on the environment in which Ty resides for the next six months, as well as what 'interventions' he receives. Sentencing may well be affected by the apparent 'treatability' of Ty, which will be more or less convincing to those sentencing him, and will be dependent on the clarity with which his current behaviour appears to be have been understood, and the extent to which its specific causes appear to be treatable.

In this situation, a practitioner psychologist might consider whether Ty presents in a way that matches a DSM-5 or ICD-10 diagnosis, although as discussed in the introduction to this chapter, these will vary in their explanatory power regarding Ty's behaviour or their helpfulness in deciding on treatment. For example, a diagnosis of conduct disorder, whilst recognising the pervasiveness of Ty's antisocial behaviour, has little explanatory value. In contrast, an assessment of general learning disability, specific learning disability, social communication needs, impulsivity, inattention and post-traumatic experiences (such as level of hypervigilance to threat) may all add far more to our understanding. Further individual assessment might also look at Ty's thinking style, attachment style, or the presence or absence of callous and unemotional traits (see Frick and White 2008 for review).

These assessments on their own, however, will have limited explanatory value without considering the environmental influences on Ty. A good assessment would be multi-systemic in nature, attending not just to the individual factors, but also to areas such as family functioning, education, peer influence, cultural and community identity (e.g. Carr 2006).

An assessment of Ty's family functioning may help us understand the family's attitudes (and thus possibly Ty's attitudes) to offending. An assessment of his relationship with his grandmother could help us understand how he would be affected (or not) by her attitudes. An assessment of her parenting skills will give us a better understanding of her ability to manage and put down boundaries around Ty's behaviour, and the history of her having been able to do so. An assessment of her own psychological functioning may elucidate why she may be struggling with managing aspects of Ty's behaviour. Further exploration of the broader extended family and social network would give a better understanding of the level of social support available to her in her parenting task. Understanding the relationships between her and the extended network may help clarify any difficulties in accessing that support.

As well as Ty's internal psychological functioning, and that of his family, Ty's behaviour can also be considered in terms of his relationship to education. Education holds a similar position for young people to that of work for adults – it is the bulk of day-to-day occupation for the majority of those operating in a pro-social manner, and provides a key source of socialisation and determination of self-worth. Understanding what has led to Ty being out of school, and the roadblocks to him returning to education or training, are also key to understanding how he came to behave in this way.

The presence or lack of peer relationships, and the quality of those relationships and lifestyles of those peers would all also be key parts of a comprehensive assessment. An understanding of the social psychology of peer associations in youth, including their role in attitude formation and risk taking, have potential to shed further light on Ty's behaviour and potential avenues for intervention.

An understanding of Ty's community and environment, for example how easy it would be for him to get from his house to another location without encountering others conducting criminal activity, or without being at risk of harm, will give us a further idea of how his internal psychological processes will be influenced when he leaves the house. Likewise, the availability of leisure resources, perceived levels of policing and attitudes towards the police may all have an impact.

In addition to considering which theoretical factors suggested by the literature may be relevant to Ty, the practitioner psychologist should use scientific methods to look for evidence backing up or refuting the likelihood of these particular factors being relevant to Ty. For any of the areas mentioned, for example, the assessor could ask herself whether those factors were present when Ty committed his other offences, as a way of helping to clarify whether they are likely to have a causative role in Ty's offending.

However, assessment on its own tells us little about what may be effective intervention – it is how these different factors are integrated into a shared understanding of the presenting difficulties (or formulation) that helps us to hypothesise as to the most likely effective interventions.

Formulation

Rather than relying on diagnostic categories or labels, that can often generate debate as to their validity and reliability (Kinderman et al. 2013), practitioner psychologists use psychological formulation to describe and understand the needs of their clients.

This 'formulation' integrates a range of psychobiosocial factors and, drawing on a broad range of psychological knowledge and theory, generates hypotheses that are open to scientific testing, and can guide interventions and action planning. As such, a comprehensive formulation should (according to Johnstone and Dallos 2006: 11):

- Summarise the [young person's] core problems;
- Suggest how the [young person's] difficulties may relate to one another, by drawing on psychological theories and principles;
- Aim to explain, on the basis of psychological theory, the development and maintenance of the [young person's] difficulties, at this time and in these situations;
- Indicate a plan of intervention which is based on the psychological processes and principles already identified;
- Be open to revision and re-formulation.

Psychological formulation differs from psychiatric formulation in that it is not based around a psychiatric diagnosis such as bipolar disorder or conduct disorder (DCP 2011). Psychological formulation is concerned with understanding the experiences that may have led to any particular presenting concern. It can be argued, therefore, that a successful and comprehensive psychological formulation eliminates the need for a psychiatric diagnosis (Kinderman et al. 2013). However, it is also important to be mindful that some young people (and their carers) may find a psychiatric diagnosis helpful, and psychological formulation can exist alongside such diagnoses if they are useful for the client. A key strength of psychological formulations is that they are created collaboratively and shared and agreed with the young person and their carers, allowing an opportunity to include their perspectives. It could be argued that psychiatric diagnosis, on the other hand, gives less opportunity for collaboration and a shared understanding of the difficulty – rather focusing on a pre-ordained 'professional' agreement of clusters of symptoms that sit together.

Intervention

Often when we think about psychological intervention, we automatically look towards the provision of individual therapy or a 'programme' to address a particular problem (e.g. 'anger management' to address violence). However, the work of a practitioner psychologist is likely to require the appliance of psychological science in a much broader variety of ways than individual therapy or set of offending behaviour programmes, which, even when indicated, may not be best delivered by a practitioner psychologist. The practitioner psychologist is expected to be familiar with the underlying principles of relevant evidence-based interventions in their field of practice, and will usually be able to deliver some of the key interventions relevant to their area of practice. However, this may not be the best use of the available resources, and there will also be others in the workplace, for example, systemic therapists, nurses trained in behavioural management, multi-systemic therapists or CBT specialists, with greater expertise in the delivery of particular interventions than the practitioner psychologist.

As well as helping to clarify what interventions are indicated by the scientific literature and what adaptations may be feasible, a key role for practitioner psychologists is in helping design treatment programmes where there is no specific intervention indicated by the evidence base, or where the indicated intervention has not produced the desired results. In medical practice, for example, if a problem presents unusually, such that: (1) there is no standard intervention, (2) the standard intervention has not worked or is unlikely to work, the medic is expected to go back to first principles of biology to tailor-make an intervention suitable for this presentation, for example to prescribe 'off-book'. Likewise, for psychological provision, where a presenting problem does not fit into a particular category with a specific evidence-based intervention, or where that intervention has been tried and not been successful, the practitioner psychologist may have a crucial role in designing and delivering or overseeing the delivery of a tailor-made intervention for that particular case, driven by psychological science and the resulting formulation.

A tailor-made intervention for a particular young person could potentially make use of any relevant information from psychological science, and this is where keeping up to date with the 'pure' as well as the 'applied' psychological literature remains important. Whilst the applied psychology literature will be an invaluable source of information on intervention methods and their efficacy, the pure psychology literature may provide information regarding likely psychological mechanisms relevant to the young person's functioning.

It is to be hoped that this encourages an understanding that practitioner psychologists are not primarily therapists – although some of them are indeed skilled therapists – they are applied scientists whose role it is to take the lead within services for the application of *psychological science* to the work of the service. As practitioner psychologists, we have an ethical obligation to keep up to date with a broad range of academic as well as applied psychology, and to use this knowledge to support services in a range of activities, from assessment and intervention to audit, research and service management. And, throughout all these areas, we have an obligation to try to scientifically deduce what would be most useful, rather than practising in a certain way simply because that is what we have always done, or what we enjoy doing. The positive aspect of this for practitioner psychologists and employers is that, as applied scientists, psychological practice will continue to vary and thus remain new and exciting, as long as scientific research in the field continues. As the science changes, so should the practice of psychology.

Consultation

In the case vignette discussed in this chapter, the main agency involved with Ty may be the YOS, or, if he receives a custodial sentence, the institution to which he is sentenced. Many of the factors that have been identified as relevant to the likelihood of his reoffending or not, getting back into education or not, living with his grandmother again or not, are not necessarily areas that would be subject to individual 'treatment' by a practitioner psychologist or other mental health professional. For example, if on a community order, but still mixing predominantly with offending peers, a consultation with the YOT staff about the pros and cons of him engaging in group work with other young offenders, versus his being supported to engage in non-offence-related activities with non-offending peers, might be part of a consultation which was looking at the relevance of these factors to his particular reasons for offending. Or, if in a custodial environment, consultation with educational staff about any learning disabilities and ways of supporting his learning may be hugely relevant to his engagement with learning whilst there. Consultation with social care staff might include emphasising the importance of supporting Grandma in efforts to be rehoused, so that she has space to have him live with her, if the assessment was that his attachment to her was the most stable, and therefore likely to be the most influential, relationship available.

Training

As well as training in specific techniques, practitioner psychologists have a key role in sharing aspects of 'pure' (as opposed to applied) psychology with other professionals involved with young people, for example, disseminating knowledge from developmental psychology, social psychology, the attachment and trauma literatures, and so on, which may be important to help them in planning their work with the young person. Lastly, practitioner psychologists can play a key role in encouraging an understanding and acceptance of the use of scientific method across organisations, from providing training to commissioners in methods for assessing the comparative benefits of various different provisions, to providing training to front-line staff on single-case design methodology for use in day-to-day practice in order to refine the efficacy of their care plans.

Competencies

In addition to the generic roles and competencies of a practitioner psychologist (HCPC 2010), we would argue that those practitioner psychologists working with young people within forensic settings should be able to demonstrate particular competencies specific to work with young people, families and forensic populations. These include:

- An understanding of the psychology of child and adolescent development and the needs of young people as different to adult and adult forensic populations.
- Knowledge and training in working with people across the lifespan, including adults, children and families.
- Understanding of legislation and service delivery as applied to young people and offending behaviour, including in forensic settings.
- Developmentally appropriate psychological provision for children and young people.
- Complex psychological assessment, formulation and intervention drawing from a range of psychological knowledge, theory and intervention paradigms relevant to children, young people and families.
- Risk assessment, risk formulation and management processes.
- Knowledge of psychological science as applied to understanding mental health needs and offending behaviour, particularly with reference to children and young people.

Outline of the chapters

Chapter 2 is unique in its scope, providing a detailed account of the real-life, 'expert' perspective of a young person, Lola-Rose. The chapter is written by Lola-Rose, in collaboration with a manager from a YOS and a practitioner psychologist. Lola-Rose provides a vivid account of how she experienced the psychological assessment and intervention process across various settings.

The chapter also includes reflections by the two professionals on their own experience of supporting young people. It concludes with the authors putting forward joint recommendations for future psychological practice.

Simone Fox and Berit Ritchie in Chapter 3 provide an overview of psychological practice with young people in community settings. The chapter provides a brief overview of YOSs and the role of practitioner psychologists within these teams. It outlines forensic child and adolescent mental health services (F-CAMHS) and the interplay such services have with the YJS. Given that many young people in looked after child (LAC) placements have a history of offending, this chapter describes LAC services (including individual placement as well as residential placements) and highlights the complex presentations of young people in care. Fox and Ritchie conclude by providing an account of multi-systemic therapy (MST) teams that have grown over the past decade, and examine the challenges and the benefits of working systemically with young people and their families.

In Chapter 4, Clare Snodgrass and Jackie Preston begin with a description of the different secure settings for young people in England and Wales, with a particular focus on the concept of imported vulnerability, and the characteristics and experiences of young people within the secure estate. They describe the various systems under which young people's liberty may be restricted (mental health, secure welfare or criminal justice) and the aims of each of these systems. Snodgrass and Preston describe a model of psychologically informed practice in secure settings, as well as exploring various aspects of psychological practice, including the provision of psychologically informed environments (PIEs). They conclude with an exploration of the practical challenges that psychological practitioners are faced with when trying to provide psychologically based services within different systems and secure environments.

Examining the evidence base in relation to risk assessment, Lorraine Johnstone and Leanne Gregory, in Chapter 5, discuss the development of risk assessment processes over time, making reference to unstructured clinical judgement (UCJ), actuarial and structured professional judgement (SPJ) approaches and the evidence of their effectiveness. Johnstone and Gregory then discuss the importance of formulating and operationalising risk assessment into effective management strategies. A case study is used to summarise the process of an SCJ approach to risk assessment and management, and a number of risk assessment tools specific to young people are highlighted and critiqued. Johnstone and Gregory conclude with a discussion on *needs* assessment and a critique of risk-based thinking.

In Chapter 6, Brigitte Squire, Tom Jefford and Cindy Cupit Swenson give a brief overview of systemic theory and then highlight the importance of taking a whole systems approach to working with young people who display high-risk behaviours. The authors highlight the limitations of intervention approaches that are solely focused on the individual or a particular offence or behaviour, and the strengths of a multicomponent approach, driven by a clear multi-perspective psychological formulation. Squire, Jefford and Swenson discuss interventions such as functional family therapy (FFT), MST and multidimensional treatment foster care (MTFC). A composite case study is used to demonstrate multi-systemic approaches in clinical practice. This chapter also carefully considers the challenges of implementing evidence-based interventions.

Wendy Morgan, in Chapter 7, examines violence among young people who come into contact with community and secure forensic settings. Morgan begins by defining violence and exploring the complex definition issue, and outlines the prevalence of violent behaviour among young people. The chapter then focuses on assessment, formulation and intervention, and includes an analysis of the evidence base when working with young people who present with violent behaviours. Morgan considers issues of engagement with the client group, the importance of multidisciplinary teamworking, and highlights the risk and ethical issues of this work.

In Chapter 8, Trudy Potter and Sarah Reeves provide an overview of the key aspects of working with young people who have perpetrated sexual offences. They begin by defining what constitutes sexual offending and inappropriate sexualised behaviours in young people, before considering the possible trajectories to sexually harmful or abusive behaviours. Potter and Reeves examine the current evidence base on the prevalence of such behaviours and the characteristics of this group of young people, including developmental and attachment factors, early trauma and history of abuse, as well as mental health problems and intellectual disabilities (ID). The authors focus on risk factors, the approaches to assessment and interventions, and use a composite case vignette to unpack the complexities of this work. Potter and Reeves consider the practicalities of working within the forensic setting, and the challenges of tackling such a taboo subject, as well providing reflections on the therapeutic relationship and the impact on practitioners.

In Chapter 9, Abigail Willis reviews the topic of fire-setting in young people, exploring the key developmental and socio-demographic characteristics of this group of young people, as well as the common co-occurring mental health problems, and intellectual and developmental disabilities. Willis uses a composite case vignette to provide an overview of the complex assessment process, including risk assessment in forensic settings and in the community, before guiding the applied psychologist through the process of assessment, formulation, clinical decision-making and intervention. Willis describes current best practice for working with young people who deliberately set fires, and highlights the ethical issues and challenges of working with this high-risk group.

In Chapter 10, Joel Harvey, Alison Sillence and Kirsty Smedley highlight the challenges and complexities of working with young people who may have thoughts of self-harm or may self-harm within the context of forensic community and secure settings. The authors begin by defining and exploring the prevalence of self-harm behaviours. Harvey, Sillence and Smedley consider the individual and systemic risk factors for self-harm, and explore the process of assessment, psychologically informed formulation and intervention, utilising a composite vignette to elucidate core aspects of practice. The authors conclude by highlighting ethical considerations involved when working with young people who self-harm and their families.

Lisa Shostak and Ben Harper examine the evidence base in relation to intervention and treatment of SM in young people in Chapter 11. Shostak and Harper explore the current evidence base on the prevalence of SM in young people, including alcohol and poly-drug use, as well as the incidence of co-morbid mental health and SM problems. Using an illustrative vignette, the author guides us through the assessment process and describes how this can contribute to a formulation in the context of forensic settings. The chapter considers the practicalities of conducting such assessments within the forensic setting and as part of the wider multidisciplinary team (MDT), and discusses approaches to treatment and intervention. Shostak and Harper conclude by highlighting the challenges and ethical dilemmas faced when providing interventions for SM within forensic settings, and during the transition between the different forensic settings and upon discharge into the community.

In Chapter 12, Charlotte Staniforth and Eve Griffin explore the complex issues around psychological assessment, formulation and interventions with young people with ID. Staniforth and Griffin begin by defining ID, as well as outlining the co-morbidities associated with this diagnostic label and the reasons why those with an ID come into contact with services. The authors discuss issues to consider when assessing, formulating and providing interventions for this population, and, using a case study, demonstrate how this translates into psychological practice.

Eve Griffin and Charlotte Staniforth then go on to examine the topic of autistic spectrum disorder (ASD) in Chapter 13. Griffin and Staniforth commence by defining ASD, and outlining the co-morbidities associated with this diagnosis. They discuss the reasons why those with ASD come into contact with forensic services, and the key issues to consider when assessing, formulating and providing interventions to this group of young people. The authors present a case study to highlight how practitioners can put theory into practice, and review the challenges of working with young people with ASD who display high-risk behaviours.

In Chapter 14, Joel Harvey and Luke Endersby examine the importance of recognising the significance of young people disclosing their personal thoughts, feelings and behaviours when in forensic secure settings, and conceptually consider the factors that might inhibit or facilitate client disclosure. The authors argue that the process of self-disclosure is significant in itself (in addition to the content of the disclosure) and outline the importance of taking a contextual approach to understanding disclosing in secure settings.

The book culminates with Chapter 15 from Andrew Rogers and Miranda Budd. In accordance with many of the themes and approaches presented throughout this book, this chapter describes an emerging therapeutic framework for working with adolescents who present with high vulnerability and high-risk behaviour towards both themselves and others. Rogers and Budd summarise an overarching framework defined as the developmentally informed attachment, risk and trauma (DART) model. The DART model is unique because it brings together an understanding of complex presentations, using an attachment and trauma 'meta-framework', and makes links between theory and practice, particularly focusing on understanding and managing risk. This chapter pulls together the key features of effective practice described throughout this text into a pragmatic psychologically informed framework that can support young people and practitioners in forensic services.

Conclusion: The importance of a developmental perspective

We would like to conclude this chapter by highlighting further the importance of taking a developmental perspective when working with young people with high-risk behaviour. We would argue that integrating this developmental perspective into a comprehensive formulation is at the bedrock of psychological thinking and practice within forensic settings.

Young people adapt to their environment with survival as a primary goal, and they develop highly adaptive strategies (reactive to their environment) to achieve this. Whilst these strategies may sometimes be unpalatable to others (e.g. the use of violence), they are often functional in terms of survival or adaptation at the time. Understanding the development, function and maintenance of adaptive strategies and high-risk behaviours cannot be achieved through a diagnostic label alone; we argue that they are best understood through a complex formulation that integrates a range of psychobiosocial factors and draws on a broad range of psychological knowledge and theory.

There is emerging evidence that significant brain development continues well into young adult life, influenced by puberty and our experiences during childhood and adolescence – breaking down the notion that we are 'adult' at the arbitrary age of 18 (Shaw et al. 2008; Blakemore, Burnett and Dahl 2010; Blakemore et al. 2010). As such, adolescents and young adults should not be viewed as 'mini-adults' and we should resist applying adult ways of understanding and intervening with young people. Evidence for efficacy of understanding and interventions with mature adults does not translate simply to working with children, adolescents and young people. Thus, we would argue strongly that understanding young people (and arguably adults across the lifespan) in terms of their early developmental experiences, and their current developmental context, is a fundamental first step in producing interventions that are truly supportive and effective.

References

Abram, K.A., Teplin, L.A., Charles, D.R., Longworth, S.L., McClelland, G.M., and Dulcan, M.K. (2004) 'Posttraumatic stress disorder and trauma in youth in juvenile detention', *Archives of General Psychiatry*, 61: 403–409.

Anderson, L., Vostanis, P., and Spencer, N. (2004) 'Health needs of young offenders', *Journal of Child Health Care*, 8(2): 149–164.

Audit Commission (1996) *Misspent Youth: Young People and Crime*. London: Audit Commission.

Bailey, S. (2003) 'Young offenders and mental health', *Current Opinion in Psychiatry*, 16: 581–591.

Barker, P. (2011) 'Psychiatric Diagnosis', in P. Barker (ed.), *Mental Health Ethics: The Human Context*. Abingdon, NY: Routledge, 139–148.

Bentall, R.P. (2004) *Madness Explained*. London: Penguin Press.

Blakemore, S.J., Burnett, S., and Dahl, R. (2010) 'The role of puberty in the developing adolescent brain', *Human Brain Mapping*, 31(6): 926–933.

Blakemore, S.J., Dahl, R.E., Frith, U., and Pine, D.S. (2010) 'Editorial', *Developmental Cognitive Neuroscience*, 1(1): 3–6.

Boyle, M. (2002) *Schizophrenia: A Scientific Delusion?* 2nd ed. London: Routledge.

BPS (British Psychological Society) (2000) *Recent Advances in Understanding Mental Illness and Psychotic Experiences: A Report by the British Psychological Society Division of Clinical Psychology*. Leicester: British Psychological Society.

BPS (British Psychological Society) (2003) *Division of Clinical Psychology Position Statement on the Classification of Behaviour and Experience in Relation to Functional Psychiatric Diagnoses: Time for a Paradigm Shift*. London: British Psychological Society.

BPS (British Psychological Society) (2011) *Response to the American Psychiatric Association: DSM – 5 Development*. Leicester: British Psychological Society.

Bracken, P., Thomas, P., Timimi, S., Asen, E., Behr, G., Beuster, C., et al. (2012) 'Psychiatry beyond the current paradigm', *British Journal of Psychiatry*, 201: 430–434.

Carr, A. (2006) *The Handbook of Child and Adolescent Clinical Psychology: A Contextual Approach*. 2nd ed. Hove: Routledge.

Chitsabesan, P., Kroll, L., Bailey, S., et al. (2006) 'Mental health needs of young offenders in custody and in the community', *British Journal of Psychiatry*, 188: 534–540.

Coppock, V. and Hopton, J. (2000) *Critical Perspectives on Mental Health*. London: Routledge.

DCP (Division of Clinical Psychology) (2011) *Good Practice Guidelines on the Use of Psychological Formulation*. Leicester: British Psychological Society.

Dolan, M., Holloway, J., and Bailey, S. (1999) 'Health status of juvenile offenders: A survey of young offenders appearing before the juvenile courts', *Journal of Adolescence*, 22: 137–144.

Farrant, F. (2001) *Troubled Inside: Responding to the Mental Health Needs of Children and Young People*. London: Prison Reform Trust.

Frick, P.J. and White, S.F. (2008) 'Research review: The importance of callous-unemotional traits for developmental models of aggressive and antisocial behavior', *Journal of Child Psychology and Psychiatry*, 49: 359–375.

Hall, I. (2000) 'Young offenders with a learning disability', *Advances in Psychiatric Treatment*, 6(4): 278–285.

HCPC (Health and Care Professions Council) (2010) *Standards of Proficiency: Practitioner Psychologists*. London: HPC.

HM Inspectorate of Prisons (1997) *Young Prisoners: A Thematic Review by HM Chief Inspector of Prisons for England and Wales*. London: HMIP.

Johnstone, L. (2008) 'Psychiatric Diagnosis', in T. Turner and B. Tummey (eds.), *Critical Issues in Mental Health*. Hampshire: Palgrave Macmillan, 5–22.

Johnstone, L. and Dallos, R. (eds.) (2006) *Formulation in Psychology and Psychotherapy: Making Sense of People's Problems*. London and New York: Routledge.

Kinderman, P. (2014a) *A Prescription for Psychiatry: Why We Need a Whole New Approach to Mental Health and Wellbeing*. London: Palgrave Macmillan.

Kinderman, P. (2014b) *New Laws of Psychology: Why Nature and Nurture Alone Can't Explain Human Behaviour*. London: Constable & Robinson.

Kinderman, P., Read, J., Moncrieff, J., and Bentall, R.P. (2013) 'Drop the language of disorder', *Evidence Based Mental Health*, 16(1): 2–3.

Kroll, L., Rothwell, J., Bradley, D., et al. (2002) 'Mental health needs of boys in secure care for serious or persistent offending: A prospective, longitudinal study', *Lancet*, 359: 1975–1979.

Lader, D., Singleton, N., and Meltzer, H. (2000) *Psychiatric Morbidity among Young Offenders in England and Wales*. London: Office for National Statistics.

Laub, J. and Sampson, R. (2003) *Shared Beginnings, Divergent Lives: Delinquent Boys to Age 7*. Cambridge, MA: Harvard University Press.

Mental Health Foundation (1999) *The Fundamental Facts*. London: Mental Health Foundation.

Moncrieff, J. (2008) *The Myth of the Chemical Cure*. Basingstoke: Palgrave Macmillan.

NACRO (National Association for the Care and Resettlement of Offenders) (1999) *Children, Health and Crime*. London: NACRO.

Shaw, P., Kabani, N.J., Lerch, J.P., Eckstrand, K., et al. (2008) 'Neurodevelopmental trajectories of the human cerebral cortex', *Journal of Neuroscience*, 28(14): 3586–3594.

Stallard, P., Thomason, J., and Churchyard, S. (2003) 'The mental health of young people attending a youth offending team: A descriptive study', *Journal of Adolescence*, 26(1): 33–43.

Teplin, L.A., Abram, K.M., McCelland, G.M., et al. (2002) 'Psychiatric disorders in youth in juvenile detention', *Archives of General Psychiatry*, 59: 1133–1143.

Vermeiren, R. (2003) 'Psychopathology and delinquency in adolescents: A descriptive and developmental perspective', *Clinical Psychology Review*, 23(2): 277–318.

Vreugdenhil, C., Vermeiren, R., Wouters, L.F.J.M., Doreleijer, T.A.H., et al. (2004) 'Psychotic symptoms among male adolescent detainees in the Netherlands', *Schizophrenia Bulletin*, 30(1): 73–86.

2
'Through My Eyes': A Young Person's Experience of Forensic Mental Health Settings

Lola-Rose Morris, Emma Jamieson and Rebecca Marshall

Introduction

This chapter is unique, as one of its authors, Lola-Rose, is a young person who has accessed psychological services within a forensic setting and chooses to share her story. It is intended that she shares her experiences to enable professionals, services and commissioners to be more aware of strengths and areas of improvement in respect of service design and delivery. Naylor, Lincoln and Goddard (2008) highlight that it is important that research on marginalised young people at risk of offending should be undertaken, since their needs are great and their use of services is low. The other two authors of this chapter are professionals from criminology and psychology backgrounds, respectively, and they have helped Lola-Rose to share and reflect upon her experiences. These authors are Emma Jamieson, a countywide manager from a Youth Offending Service (YOS), and Rebecca Marshall, a practitioner psychologist who is a multisystemic therapy (MST) consultant. The young person's experiences of these two services are shared, along with her experiences of a substance use service, Child and Adolescent Mental Health Services (CAMHS), Adult Mental Health Services (AMHS) and National Health Service (NHS) hospital admissions.

Method

This chapter focuses upon what has been seen, heard and experienced by Lola-Rose. It also includes reflections made by the two authors (Emma and Rebecca) who work in the youth services involved. This process forms a detailed

---

The names of authors are pseudonyms in order to ensure confidentiality. However, those who would like further information can contact the editors.

exploratory case study. At the beginning, there were no expectations about what we would learn and there were no hypotheses set out. It was intended that our learning would develop during the process. To enable us to describe the detail of complex experiences and the depth of those experiences, a descriptive process was needed. King and Wincup (2008) argue that where little is known, exploratory case studies offer the best way forward. At the start of the process we met together and came up with the following questions:

- Why did Lola-Rose access services, and what was going on in her life during this time?
- What helped her to engage with services or would have impacted on her not engaging?
- How did she feel about the services and the workers she was involved with?
- What was helpful and not helpful in influencing change for Lola-Rose, and what helped her to improve her life?
- What can services learn from this young person's experience?

This chapter explores Lola-Rose's thoughts and experiences using a single qualitative method. To enable the chapter to be written we discussed a number of different methods that may have been useful. These included timelines, semi-structured interviews, writing separately and then bringing together the different aspects of the chapter. We decided to use a timeline and semi-structured interview. To identify the different services that the young person had experienced, we started by completing a timeline of the different periods of need and services accessed. We then went on to complete semi-structured interviews focusing on each stage of intervention identified. King and Wincup (2008) describe how such interviews can provide a degree of control over topics discussed, but still allow freedom to offer prompts. Individual interviews allowed the opportunity for us to develop a rapport and good relationship, and helped Lola-Rose to feel comfortable sharing her views and experiences. King and Wincup (2008) argue that the ability to develop a rapport with participants in this way, and to listen carefully to their responses, is the key to successful interviewing. One of the authors (Emma) then analysed the transcripts and discussed the key themes with the young person before they wrote the chapter together. The professional authors (Emma and Rebecca) then both added their reflections and interpretation on what had been written.

When thinking about who to ask to write the chapter, the two authors who work in youth services looked at what would make the ideal young author and were very lucky to find Lola-Rose. It was important that the young person had accessed both youth justice and psychological services, that they were aged 18 or above and were currently stable, and that they were able to reflect without it having a negative impact. Lola-Rose also needed to be motivated to engage throughout the process and share her experiences. Emma and Rebecca identified the young person who would co-author the chapter by looking at previous clients who had exited services. Lola-Rose was identified through her previous MST therapist, and from the outset she was extremely motivated and positive about being involved. She received strong support from her parents, who had also accessed MST services, and her mother also agreed to share her experiences. One of the ideas that was developed early on during the interviews was that Lola-Rose's parents may have different views of services than hers. It was therefore agreed with Lola-Rose to include an interview with her Mum, which she then conducted with support from one of the other authors.

Ethical considerations

To write the chapter, it was essential to explore any ethical considerations. It was, firstly, important to ensure that Lola-Rose was feeling psychologically secure enough to discuss her previous experiences, and that support was put in place if she felt the need for it. All planning and interview sessions took place at a location of her choice. Both the planning of the process and the writing were also strongly led by Lola-Rose. Consent was sought from both Lola-Rose and her parents, and they were made aware that they could withdraw from the process at any point. Vouchers were used as a way of thanking her for her time, involvement and commitment. After long deliberations, it was agreed that Lola-Rose would use a pseudonym to enable her identity to remain anonymous. Lola-Rose was initially keen to share her real identity as she said that she was not ashamed of her past, wanted to help others by sharing it and get full credit for her contribution. However, after careful discussion it was agreed that a pseudonym would be used to prevent the risk of prejudice against her, which could become a possible disadvantage to her later in life. It was also decided that Emma and Rebecca would not interview the primary author about her involvement with their own services, in order to try and encourage an honest and balanced reflection of the service provided. The final consideration in respect of ethics was being sensitive to how Lola-Rose and her mother might feel during the interview process and making sure they were supported. Therefore, a debriefing and support system was put in place, including access to a YOS psychologist and access to the County Council Youth Support Services Head of Service if needed.

Lola-Rose: My background, how it started and what I expected

When I decided to share my experience I was asked about all the different services I had been involved with and that made me start thinking about what was going on back then. To start with, it felt a bit embarrassing talking about the things I had done and what I must have been like. It felt like someone else that I was talking about. I remember it all clearly and I remember how horrible it felt, but it seems like a million years ago. Like it was someone different, because it was really.

We started working on the chapter in August 2013 and I hadn't been involved with any service for just over a year at that point. Altogether I'd been in touch with six different mental health and youth justice services over a period of just under four years. I found it really hard to remember all the people I'd been involved with, but my Mum had lots of notes and letters that helped me to remember. Six different services in four years isn't bad going!

During those four years there was a lot happening for me and I'd been involved with friends and boyfriends that weren't good for me. I was drinking and taking different drugs, getting into trouble with the police and going missing from home. I went into foster care. I was hurting myself and in the end I tried to commit suicide too. Basically, I was doing loads of stuff that meant I just wasn't safe.

At the start, in about 2008, I was seeing CAMHS and was referred to them by my GP because I was cutting myself, drinking and taking drugs. I also ended up having to go to hospital quite a lot for drinking too much. Things then got worse and I started to get in trouble with the police and then I started to see the YOS too. My family then got referred to MST, and in December 2009 I went into foster care and took an overdose so I ended up in hospital again. I carried on doing drugs and doing things that were unsafe, and in 2011 got involved with the local substance use service. In 2012, I ended up trying to commit suicide again and went back to hospital where I saw the Adult Mental Health Crisis Team. In December 2012, I went back home to live with my Mum, Dad, brother and sister. I'm doing really well now, feel much closer to my family, have a boyfriend and also have a permanent job as an assistant manager in a retail store. I also have a Diploma in Health and Social Care and would like to work in this field one day. It's amazing to think that I kept my college course going through some of these really hard times, and I'm so pleased I did.

I usually first got involved with services because my Mum and Dad would contact them, and I'd end up doing it to try and keep them happy and off my back. That was how it happened with CAMHS, MST and the substance misuse (SM) service. Getting involved with the YOS, hospital and Adult Mental Health wasn't planned though, and happened because I was in a bad way and never quite knew whether I was going to wake up in a police cell or at hospital. I suppose with those services I had less of a choice because it happened in a crisis as a result of things I'd done.

With CAMHS, MST and the substance use service, I just wanted to be left alone to start with, it wasn't really for my benefit and I was doing it to keep my Mum and Dad happy. I wasn't really that bothered about it, but thinking back now I think I needed it. So it was all about humouring my parents and there were times when I just thought it was a bit of a joke. I wasn't looking at the whole thing as a serious issue, but then sometimes I actually ended up getting more out of it than I thought I would.

When MST turned up it was kind of sprung on me. I was really unhappy about it in the beginning. They were kind of just there in my house one day and my Mum was like – this is MST... and I was like oh! Nobody told me about this.

Services weren't always like I expected them to be and I remember thinking that people were going to be snooty and that they wouldn't understand me. When I got involved with the YOS I thought that it would all be about punishment and teaching me a lesson, but they wanted me to realise the consequences of what I had done and prevent me doing something else. I also thought that the people I spoke to would be really shocked about what I told them and I thought they would just tell me to stop self-harming and tell me all the things I'd done were wrong and would keep going on about things. When I went to CAMHS I expected them to just back my Mum and Dad up and that they wouldn't understand from my point of view. This did happen with my first worker, but when I got a worker that tried to understand me it wasn't like that at all. I think I had a better understanding about what some services would be like, especially the drug service, because my Mum had sat down with me and told me a bit about them and what they did, but I still worried about what they would be like when I met them. It was really helpful that this information was available though and that I knew what to expect.

Adult Mental Health was a bit different though and I was more scared by them than anyone else because I thought it was more serious and I worried that they were going to think I was crazy and section me. I think this was because they had some serious discussions with me about hospital admissions early on and that scared me. You also have this idea that AMHS deal with really crazy people and I think I was really scared they might give me a diagnosis that would mean they would take my control away. Going to hospital was also different, as I thought that when I got admitted to hospital for drinking too much and trying to commit suicide they'd be caring and supportive but it wasn't always like that.

When speaking to Mum, she thought that people didn't respond quickly enough. She said that when they first contacted services they were calling them for about a year before they actually stood up and said, 'Yes there is an issue'. Mum has quite strong views around that area because she felt that they could have helped us a lot more quickly, and if they had listened a bit more they could have understood more. The reason my parents asked for help was because I was going missing quite a lot, was drinking, taking drugs, and they weren't sure at that point in time how much or what I was taking. Mum felt as though she and Dad just needed some reassurance really, that they were doing the right thing as parents, and just to get some support and know what the wrong thing to do was. When I asked Mum she'd say that:

> I feel they could have listened a bit more and tried harder to understand. I think from our point of view they were waiting for something serious to happen to believe what we were actually saying. I would like services to have taken it more seriously and to assess it quicker than they did. It took a long time to get an assessment done and by which time it had gone past the point of assessment and that is when we started having the Child in Need meetings and it got more serious and I think if they had listened quicker, I am not saying that Lola-Rose would have behaved herself more, but from a parent's point of view seeing your child go through that and nobody is listening or helping you, it is really hard and there is only me and my partner actually seeing it from a parent's point of view and you tell people these things that happen and it is almost as if they are not believing you.
>
> (Lola-Rose's Mum, 2014 interview)

The psychologist's reflections

From my experience as a psychologist, young people in Lola-Rose's position are rarely the ones to first request help themselves. They often do not see their behaviour as problematic and just want everyone else around them to leave them alone and 'get off their backs'. It is no surprise that Lola-Rose admits that she initially went to services because her parents wanted her to, which demonstrates that, in spite of the difficulties they were having, she still valued their concern. Once there, she did gain more than she expected, but this did not necessarily lead to any lasting change at that time. We know that parents are a common and important influence for children and adolescents in regard to seeking help from mental health services (Logan and King 2001) as they are often the ones who can see the issues where the young person is unable to do so themselves. This made me think how fortunate Lola-Rose was to have parents who were so concerned and pushed things forward. Her parents were able to keep asking for help in spite of the knock-backs they received. However, it also raises a concern for me around what happens to young people whose families are less resilient and have less perseverance, for what may be a whole variety of reasons. Maybe these parents are less vocal, less able to navigate the complex systems we have in place, or perhaps they are occupied in managing issues of their own, such as financial or mental health concerns. It makes me wonder what happens to these families and young people. As professionals and services we need to strive to be open and listen more effectively to what parents are saying when they say 'I can't cope' or 'I'm really worried about my child'. We need to be willing to explore this further and offer more timely assessments. We can also be more vigilant in our different roles, whether that be as social worker, schoolteacher, youth worker or practitioner psychologist, to notice when a young person or family is struggling, and take responsibility to ask more about this and support them in gaining the help they need.

The youth justice manager's reflections

As a manager of a youth justice service I think is really important to reflect on what it must have been like for Lola-Rose and her parents during that first year, when they felt desperate and didn't get the help they felt they needed. Kadzin and colleagues (1997) argue that barriers to treatment could be overcome by explaining clearly the reason for referral, the role that the service would play and being clear about what would happen next. Hindsight is always a good thing, but if services had intervened earlier and made Lola-Rose and her family more aware of what to expect from them, then her engagement would have been different and possibly better. Also, we might have prevented things like her going into care, her substance use getting worse, and, most important of all, prevented some of those hospital admissions and suicide attempts. It has been argued that:

> [Y]oung people often faced persistent problems accessing support from mainstream specialist health and social care services. This appears due in large part to inflexible exclusion criteria, failure to recognise multiple and safeguarding needs, and poor design of services that are not experienced by young people as accessible or engaging.
>
> (Khan and Wilson 2010: 7)

It is important for services to ensure they are accessible and to have screening processes for risk and need factors that identify that young people require early intervention. Ensuring young people are involved in service design and evaluating service effectiveness is an effective way to do this. This could prevent escalation of problems for service users and their families, and ensure that we intervene early to save later, which benefits us all.

Lola-Rose: My relationships with professionals

My experience of my relationships with my workers was really different from worker to worker and from service to service, depending on how I felt they treated me. There were two workers that I would say I had a really good relationship with, and that's because I felt they really understood me and listened to me. They also really stuck by me and tried to not let me down, which I respected, and this made me feel as though I could go to them when I needed to and I knew I could always rely on them. Having one person to go to share things with made me feel like I had stability. It was difficult for me to continue seeing someone for a long period of time and not get fed up or angry with them eventually. Although I did, a couple of times, lose my rag, the worker still stayed and still stuck with me. So I think she did pretty much hang in there. She seemed to understand me and know where I was coming from, and I also felt like she really cared about her job and wanted to get to know me more and help.

There were other workers that I also think were good for me, and the things that I liked about them were that they were empathetic and seemed to show that they cared. I was finding it really difficult because I felt quite hateful towards men, but there was this guy that was really nice to talk to. He was the only bloke I ever spoke to, because he was so easy to talk to and I felt comfortable sharing things with him, and felt as though he wasn't going to judge me. There was also a worker who was involved with my family and she put so much effort in and really had staying power and never gave up. This was important to me because she stood up to me and I really respected her for that, and it also made me feel like she wasn't going to give up on me. I remember this one time when I walked out of a session with her and my parents and went for a long walk to cool down for about 30 minutes. I then came home and couldn't believe she was still there. It felt as though she wasn't reacting to me, but still stayed to help. I also had a similar experience when I was working in a group of young people and I was really surprised how good the workers were at putting boundaries in place with us. I had real respect for how well they kept the group together, but they were really caring and warm towards us. This surprised me because I thought they might lecture me and tell me off. Some people would just trigger me off but if you got the right worker they had a way of approaching things that didn't make me kick off.

It wasn't all good with the people I worked with and there were a few workers that wound me up and came across as being really snooty. I actually asked for one of my workers to be changed because she made me so angry: she just stuck up for my parents and I felt as though she was never on my side. She didn't show me any empathy and I thought she was judging me and didn't respect me at all. I wondered whether she really cared about her job and was just there because she wanted to get paid. I had a really similar experience when I was in hospital and I had this one incident when a nurse just told me off for wasting their time, which made me feel really judged because they knew nothing about me. It was hard because you always saw a different face each time you got admitted and people always seemed like they were so busy and didn't have the time to understand what was going on. It was hard feeling judged by someone who didn't know me because I already felt really ashamed and as though I'd let my family down. It felt as though there was a lot of stigma attached to what I had done.

There was one service I worked with and it felt like they never really wanted to develop a relationship with you because I didn't see the same person more than twice. You could also tell they didn't have a lot of time on their hands and it felt like they just wanted to get you sorted quickly which meant I didn't tell the truth about what was going on. Not helpful hey! I think I was really scared about what would happen to me if I told the truth and I thought they might section me and that made me really scared and feel like things were getting serious. It would have been helpful to have someone I felt like I could talk to and was there for me at this point.

I think relationships with my workers were really important and impacted upon how much a service was able to help me. There was something about getting a good match with my worker and I felt it was good to have someone a bit younger and closer to my own age or someone who had a young outlook on things. I think this helped me to relate a bit more and made me feel like they might get me.

When I asked Mum, during the interview, about our relationship with my workers she said that it just seemed we were doing the chasing and every time you phoned to speak to a certain person you would go through so many different people and then the person that you wanted to speak to was off sick. Eventually she was really forceful, but at that point she'd had learnt that she had to be like that, because nobody was listening otherwise. Mum remembered that there was only one service that contacted me in-between visits. The worker would always phone to see how things were, whereas nobody else did that. So just to have that phone call and know somebody was actually thinking about you was quite nice. During the interview Mum also said that:

> There were a few workers I liked because I think that they worked for both of us fairly, they listened to what Lola-Rose wanted and what we wanted and tried to compromise. There was no, 'I am working for Lola-Rose and I am not working for you', it was very together, you know, and I think those two in particular could see that Lola-Rose was quite a bright intelligent girl and she shouldn't be doing what she was doing.
>
> (Lola-Rose's Mum, 2014 interview)

The psychologist's reflections

As a psychologist, it comes as no surprise to hear how the quality of the relationship Lola-Rose had with a worker impacted on how she felt about the service she received, how helpful it was to her and how likely she was to continue to engage with the service. A number of studies have shown the importance of the quality of the therapeutic alliance between a worker and young person in the engagement and outcome of therapy (e.g. Green 2006; Chiu et al. 2009).

To summarise, the qualities Lola-Rose mentions that she felt facilitated her engagement with workers included: effort to understand and listen to her, reliability and stability, absence of judgement, genuine care about their job, perseverance and a desire to help, implementation of clear boundaries and not being put off by her difficult behaviours. Lola-Rose's Mum also mentioned reliability and continuity, along with someone being proactive in helping, as important qualities. These reflections generally fit with what research has shown to be important to young people in seeking and engaging in help. It has been found that it is important to young people to have staff that they feel they can trust, who are good at listening to them and understanding their needs (Frydenberg 1997; Rickwood et al. 2005). Staff who fail to understand adolescents, are not sensitive to their needs and realities, and don't know how to listen to them have been cited as barriers to young people using some health services (Newton 2000). Past experiences where a young person has sought help and had a negative response or not felt they were taken seriously have also been identified as substantial barriers to seeking future help (Rickwood et al. 2005).

So what does this mean for practitioners working with families and young people? Over the years, I have had contact with numerous young people and families who have felt let down by practitioners or services because they felt they did not listen, were not sensitive to their needs, and didn't follow through and do what they said they would; they were ultimately viewed as unhelpful. I have also myself had the experience of sitting in front of a young person and family and them confront me along similar lines: 'how could I possibly know what it is like for them' and 'how am I going to do anything different to what has already been offered and been unsuccessful'. It is rarely helpful to challenge such views directly, instead it is important to be open and willing to listen to their concerns, careful to not make assumptions and, most importantly, be prepared to follow through with any actions you say you will take. We also need to be willing, as professionals, to take that 'one-down' position and acknowledge our part in things which don't go as planned, then step up and do something differently. Cunningham and Henggeler (1999) remind us that when we are trying to understand any challenges with engaging 'multiproblem' families and youth we should pay consideration to potential barriers in three general domains: caregiver factors, including personal attributes and characteristics and family and social influences; therapist factors, including personal characteristics and environmental factors such as the culture of the treatment team and influences of the provider organisation and other stakeholders; and therapist–caregiver interactions, such as the way therapists responds to resistance. Being reflective and identifying the specific factors that may be impacting on engagement for any individual or family then leads to the identification of strategies to work towards overcoming these. This process is ultimately viewed as the responsibility of the clinician and the service within which they work, rather than viewed as resulting from some failing of a young person or family to engage.

The youth justice manager's reflections

As a service manager, I can see how important it was for Lola-Rose and her Mum to feel that they had a good relationship and alliance with their workers. This can be such an important and influencing factor to a young person engaging with a service, and it must have been really hard when she felt as though some of the staff weren't listening, showing her empathy or trying to see how things were from her point of view. To sit in a room with a worker and feel like they don't even like their job is just not acceptable. All services should have processes in place to evaluate practitioner interaction with young people and observe what their engagement skills are like so this can be improved upon or addressed. Lola-Rose talks about positive relationships with workers and how she felt that they listened, didn't judge and really stuck it out when she was being hard to work with, which I'm sure influenced her making progress and helped her to change in the end. Research conducted by Naylor, Lincoln and Goddard (2008) found that young people expressed appreciation of their practitioner's manner towards them, felt that they might not have attended if they had disliked their worker or if the worker had failed to show them 'respect', and that it was important to feel the worker genuinely wanted to help them. Wells (2001) suggests it's important to young people that services and practitioners understand what it is like to be them.

Motivation, access and engagement

Lola-Rose's reflections

I think it was hard for services because I really didn't want to engage and wasn't very motivated at all a lot of the time. Although I wasn't really interested in changing much about my drug use, how I was feeling and the things I was doing at the start, services did really stick with me most of the time. It was strange because although I never started out thinking that I was going to change anything I think things did without me even realising it. Even though I wasn't motivated to change much I was good at turning up because I thought it would keep my parents happy, and then sometimes I started to develop a good relationship with a worker and ended up wanting to do some things differently.

   I remember going to see a mental health service and it felt a bit like a doctors' waiting area, but it wasn't really a scary place and one of the workers I saw there was really good. Another service I went to you could just drop into whenever you wanted, which was really good, and I used that all the time when I was feeling really stressed and just needed to talk. I could just go and nip in even without an appointment and then still see her once a week as well, which was really good because I didn't have a lot of support at this point at time and was living in a hostel. It was good to have somewhere to go and get someone to listen, as the other alternative would have been to go and do something stupid, like go and get drugs and sit in my room.

Other services would come out and see me in my home and most of the time I liked that, apart from when they were supporting and working with my parents to put boundaries in place and then I just wanted them to go away full stop. It was my environment, it was my home and they were coming into it telling me how to do things and I think perhaps that wasn't so beneficial. Perhaps if it was somewhere else I would have felt that they had the right to tell me how to live. I think this felt like they were trying to take my control away in my own house, but then I know that needed to happen and maybe that's why I didn't like it. I remember there was the YOS Officer who came to see me here at home and with the group at a community centre and that was ok, but they were just here to see me and not my family.

With one service it was really hard, because at the point I'd decided that I wanted to stop feeling the way I did and wanted to change the help seemed less available, and I got scared about telling them about how I was feeling because I thought they were going to section me. This one worker did see me in hospital and then at home, but it all felt really rushed and as though it focused on me trying to commit suicide and not how I was feeling in general. They just referred me on to somewhere else and I didn't go for two appointments and they closed the case and just shut me off. It felt a bit like 'we'll just see you in hospital next time' and I didn't want to tell them what was going on all over again because I was scared about what they might do. In fact, I wanted them to realise how crap I was feeling and do something different. I wanted someone to take the time to understand why I was feeling shit, not just brush me off and that is exactly what they did – brush me off. This was when I decided I needed to change and I think I used lots of the things I'd learnt with previous workers to help me with this, and it all finally started to make sense because I was growing up.

When I talked to Mum when writing this chapter she remembered one worker saying:

> 'If you ever want to come and have a rant we are always there' and I can remember one day me and my partner had a massive row about something Lola-Rose had done and I phoned the worker up and said, 'Are you busy?' And she said 'no, what is the matter?' So, I said 'me and my partner have had this huge row' and she said she would drop everything and for me to come down to the office. Just like that she just dropped her whole workload and we went and sat out the back in the big garden area. We just sat there and I ranted for an hour and she said 'Do you feel better now?' And I said, 'Yes, I do thank you.' You know, it was just nice to have somebody like that really.
>
> (Lola-Rose's Mum, 2014 interview)

The psychologist's reflections

When thinking about this as a psychologist it comes as no surprise that, for Lola-Rose and her Mum, it was important that services were accessible, not just at pre-arranged appointment times, but at other times when they felt they needed support. Accessibility of services has been linked to young people's help-seeking behaviour (Barker 2007). Rickwood and colleagues (2005) state that services need to be very easy to access and be provided to young people in settings in which they feel comfortable. This seems somewhat obvious, but the dilemma Lola-Rose presents is that she was looking for different things at different times from services depending on her level of motivation and what was going on for her at the time. Services need to be open and willing to provide a number of options for young people and, more importantly, be open to listening and gaining feedback about how they are experienced. It is not acceptable to have a rigid view of intervention taking place within a specific clinic during set times for a specific length of time. This just doesn't work for many young people and their families. In Weisz and Kazdin's (2010) review of evidence-based psychotherapies for children and adolescents they specifically mention the challenge faced in developing and evaluating intervention programmes with a whole array of intervention delivery strategies, including working in other areas of the families' environment, such as school and home, and using wider methods, such as DVDs and stories. With the increase in modern technology and the role that social media plays in young people's lives, services should be willing to incorporate these into the way services are designed and offered, to increase accessibility and credibility in young people's lives.

The youth justice manager's reflections

When I thought about Lola-Rose's experience of services and what it was like to access and engage with them, the thing that really stood out for me was how one service was very flexible in the way they allowed her to have appointments at home and also just drop in whenever she felt she needed some additional support. I think ensuring she had venues that she felt comfortable with, but also fitting in with how she was at different motivational points, was really important for her and helped her to engage and benefit from the service when she needed it most. It has previously been found that accessibility and flexibility can impact upon young people with conduct disorder engaging with interventions. Wells (2001) conducted a randomised controlled trial (RCT) using a specific intervention programme for young people, with measures used to identify effectiveness. During the process of this trial, he claimed that it was not reasonable or realistic to expect young people to take on the responsibilities of a young adult, and that, whilst we should not be too flexible, we need to ensure we respond to the needs of young people. It has also been argued that:

> [Y]oung people often faced persistent problems accessing support from mainstream specialist health and social care services. This appears due in large part to inflexible exclusion criteria, failure to recognise multiple and safeguarding needs, and poor design of services that are not experienced by young people as accessible or engaging.
>
> (Khan and Wilson 2010: 7)

It is important that services are able to understand what life is like for young people with mental health needs and make services fit with what they need. Naylor, Lincoln and Goddard (2008) found that services need to be flexible to their needs, not just in respect of location, but also with regard to the structure and timing of sessions.

Methods used and outcomes for me and my family

Lola-Rose's reflections

There were so many different things that people tried with me over those few years and I do think that some things helped me, some more than others. At the start, I was working with one service and it didn't really feel like I was getting anywhere at all. I had this one worker that just kept going over the same things and I'd just end up venting and leaving feeling upset and angry. It was talking a lot about my parents and how they made me feel and she just seemed to support them and that would upset me. I didn't really understand what she was trying to do and I just ended up getting angry and venting at her.

When my worker changed it was good because the new worker focused on my parents in a different way, and introduced group sessions with my Mum and Dad and got them more involved. I then had sessions with her on my own and with Mum and Dad, which helped to separate things out a bit, and I think it was more effective because when I saw her by myself I was just able to have time for me. It was really hard doing the group bit with my parents, but things improved a lot with them at that point, and whilst the sessions were quite stressful and everyone let their feelings out, things were much better at home and we were able to communicate better. This was even though I was still doing things that I shouldn't, like taking drugs, but I was just learning how to get on better with my parents.

When I did group work with the YOS, even though it was a bit intimidating, I did learn stuff and it helped me to communicate and be sociable without being wasted on drugs. I think this helped with my confidence too. It also made me realise that I was really lucky compared to some of the other girls, because they had problems that were much worse than mine. There was this one weed incident though with one girl smoking. The workers didn't pick up on it and that wouldn't have been good for me if I'd been offered some as I'd probably have smoked it.

Doing one-to-one work around my offending also made me learn more about the consequences of crime and getting into trouble with the police and where I would be heading if I didn't stop. We did things like card games that looked at the seriousness of crimes and types of punishment, which really made me more aware of things. It was good that it wasn't just focusing on what I'd done, but also tried to help me to prevent getting in trouble again by looking at how I thought about things. I didn't end up having to go to court after this, so I suppose it did work even though I carried on doing things. It made me avoid really serious stuff with the police.

Even though I really hated it and wanted them to go away, MST with my family really helped my Mum and Dad to keep me safer. I had this behaviour plan that involved my Mum and Dad contacting the police if I went out when I wasn't supposed to. The police would then turn up at the parties I was at and take me home, which wasn't cool, so I stopped going as much. I think MST helped my parents to take some control back and even though I didn't like it, I think it was what I needed. They also helped me to see things from the rest of family's point of view and I remember starting to think more about how my sisters might feel and I hadn't even thought about that before. Even though at the time it felt like that they were never going to go away, maybe six months was a bit short for me and it could be a bit longer for some young people who are really out of control.

I also worked with this service that helped me with my drug use and how I was feeling about myself. I think it really helped and it was all about me getting a better understanding of what I was doing and the drugs I was taking. They tried to help me to understand more about the effects of what I was taking and keeping myself safer. They also tried to help me to understand how my drug use was impacting upon how I was feeling and vice versa. I did a drug and drink diary and a mood diary, which really helped me to understand why I was feeling the way I was and how drugs were helping or not. I also started to take an anti-depressant at this point because I was really low and self-harming a lot. It felt as though this was done in a really careful way and the psychiatrist really explored with me which would be the best one for me and the dangers of taking drugs with medication. I felt as though I was really in control of this choice and thought it was worth it to try and help me to feel better. My drugs use did dwindle and I was taking less drugs, less often, and sticking to three types, rather than anything I could get my hands on. Although I didn't stop taking drugs completely it did really help me to stay safer and change things.

When I ended up in hospital I'm not sure what they really did to try and help me. They treated me in a physical way and put me on a drip and things to make me better and I was also assessed by a psychiatrist. They then referred me on to other people and just lectured me about how I was taking up the space of other ill children. I don't think my experience in hospitals really helped me to change or learn anything. Apart from one time when someone really did just listen to me and try to make me feel better they just made me feel more ashamed than I already was. I also kind of felt awful after it all blew over and I was feeling better, because they put me on a ward where there was loads of really sick children and I was sitting there in bed thinking I did this to myself but they didn't, so I don't know whether they did that deliberately. One of the services that the hospital referred me to was an adult mental health crisis service, but I didn't really do anything with them. This was when they talked about sectioning me and then just closed the case.

I think all of the earlier services I mentioned did help me in different ways when I was working with them. Although I didn't stop taking drugs, going to unsafe parties, doing illegal things or start feeling better about myself immediately, things did change. Also, when I was ready and motivated to change, my family, college and real friends really helped me, and these were all things that those services encouraged me to try and get right.

When talking to Mum about things she said that MST gave her and Dad a bit of power back. She worried that this might sound awful, but said it was almost like someone standing behind them saying 'you are doing it exactly how you should be, you know, don't back down from Lola-Rose', and that almost gave them their role as a parent back, rather than just being these people who had been knocked back so many times by my behaviour. Back then, Mum said that she and Dad didn't want to go out a lot as a couple. Mum said that this was 'because we never knew what the situation, especially on a Friday and Saturday, was going to be', so they lost their social life. The MST worker worked with them to help them see that they must go out and said they were on the end of the phone if needed. When I asked Mum what made the biggest difference for her, she said:

> Confidence made the biggest difference for me as a parent, the more you go down the line the more confident you get and you actually start to think, actually this is my child and you have to remind yourself that they didn't get involved with us, we phoned them and we were the ones who wanted the help so we are not the bad people. I think we felt quite guilty for a long time and then all of a sudden you get this little bit of power back and you think, actually, no, we have asked for the help, we have done the right thing.
>
> (Lola-Rose's Mum, 2014 interview)

The psychologist's reflections

As a psychologist, I thought about how many different approaches were used by services to support Lola-Rose and her family and how these all had an impact in different, but not always immediate, ways. Lola-Rose's comments around group work are interesting, as one of the concerns about work like this is the potentially negative impact of putting together groups of young people with antisocial behaviour difficulties. Leading researchers in understanding the determinants of delinquency point out that, due to the often mutually reinforcing effects of peers with difficulties on one another, groups and activities which place them together can exacerbate rather than ameliorate the difficult behaviours they demonstrate (Elliot, Huzing and Ageton 1985). Lola-Rose mentions her concern that this could have happened for her (especially relating to the cannabis use), but also points out some positive things she feels she gained, such as realising the harder situation some of the young people who also attended seemed to be facing in comparison to her.

Lola-Rose also talks about the importance and usefulness for her of involving her parents and wider family in a sensitive way in the interventions, especially at points at which she seemed rather resistant or ambivalent to getting help. This points to the importance of models and approaches which view young people within their naturally occurring context, rather than solely individual interventions. Interventions such as MST or family therapy rely more heavily on the engagement of concerned others (i.e. the parental figures) than the young person to support the process of change. For example, MST usually places the caregiver as the 'main conduit of change':

> The therapist collaborates with the family, using family strengths (e.g. love of the adolescent, indigenous social support) to overcome barriers to caregiver effectiveness (e.g. caregiver substance abuse, debilitating stress, hopelessness). As caregiver effectiveness increases (e.g. ability to monitor, supervise and support the children) the therapist helps the caregivers design and implement interventions aimed at decreasing youth antisocial behaviour and improving youth functioning across family, peer, school and community contexts.
>
> (Henggeler and Scaheffer, 2010: 261)

However, although Lola-Rose acknowledges the importance of involving her parents and wider family she also talks about how she valued privacy and confidentiality within services. This is consistent in research investigating conditions which young people require to successfully engage with mental health services (e.g. Street and Svanberg 2003; Hart, Saunders and Thomas 2005; Day, Michelson and Hassan 2011).

The youth justice manager's reflections

As a service manager I was initially disappointed by how many different services Lola-Rose had been in contact with and how many different types of approaches had been used with her and her family. It felt a little like everything had been thrown at them without a lot of thought going into what they needed and what would be most effective, but when I think about all the interventions I think they did have some impact even if it wasn't immediate. It was also interesting that although Lola-Rose didn't really enjoy certain interventions and took part because she felt she had to, they were still effective in some way and bought about change for her.

Ensuring effective interventions and treatment is important to ensure successful outcomes for young people, especially those with mental health needs who have offended. Harrington and Bailey (2005) reviewed four types of intervention that included psychological treatment, pharmacotherapy, systematic/family therapy and multimodal treatments. Lola-Rose had received all of these types of interventions and I think some were more successful than others. The Harrington and Bailey (2005) review established that cognitive behavioural, family therapy and multimodal treatments such as MST were most effective. Pharmacotherapy was also considered appropriate for short-term benefits, but was rarely effective alone. I think that the timing of Lola-Rose going on medication with the Community Substance Misuse Service was effective, as it happened alongside other psychological intervention and support and enabled her to both reduce her substance use and, at the same time, start to feel better about herself. Also, MST appeared to have a successful outcome for Lola-Rose's parents, and ultimately her in the end, even though she did not like it at the time.

Holistic approaches, joined-up services and transitions

Lola-Rose's reflections

I worked with seven different services, including all of the ones I've mentioned and social care, and it felt like I was always having to go over things and that there was no real handover from one service to the next. Sometimes there was more than one service involved at a time too, and some of them also worked with my parents and some didn't.

When I was working with the YOS it felt like it was the right time to end my work with them because I had CAMHS involved, so I was just relieved because it was one less person to speak with. Then my family started working with MST and CAMHS were still involved, but I think I was probably getting too much at that point and didn't want to see anyone else. At the point I finished with CAMHS, eventually I remember thinking, 'well who is going to listen to me next and hear me go over things again?' I think that was the problem when I started seeing AMHS because I just didn't want to have to go over things again, and didn't feel like they had the time to get to know me and find out things from me or anyone else. I think I did need more than one service working with me, but it just felt like they didn't really talk to each other, so I had to keep telling my story time and time again.

Some services worked with me and my family too. When MST started it was good that they spoke to us all, as there was a lot going on and I think my Mum just needed some help to get control. I didn't really like the fact that they were helping my parents to do this, but it did feel like they were there for everyone. It was all very well and good with CAMHS speaking to me and stuff, but I was out of control at home. I think my Mum needed support rather than me because I didn't care. My parents definitely needed support at that time, I don't know if they'd been able to do it on their own.

The YOS didn't work with my family and were happy to just leave me to it, and I felt happy that I had someone to speak to. I think when my parents weren't involved they were worried that I'd be able to manipulate people and there might have been some truth in that, so it was good to have everyone taking part. It was also really helpful when the worker at CAMHS got my parents coming to sessions. I was quite bitter towards my Dad at the time, so it was a good move to get him involved because, when he didn't come, I thought he didn't care. Those sessions, I think, helped us all, and she was like let's get your Dad here and you can tell him that and see how it feels for him.

I think the worst time when services didn't communicate with everyone was when I was in foster care and took an overdose. I ended up in hospital, and although my foster carer was there, no one told my parents and I thought because they hadn't come they didn't care about me. I was so upset and ashamed at that point. They weren't there to start with because they didn't know, but I didn't know that. I can't believe how bad that is – surely someone should have told them! They didn't even involve my Mum and Dad in the psychiatrist appointment and my parents were like 'she needs help' and he said 'she's told us she doesn't' and that was that. Even adult mental health involved my Mum and said I need to go home to keep me safe, even if that was all they did.

I do think it's really important that services talk to each other and your family. This means you don't have to keep going over things, and it might help workers to feel they know you a bit more. It also helps your family because, let's face it, I went home in the end and managed to get things sorted with their help and I'd never have been able to do it without them. Now when I feel rubbish I just spend time with them and it's a real pick-me-up spending time with my little sisters: they make me feel good and special if I'm having a bad day.

When I interviewed Mum about how joined-up and holistic things were she said it felt like communication was one of the biggest problems. She said that this was the biggest thing she would change, because none of the services seemed to communicate with each other and it was her that was always phoning everybody and making things happen. Mum also felt that the thing that made the biggest difference for me was coming home and us working on things together. She said that if I hadn't come home I possibly wouldn't be here now.

The psychologist's reflections

As a psychologist, and thinking about my previous experiences with young people, families and services, it sadly comes as no surprise that both Lola-Rose and her Mum mentioned 'communication' and lack of joined-up working as one of their biggest concerns here. Just take a moment to consider how many serious case reviews mention agencies failing to communicate effectively with each other as a factor in things going wrong. Lola-Rose and her Mum remind me that we still have so much work to do here. It is not enough to develop the working protocols and sharing of information protocols between services. We also need to make sure we have methods in place to constantly review these and gain feedback from families and young people as to how well they are working, and make changes accordingly.

The youth justice manager's reflections

As a service manager, this made me reflect on Lola-Rose and her Mum's experiences, and how important it is for each service to make sure that transitions and joint working are effective across services. We really can't underestimate how much of a difference it makes to young people if we are good at sharing information and communicating better with each other. Simple things like a joint handover and planning meetings, and sharing assessments so young people don't feel like they have to go over things time and time again are essential. It's clear that the systemic approach that both CAMHS and MST took had an impact for Lola-Rose and her family, and that involving those in the system around her helped them to make small changes at the time and in the long term.

Learning for services

We will now look at what services can learn from Lola-Rose's accounts, and identify any areas of strength and recommendations for future development. It is important to highlight that Lola-Rose had some very positive experiences with services that were based on her having a positive introduction, excellent relationships with her workers, effective methods and interventions, flexible access to services and a holistic approach. However, this wasn't always the case.

The key strengths for services that need to be retained are detailed below.

- Having skilled workers that understand the importance of engaging, respecting and understanding young people.
- Services responding to resistance and being persistent even when young people are reluctant to engage or make changes.

- Services being accessible in respect of physical geography and ensuring they meet with young people in an environment where they are likely to feel comfortable and engage.
- Services being adaptable and willing to change a young person's worker if a young person and professional are not compatible.
- Services using methods and interventions where outcomes and success can be monitored.

The key areas for development and areas of learning that may be of interest to commissioners and those responsible for service design and delivery are detailed below.

The key learning that we propose to be considered for the future are:

- Development of pathways and criteria to ensure that services are accessible to young people so interventions can be identified when required and support accessed earlier.
- Exploration of how agencies can more effectively ensure that the aims and outcomes of services are explained and represented to young people and their families at referral stage.
- Consideration of how treatment can be based upon and effective alliance with workers and remain young person-focused.
- Structuring services to have a flexible approach that is led by the needs of young people and provision of a non-clinic-based approach.
- Implementation of effective evidence-based programmes for young people with mental health problems who offend (or those at risk of offending), and systems for success to be measured.
- Holistic involvement of parents and other professionals in treatment in a systemic way.

Reflections on the experience of writing the chapter

We would like to end by reflecting on the experience of writing this chapter. As professionals we (Emma and Rebecca) felt very privileged to meet with Lola-Rose and her Mum and have the opportunity of sharing the experience of writing this chapter. To meet a family four years after they have first accessed services is not something we have the opportunity to do very often, especially not in such an intimate way. It felt very different to a professional and service user relationship, because we worked very closely over a long period of time and professional boundaries were less of an issue, and this felt fine.

What struck us most was the fact that Lola-Rose had developed into a mature and responsible young adult, despite the relatively recent trauma that had occurred within her life. It felt as though she had grown up very quickly and was really able to reflect on experiences in her past and respond to these in a very positive way. Looking back at the treatment and intervention outcomes from our services, we certainly didn't think this was a case where we would expect the issues to be resolved in any shape or form, and this is backed up by the further support and services she continued to access into the first few years of her adult life. However, her story makes us wonder about the cumulative impact of interventions, particularly that their true impact may not be immediately apparent, but may be more evident at some point further along the line. The fact that, at a time of real need, Lola-Rose was able to return to her family home and develop positive relationships with family members, and that her family were able to accept her back, is a testament to their strength. As professionals, this made us ever more aware of the importance of a supportive family environment, and that the support of services offering help to families to make changes is key. What was very clear with Lola's case was that, whilst services helped her and her family, she made the choice to make changes and sustain them in the end.

When, I, Lola-Rose, think about this process, it's been really good working with the two other authors and I think they've been really aware of how I'm feeling and have responded and helped me get things done when they've sensed I've felt a bit stuck and out of my depth. I've felt equal to them throughout the process and it really feels as though I own this chapter and have played an important part in making it happen. During the process, I looked back at my diary entries and they were really depressing. I couldn't believe how my life completely revolved around the drugs I was taking and how I was always writing about how rubbish I felt. I'd almost forgotten about how bad I was feeling and how depressed I was back then. The process of looking back at my diary was helpful and re-enforced how much better life is now. Sometimes I would feel a little bit stressed out after the interview sessions, but I would always talk to my Mum about this and she would reassure me. I knew that I could contact the professionals to talk to them if I needed to, but my relationship with my Mum is really good now and doing this with her worked really well. It was also good to do the interviews in small sections and space them out, as this gave me time to talk to Mum, reflect, and get myself prepared and think about what was next. I think all services helped in some way, but the biggest thing for me was making my mind up to make things change and going home and getting the support from my family.

It's been really good for me having a project in life that is different to work and I'm really grateful that I've had the opportunity to be involved. I feel very happy that someone has wanted to hear about my experiences, and proud that I've contributed and that the other people involved picked me for this project. I know that my Mum feels really proud and so pleased that I have been able to take part and share my experiences too.

References

Barker, G. (2007) *Adolescents, Social Support and Help-Seeking Behaviour: An International Literature Review and Programme Consultation with Recommendations for Action*. Geneva: WHO Press.
Chiu, A., McLeod, B.D., Har, K., and Wood, J.J. (2009) 'Child-therapist alliance and clinical outcomes in cognitive behavioural therapy for child anxiety disorders', *Journal of Child Psychology and Psychiatry*, 50: 751–758.
Cunningham, P.B. and Henggeler, S.W. (1999) 'Engaging multiproblem families in treatment: Lessons learned throughout the development of multisystemic therapy', *Family Process*, 38: 265–286.
Day, C., Michelson, D., and Hassan, I. (2011) 'Child and adolescent service experience (ChASE): Measuring service quality and therapeutic process', *British Journal of Clinical Psychology*, 50: 452–464.
Elliot, D.S., Huzing, D., and Ageton, S.S. (1985) *Explaining Delinquency and Drug Use*. Beverley Hills, CA: Sage.
Frydenberg, E. (1997) *Adolescent Coping: Theoretical and Research Perspectives*. London: Routledge.
Green, J. (2006) 'Annotation: The therapeutic alliance – a significant but neglected variable in child mental health treatment studies', *Journal of Child Psychology and Psychiatry and Allied Disciplines*, 47: 425–435.
Harrington, R. and Bailey, S. (2005) *Mental Health Needs and Effectiveness of Provision for Young Offenders in the Community and Custody*. London: Youth Justice Board.
Hart, A., Saunders, A., and Thomas, H. (2005) 'Attuned practice: A service user study of specialist child and adolescent mental health, UK', *Epidemiologia e Psichiatria Sociale*, 14(1): 22–31.
Henggeler, S.W. and Scaheffer, C. (2010) 'Treating Serious Antisocial Behaviour Using Multisystemic Therapy', in J.R. Weisz and A.E. Kazdin (eds.), *Evidence-Based Psychotherapies for Children and Adolescents*. 2nd edn. New York: Guildford Press, 261.
Kadzin, A., Holland, L., Crowley, M., and Breton, S. (1997) 'Barriers to treatment participation scale: Evaluation, validation in the context of child outpatient treatment', *Journal of Child Psychology and Psychiatry*, 38: 1051–1062.
Khan, L. and Wilson, J. (2010) *Just Get on and Do It: Health Care Provision in Youth Offending Teams*. London: Centre for Mental Health.
King, R. and Wincup, E. (2008) *Doing Research on Crime and Justice*. New York: Oxford University Press.
Logan, D.E. and King, C.A. (2001) 'Parental facilitation of adolescent mental health service utilization: A conceptual and empirical review', *Clinical Psychology: Science and Practice*, 8: 319–340.
Naylor, C., Lincoln, J., and Goddard, N. (2008) 'Young people at risk of offending: Their views on a specialist mental health service in South East London', *Clinical Child Psychology and Psychiatry*, 8(2): 227–286.
Newton, N. (2000) *Applying Best Practices to Youth Reproductive Health: Lessons Learned from SEATS Experience*. Washington, DC: JSI.
Rickwood, D., Deane, F.P., Wilson, C.J., and Ciarrochi, J.V. (2005) 'Young people's help-seeking for mental health problems', *Australian E-journal for the Advancement of Mental Health*, 4(3): 1–34.
Street, C. and Svanberg, J. (2003) *Where Next? New Directions in In-patient Mental Health Services for Young People*. London: Young Minds.

Weisz, J.R. and Kazdin, A.E. (2010) 'The Present and Future of Evidence-Based Psychotherapies for Children and Adolescents', in J.R. Weisz and A.E. Kazdin (eds.), *Evidence-Based Psychotherapies for Children and Adolescents*. 2nd edn. New York: Guildford Press, 557–572.

Wells, C. (2001) 'The Treatment of Severe Antisocial Behaviour in Young People', in G. Baruch (ed.), *Community-Based Psychotherapy with Young People: Evidence and Innovation in Practice*. New York: Brunner-Routledge, 125–137.

3
Psychological Practice in Community Settings

Simone Fox and Berit Ritchie

In the UK there are various points within the criminal justice system (CJS) where young people who have offended may come into contact with community forensic services. These include point of arrest, through community sentences, to release from custody back into the community (Williamson 2006). Some young people may be in contact with statutory services such as the youth offending team (YOT), and others may be referred to forensic child and adolescent mental health services (FCAMHS), which is currently provided by the National Health Service (NHS) (Harvey 2014). The mental health service provision in the UK that supports young people in the CJS has grown rapidly over the last 10 to 15 years. Not only have FCAMHS expanded (Dent et al. 2013), other models of intervention, such as multisystemic therapy (MST), functional family therapy (FFT) and multidimensional treatment foster care (MTFC) have developed to work with young people with antisocial behaviour. There is a predominant role and need for psychological practice and thinking within each of these systems.

The aim of this chapter is to provide an overview of psychological practice with young people who have offended and who are in contact with community services. The high level of psychological and mental health needs of this population will be highlighted. The chapter will then outline FCAMHS and the interplay such services have with the youth justice system (YJS). Given that many young people in looked after child (LAC) placements have a history of offending, this chapter will describe LAC services (including individual placement as well as residential placements) and highlight the complex presentations of young people in care. The various evidence-based specialist services that have recently developed will be highlighted. The chapter will examine the challenges and the benefits of working systemically with young people and their families.

The psychological needs of young people in the youth justice system

In 2009, the UK Department of Health (DH) published a strategic document addressing the complex needs of young people in or at risk of entering the CJS. They reported that young people in this group have far more unmet health needs than other children of their age. They also have a high chance of experiencing a range of other difficulties, including school exclusion, substance misuse (SM), fragmented family relationships and unstable living conditions. Furthermore, contact with the CJS could bring additional problems for some children and young people, including those with learning difficulties, communication needs and mental health problems. Organisational and negative attitudes towards young people who offend were seen as barriers to progress. The DH (2009: 6) stated that: 'The task is to intervene more effectively, providing the right help at the right time and in the right place. When diversion from the Youth Justice System (YJS) has failed, we need to use the opportunity of young people's contact with it to give them better support.' The key principles for action from the DH were to have established policy and legal commitments for all children, based on the UN Convention on the Rights of the Child and on related legislation in England, in particular the Children's Acts 1989 and 2004 and the Human Rights Act 1998.

In 2006, Chitsabesan and her colleagues evaluated the mental health and psychosocial needs of a nationally representative sample of juvenile offenders in England and Wales. They used a cross-sectional survey of 301 young offenders, 151 in custody and 150 in the community, conducted in 6 geographically representative areas across England and Wales. Each young person was interviewed to obtain demographic information, mental health and social needs, and psychometric data. They found that young offenders had high levels of needs in a number of different areas, including mental health (31 per cent), education/work (36 per cent) and social relationships (48 per cent). Young offenders in the community had significantly more needs than those in secure care and their needs were often unmet. One in five young offenders was also identified as having a learning disability (IQ<70). Chitsabesan and colleagues (2006) concluded that needs for young offenders were high, but often unmet.

There is further empirical evidence to support the vast psychosocial needs of young people in the YJS (Lader et al. 2000; Kroll et al. 2002; Harrington et al. 2005). Children and young people in the YJS are at least three times more likely to have mental health problems than their non-offending counterparts (Hagell 2002). In the population as a whole, around 20 per cent of children experience some form of mental health problem (Mental Health Foundation 1999). Though these are helpful studies that identify important mental health needs in such a population, they still categorise such needs through a mental illness model, utilising diagnostic labels such as conduct disorder, depression, anxiety and attention deficit hyperactivity disorder (ADHD) as examples.

Van der Kolk (2005: 3) stated that 'people with histories of childhood trauma, abuse and neglect make up almost our entire criminal justice population'. It is important for psychologists working in the YJS to consider trauma, and the concept of complex developmental trauma (in which post-traumatic stress disorder (PTSD) symptoms may, or may not, be present) when working with young people. The causal links between childhood trauma and offending are not clearly evidenced in the available research, although some types of traumatic experience are suggested as predictive of offending, such as chronic bullying (Farrington et al. 2012). Whether direct links between trauma and offending behaviour can be established, the impact of childhood trauma is certainly relevant (and, in the experience of the authors, critical) to the engagement and effectiveness of clinical work with young people who have offended. It also has implications for the way we understand a young person's treatment needs, their subsequent progress (or lack of) and their longer-term outcomes (Ardino 2012). We would argue that a diagnostic framework has proved to be of little utility in understanding and intervention with young people who have experienced complex trauma, and that they are better served by utilising a psychological formulation-based approach, drawn from multiple theoretical perspectives. Formulations, on the other hand, explain the background development and maintenance of any presenting needs.

Community forensic services

Youth offending teams

In England and Wales, YOTs have undertaken the main forensic role in community settings and have been doing so for many years (Bridges and Torchia 2014). There are around 100,000 sentenced offenders under the age of 18 years who are managed by 158 YOTs (YJB 2014). YOTs use a structured risk assessment tool called the Onset and the Asset (YJB, 2000). The Onset referral and assessment framework was designed for the Youth Justice Board (YJB) to promote their prevention strategy by helping to identify risk factors to be reduced and protective factors to be enhanced in young people aged 8–13 years. The Asset is completed for all young offenders who come into contact with the CJS. Information from these assessments can be used to inform court reports, so that appropriate risk management and intervention needs can be recommended.

Some YOTs also offer accredited offending behaviour programmes, which are often implemented in a group format by YOT workers. Whilst strengths of these programmes are that they are evidence-based and operate manually, and can thus be offered by a range of professionals with specific training in their implementation, such programmes do not meet the needs of all young offenders.

Those with complex presentations, which may include factors such as learning difficulties, traumatic brain injury, complex trauma or mental health concerns, may not benefit from such programmes. Complex cases often have a multitude of difficulties that include individual as well as wider systemic needs, such as peers, family and education. Such cases may be subject to 'scattergun' referrals to a multitude of services at the same time, resulting in different services working with the same case. Practitioner psychologists have a role within YOTs, helping staff with complex assessments to develop a shared psychological understanding of the needs of each individual case (formulation), and helping co-ordinate the most efficient treatment plan, starting with the most critical issues. The priority interventions are often focussed on supporting and stabilising a young person's systemic context through safety planning and risk management, prior to embarking on any specific individual therapy.

Forensic child and adolescent mental health services

The remit of FCAMHS is to assess and provide intervention for young people under the age of 18 who are either in, or pose a significant risk of, entering the YJS. FCAMHS have evolved in an ad hoc manner across the country, and there are still areas in the UK where no such provision is available for young people (Dent et al. 2013). The configuration of these teams is also varied, ranging from locally funded services, to regionally and nationally funded provisions.

At present, there are no set government frameworks for what FCAMHS should offer, and thus the service delivery models vary greatly. Equally, the size of the team compared to the population it is trying to serve is also inconsistent. In 2013, Dent and her colleagues published a paper in which a national overview of existing FCAMHS community provision and commissioning arrangements were outlined. A community FCAMHS might broadly be defined as a service designed for young people about whom there are questions regarding mental health or learning disability, and who:

- present high risk of harm towards others and about whom there is major family or professional concern
- and/or are in contact with the criminal justice system.

(Dent et al. 2013: 6)

The needs of this population have been recognised within legislation and through community sentences, and include arrest referral schemes and the court diversion initiative, which involves rehabilitation and intervention. This is where practitioner psychologists can be helpful, whether this is providing direct or indirect work through training other professionals and providing supervision of their psychologically informed clinical work. Practitioner psychologists can also develop intervention programmes, based on psychological research findings that tap into the various factors contributing to antisocial and criminal behaviour.

FCAMHS are often multidisciplinary, with professionals from backgrounds such as psychology, psychiatry, occupational health, speech and language therapy, mental health nursing and social work. The services offered range from consultation, teaching and training, assessment and intervention for a very complex group of young people. Whilst often community-based services, many FCAMHS offer consultation and support within the secure estate, providing assessment and advice in relation to management and release planning.

Dent and colleagues (2013) found that the services undertaking work with young people in the YJS occurred across a range of settings, such as the community and the secure estate. They identified around 57 services from across the UK that were involved with some kind of work related to young people in contact with the YJS. Forty-four out of the identified 57 services responded to the survey and these were grouped into four broad categories:

1. Comprehensive specialist community FCAMHS provision. These were services with a clear Tier 4 specialist FCAMHS focus, including dual trained staff and functions supplementary to those of generic Tier 3 child and adolescent mental health services (CAMHS).
2. Specialist FCAMHSs Tier 4 inpatient services providing some ad hoc community input.
3. Local services clearly linked to Tier 3 CAMHS or mental health trusts, providing some but not comprehensive forensic functions.
4. Other arrangements providing some input to high-risk young people with mental health needs (stand-alone therapeutic provision within independent care organisations or specialist education providers and national spot-purchase forensic psychology services).

Dent and colleagues (2013) found significant consistency across specialist community FCAMHS regarding the need for senior psychiatric and psychological input to the teams. Involvement of nursing staff, social workers and therapeutically trained staff was less consistent.

In addition to the high levels of mental health need, young people presenting with high risk experience high levels of psychosocial adversity, multiple transitions between services, and high levels of geographical and domiciliary displacement (Dent et al. 2013). They can also be subject to a complex range of statutory educational, social care, mental health and criminal justice legislation. Dent and colleagues (2013) concluded that it was crucial that any attempt to meet the well-documented needs of these young people should seek to address the consistent provision of accepted interventions, but also to offer a coordinated response to complexity.

Psychological work

The psychological work undertaken within FCAMHS is diverse and challenging. It is the role of the practitioner psychologist to bring a broad psychological understanding to the presenting issues of a young person and family, including understanding and formulating the variety of reasons that may have led a young person to enter or be at risk of entering the YJS. Whilst not the key part of their role, many practitioner psychologists are able to undertake cognitive and neuropsychological assessments and utilise psychometric assessments that are useful in aiding formulation, intervention planning and meeting educational needs for young people, based on their current functioning. There is emerging evidence around the high prevalence of neurocognitive difficulties and head injury for this population (Davies et al. 2012). However, whilst the importance of understanding the individual needs of the young person themselves is clear, it is key for therapeutic intervention to also understand and formulate the wider systemic context and recognise how changes in the system could directly affect change in the individual.

Due to the complexities within this population, rather than taking a reductionist diagnostic approach, it is argued that the best interventions appear to be grounded in solid multifactorial formulations that draw on a broad range of psychological knowledge and theory and have clear goals and aims that fit with the wants, as well as the needs, of the client. Formulations involve the creative application of sound scientific psychological knowledge and can include (but not be driven or underpinned by) biological and social factors as well. Within CAMHS, clinical psychologists (and other practitioner psychologists with competencies in assessment and intervention of mental health need) are well placed to promote an overarching therapeutic approach based on promoting system changes and improving the quality of interactions. The core of training is to develop sound formulations; to apply a wide range of valid psychological knowledge and theory, flexibly and creatively, to build a rational understanding of the difficulties with which our clients present. From these formulations, along with the client's wishes and goals, comes an understanding of the therapeutic task. We can then select from/advise on, the possible, evidence-based ways of completing the task (Rogers, McMahon and Law 2011).

Case vignette

We will now use a case vignette (Tom, aged 11) to highlight the role of the practitioner psychologist in a FCAMHS team.

Tom was referred to FCAMHS from the local CAMHS due to an allegation of sexual abuse towards his 9-year-old sister. The allegation was investigated by the police, but the charges were dropped due to lack of evidence. There was a long-standing history of inappropriate sexual behaviour between siblings in the family, and more recent problem sexual behaviour (PSB) at school exhibited by Tom. This behaviour included talking about having sex, referring to pornographic material, and sexually touching female staff and pupils. Furthermore, concerns around Tom's educational achievements were raised.

Tom was one of ten children who grew up in a household described as emotionally, physically and possibly (nothing evidenced) sexually abusive. His mother was addicted to heroin and had a history of volatile and violent relationships with men. The supervision and care of the children in the household was extremely neglectful at times, and reports of the children stealing from the local shop in order to get food were given in their social care history. It was believed that Tom's mother would have sex with men for money in order to fund her drug addiction. The children in the family were thought to have observed such activity whilst in the care of their mother. At the age of 6, Tom and the other children were taken into local authority care under the category of neglect. Tom initially went to live with his maternal grandparents (all the other children went into foster care). He lived with them up until the point of referral to the FCAMHS, when he went to live with his maternal uncle. The reason for this move was due to the grandparents reporting that he was impossible to care for and having described him as 'evil'.

From the clinical formulation, Tom was understood from a complex developmental trauma framework perspective (Van der Kolk 2005), with a categorisation of his attachment pattern as disorganised. Tom's caregivers did not consistently provide for his basic needs, both physiologically as well as psychologically. Instead, he experienced a life of chaos and frightening events. Those experiences left him with difficulties in managing emotions, impairments in interpersonal relationships, impaired systems of meaning about self, others and the world, as well as cognitive difficulties around attention, concentration and memory. He had limited experience of healthy and appropriate interpersonal relationships, and lacked an understanding of boundary setting within such relationships, including peers and adults. He had a clear lack of trust in adults, and would often dissociate or 'cut himself off' from emotional experience when distressed. His PSB was understood from a perspective that Tom self-soothed and sought intimacy from others, combined with a lack of understanding of interpersonal boundaries. It was also hypothesised that it was a way of Tom feeling in control or being in charge, as most of his sexual behaviour was directed towards younger peers. His lack of age-appropriate peer relationships or ability to form such relationships were also deemed important in his exploratory sexual behaviour, as opportunity to explore his sexuality in a developmentally appropriate way was limited.

The first stage of the intervention for Tom was to convene a strategy meeting to share the psychological formulation with all other agencies involved in his care. This also included sharing a safety plan, both in terms of managing his risk of violence and PSB. Due to the lack of positive parental caregiving and frequent change of placement, the first step of the intervention was focused on stabilising the current placement arrangements for Tom. At this point, he had been moved into long-term foster care. The safety plans were shared with his foster carers, and parental support was provided from the local CAMHS. Specific intervention was undertaken with the parental caregivers around creating a safe environment, managing emotional dysregulation and setting appropriate boundaries (including sexual) within the household. The same strategies were shared with school staff to try to create more consistency. Furthermore, recommendations were made around supporting Tom to engage in positive activity, and helping him develop and maintain a positive peer group, as long as this was done within the remits of the safety plan and with appropriate monitoring and supervision. The case was discharged, but with the clause that Tom could be referred again if more specific harmful sexual behaviour work needed to be undertaken following stabilisation of the case.

Interventions

Multisystemic therapy

MST is a community-based, family intervention for young people with complex social, clinical and educational problems, such as violence, SM and offending behaviour. The main aim of MST is to reduce further antisocial behaviour in order to prevent the risk of out-of-home placements, either in care or custody. MST was developed in the United States in the late 1970s by Scott Henggeler and his colleagues to address the limitations of traditional services (Henggeler and Borduin 1990).

MST focuses particular attention on the multiple factors in the young person's and their family's environment that are linked with antisocial behaviour. It is based on the assumption that delinquency is multi-determined and is related not only to the characteristics of the individual, but also the risk factors in the family, the peer group, the school and the community (Henggeler et al. 1998, 2009). In order for interventions to be most effective at reducing antisocial behaviour, they need to be comprehensive and be able to address all of the relevant risk factors within the young person's ecology. In MST, the caregivers are viewed as the primary catalysts for change. The interventions are thus focused on empowering the caregivers, through the acquisition of skills, to effectively manage their child's behaviour (Henggeler et al. 2009). According to the MST theory of change, the MST therapist works with the family to overcome barriers that prevent effective parenting and management of child behaviour (e.g. the introduction of consistent boundaries). As the parents' effectiveness increases, so will their impact on the other systems around the young person, thus reducing the risk of antisocial behaviour.

MST is implemented by therapists from different professional backgrounds, including psychology, social work and family therapy. MST supervisors, again from varying backgrounds, provide weekly group supervision focused on reviewing cases, and there is a strong emphasis on drawing upon evidence-based psychological approaches to intervention development, such as behavioural, cognitive and structural/strategic family therapy models.

MST has a good evidence base, especially from the US, but increasingly across other countries (Borduin 1999; Fonagy et al. 2002; Henggeler et al. 2009). Numerous randomised control trials in the US and, more recently, in Norway and the UK, have found that it is effective, both in the short and long term, in reducing 'out-of-home' placements and antisocial behaviour and improving family relationships (Schaeffer and Borduin 2005; Ogden and Hagen 2006; Butler et al. 2011). However, Littell, Popa and Forsythe (2005) have criticised these conclusions and reported that results were inconsistent across studies and that there was a variation in quality and context. The MST research was also criticised in that it was carried out by the programme developers, and they questioned the transportability of the intervention. Despite criticisms of MST, the National Institute of Clinical Excellence (NICE 2013) guidelines now recommend multimodal interventions, such as MST, as the treatment of choice for 11 to 17-year-olds who may attract a diagnosis of conduct disorder.

MST standard

Standard MST intervention works with families and young people aged 11 to 17 years for three to five months. The frequency of sessions vary, and are tailored to the needs of the family and can be daily to once or twice a week, at times that suit (e.g. evenings). There is also a 24-hour/7-day per week on-call service to families for managing crises. The intervention is delivered within the family home and other community locations (e.g. the school or extended family home).

Multisystemic therapy – child abuse and neglect (MST-CAN)

MST-CAN is an adaptation of MST that was developed to treat families who have come to the attention of social care services due to physical abuse and/or neglect, have a target child in the age range of 6 to 17 years, and have had new reports of abuse or neglect in the past 180 days. MST-CAN includes the core components of standard MST as well as several adaptations for treating maltreated young people and their families (Swenson et al. 2010). The adaptations take into account serious child safety concerns and the severity of parental difficulties identified in families of physically abused and neglected young people. The length of treatment can be extended beyond three to five months.

Multisystemic therapy – problem sexual behaviour (MST-PSB)

MST-PSB is another adaptation of standard MST that targets chronic and violent juvenile offenders who engage in criminal sexual behaviour, including sexual assault, rape and sexual abuse of younger children. As with standard MST, MST-PSB therapists have a small caseload and see the young person and their family in their home setting. MST-PSB aims to: address the denial by the young person and family that there is a problem; focus on the components of the young person's environment that contribute to the sexual delinquency; help parents or carers to build support networks; and enable the parent or carer to provide boundaries and guidance to enable the young person to develop social skills in order to establish healthy relationships with peers.

Multisystemic therapy – substance abuse (MST-SA)

MST-SA (also known as MST-CM for MST enhanced with contingency management protocols) works with young people who are abusing drugs and alcohol. The main focus of the intervention is on the SM, and at every session the therapist determines whether the young person is using. If they are using, the underlying reasons for use are explored and these inform the intervention. If the young person has not used that week then the factors that have led the young person to stopping are leveraged to influence future behaviour. The young person is given specific training on drug-refusal skills, which include role-playing scenarios. The parent/carer is also an integral part of the treatment process.

Formulating referral behaviours in MST

In MST, referral behaviours are formulated in terms of 'fits' or 'fit circles'. The main purpose of the assessment is to understand the fit between the identified problem (such as aggression, theft or SM) and their broader systemic context. Hence, the 'fit circle' is the term given to the process therapists use to develop hypotheses around potential causes (or drivers) of the problematic behaviours. MST interventions lead on from the prioritised drivers of the fit (those in bold in Figure 3.1).

MST case vignette

Jason, aged 12, was referred to the MST team by the local YOT. His family had been known to children's services for the last six years for issues mainly related to Jason's antisocial behaviour, such as throwing stones, being verbally abusive and exposing his bottom and genitalia to members of the public. He had a diagnosis of ADHD and was being seen by CAMHS to manage this. The referrer noted that Jason's mother was finding it increasingly challenging to parent her son and she was 'at the end of her tether' and 'at a complete loss as to what to do'. Jason was reported to have poor attendance at school. At the time of the referral, the home environment was very chaotic, and although his mother attempted to set boundaries, Jason was not abiding by them. Any attempts to set boundaries would lead to verbal and, on occasion, physical aggression, towards his mother. She was concerned that her inability to parent her son meant that

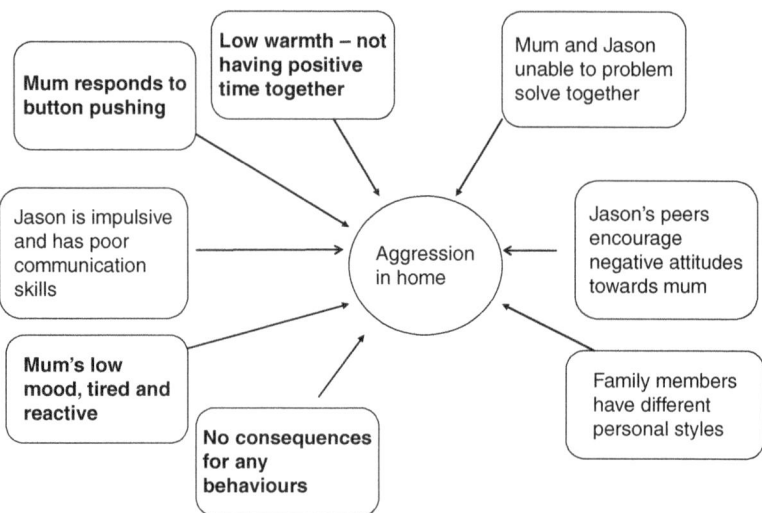

Figure 3.1 'Fit' for aggression

she was unable to keep him safe from harm. Without an intensive intervention this family was at risk of breakdown.

Figure 3.1 shows the assessment of 'fit' of aggression for Jason.

During MST, a safety plan was developed, as well as strategies for Jason and his mother to manage the aggression. There was a clear behavioural plan with rules, rewards and consequences. Work was done with his mother in relation to her awareness of triggers and 'button pushing', and how she needed to respond appropriately to her son's behaviour. Some cognitive behaviour therapy (CBT) was undertaken with her, focussing on her negative cognitions and low mood, as this was identified as a key 'driver' for how she responded to the 'button pushing', thus escalating Jason's aggression. There was work done with Jason and his mother around developing a routine/activities and structure for both inside and outside the home, and his mother increased her levels of monitoring and supervision, thus reducing Jason's association with his antisocial peers. Work was also aimed at increasing positive interactions and relationships within the family and extended family. There was also work done to increase communication between the mother and school and generalise the plans at home to work on improving school attendance.

Other evidence-based interventions

In addition to MST there are a number of other evidence-based interventions for young people displaying antisocial behaviour, as well as those either on the edge of, or already in, care. Many of these interventions work with younger children, but those that target adolescents include FFT and MTFC. FFT addresses the needs of 11–18 year olds and their families, where there is antisocial and violent behaviour. It is office and home-based, but can also be done in schools and other community settings. All practitioners are trained family therapists and it uses a strength-based relational focus, with behavioural components. The intervention is undertaken for 3 to 6 months in duration, with 8 to 12 sessions for those with moderate needs and 26 to 30 sessions for those with high needs. There is good evidence from outcome studies to suggest that FFT, when applied as intended, can reduce recidivism and/or the onset of offending from 25 per cent to 60 per cent compared to other programmes (Alexander et al. 2000). There have been several randomised controlled trials (RCTs) of FFT conducted in the States and Sweden, and one in the UK (Roberts, Jones and Scott 2005). A meta-analysis of 24 studies of MST and FFT has provided additional evidence that these interventions had a significant and substantial effect on adolescent delinquency relative to control groups (Baldwin et al. 2012). However, these effects were smaller when MST and FFT are compared to alternative therapies (Baldwin et al. 2012). One recent study found that FFT, when used with juvenile offenders and their families in community justice settings in the USA, reduced the likelihood of violent crimes by 30 per cent (Sexton and Turner 2010).

MTFC is designed as an intervention for children already looked after in three age groups – young children, primary-school-aged children and adolescents – with a range of complex behaviours which may lead to placement disruption, including conduct problems and offending in older children. MTFC uses social learning theory, delivering intensive support to the child, foster carers and birth/adoptive family through a very close team around the child approach. Foster carers are recruited, trained and receive professional support in providing single family placements for these children and young people. They remain in contact on a daily basis with specific members of the clinical team, are provided with a clear treatment programme, which they deliver with the child or young person, and have access to 24-hour support. The intervention is 6 to 12 months in duration. There have been a number of RCTs of MTFC that have demonstrated the positive effect of the intervention for high-risk young people in foster care (e.g. Fisher, Burraston and Pears 2005; Chamberlain, Leve and DeGarmo 2007; Westermark, Hansson and Olsson 2011). Eddy, Whaley and Chamberlain (2004) found that adolescents who received MTFC services were less likely to commit violent offences (21 per cent) than young people who lived in group homes (38 per cent).

Looked after children

In 2013, there were over 92,000 children under the age of 18 years in care in the UK (NSPCC 2015). The majority of these children were in foster care, around

10 per cent were in children's homes, and a small percentage were cared for in settings such as residential schools or placements with parents (Munro 2011). It is well documented that the outcomes for this group of young people are much worse when compared to children living at home, and they are much less likely to be in full-time education (Harker 2012). They are also more likely to have serious behavioural problems, misuse alcohol and illicit substances, and be involved with the YJS (Meltzer et al. 2003; Jones et al. 2011). It is important to note, however, that not all children who end up in care will exhibit significant behavioural disturbance. Whilst many may suffer from emotional problems (such as anxiety and depression), there are also those who do not develop difficulties and are able to function well in placement settings and school.

In June 2010, Graham Allen, MP, was commissioned to undertake a comprehensive review of the evidence base for early intervention programmes for young people and families with complex presentations, with the aim of making recommendations for the UK government spending review. The review built a strong argument in favour of investing in early interventions and highlighted the large costs to society if investments were not made at this stage (Allen 2011a). There are a wide range of interventions in the UK available for families where the young person is either at risk of entering care or is already looked after. These interventions vary in terms of the evidence base for their effectiveness and the quality of the research evaluation of the programme. Some current models of practice in local authorities and partner agencies in England and Wales to divert young people away from care include family intervention projects (FIPS), family group conferencing (FGC) and MST. A report in 2011 published by the Office for Standards in Education, Children's Services and Skills (OFSTED) that sought young people's views, highlighted that increased family support may be useful in preventing young people going into care (OFSTED 2011). However, the report did not identify or evaluate any specific intervention.

Since 2008, the Department for Education, in partnership with the DH and the YJB, has supported a range of pilots of intensive interventions for LAC and children on the edge of care or custody. The interventions include: MST, MTFC, KEEP (parenting skills for foster carers) and FFT. Whilst different in the specifics of their delivery, these interventions all have general requirements of model fidelity, clinical supervision and psychological consultation, as well as an investment of finance. There is increasing evidence that, if delivered with fidelity to the appropriate population, they can reduce the need for a child to enter care or custody, or to move into more intensive or costly placements (Fox and Ashmore 2014). For some children they can reduce the length of time they are placed away from home (Fox and Ashmore 2014).

Following initial positive evaluations, there has been a commitment to continue their development over the next spending review period, at least until

March 2015. The programmes draw on the expertise that has been developed within local authorities and their sector partners, as well as a national team/network partnership that provides clinical support and supervision, or other centrally provided support. Several of these programmes, such as MST and MTFC for adolescents, are also suitable for young people in youth justice services, and further expansion of these programmes will support the government's agenda to devolve more responsibility for these services to the local authority level.

Challenges and benefits of working systemically

Challenges

These systemic, evidence-based interventions provide a number of challenges for those implementing them. The families referred are often chaotic and disorganised, and engagement can take several weeks and may be an ongoing issue. Addressing some of the key referral behaviours, such as aggression and offending, may be secondary to working on engagement and trust, and helping families manage crises may be prioritised. The therapist–parent relationship is a key focus of the intervention, and there is a strong ethos on collaborative working and seeing the parent as the expert in their own lives, thus empowering them to take responsibility for enabling their child to make positive changes. Due to the time-limited nature of these interventions, the therapists may feel that they have not been able to achieve the overarching goals by the time treatment has come to an end.

The delivery of traditional services for young people and their families in the CJS has typically meant services for individual young people, in groups in custody, or in the community with others who have offended or are behaving antisocially (Fox and Ashmore 2011). Furthermore, the cultural context still considers therapy to be 'individual' and targeted at the young person, rather than at the systems within which they are embedded. It is often a challenge, when trying to engage a family, to help them align to an understanding of how their behaviours may have a reciprocal effect on their child and the role that they may have in maintaining, or even increasing, negative behaviours. Parents and carers may want the intervention to be just with the young person, as they are viewed as 'the problem'. It may not be just the parent/carer who feels that the intervention should focus only on working with and involving the young person. It is our experience that there may be pressure from referrers and professionals within the CJS, such as judges or the police, to engage the young person. The young people referred may not engage well and refuse to participate in sessions, and this can be a source of frustration for therapists, who may feel that they are not able to address the desired outcomes of key stakeholders. Rogers, McMahon and Law (2011) further discuss the challenges of the dominant discourse of individual therapy for this population, and conclude by suggesting that the most helpful role as practitioner psychologists may be around translating formulations and interventions into everyday therapeutic interactions that optimise the possibility of sustainable change in young person's lives. They recommend a more balanced approach to working with young people, which includes the system around them.

Additionally, there may be pressure from other services to take cases that might not meet criteria. Each intervention has clearly defined target populations and explicit inclusion and exclusion criteria, based on what is known to work. However, referrers may be unfamiliar with these and, due to limited availability of other interventions, there may be pressure on those existing services to take on these referrals. For example, MST teams typically have a lot of referrals for young people with significant issues, including self-harm and suicidal thoughts and/or pervasive developmental disorders, when these may be exclusion criteria. Referrers may feel that MST is the only option, as other services may not be able to address the intensive systemic needs of the young person, or the young person has a history of non-engagement with CAMHS. It is therefore important to have clear and consistent referral pathways to specific services. As well as the experience and training of the staff delivering the intervention, having a strong multi-agency board working both operationally and strategically is essential in supporting the provision and sustainability of the service. This involves strategic analysis and understanding of the needs of this cohort of young people, accompanied by investment in services to address these needs (OFSTED 2011).

Many of the interventions discussed in this chapter are seen as resource-heavy services. This presents a commissioning challenge. Commissioners need to consider reallocating resources in favour of robust, evidence-based practice, which has been shown to have an impact on reducing the costs of care and custody (Fox and Ashmore 2014). The implementation of any evidence-based model requires careful design, and strong project management and support, especially in the early stages. Effective stakeholder engagement, both operationally and strategically, is key to success.

Another unique role of practitioner psychologists within services in which complex clinical presentations frequently present is around the skill of individual formulation and intervention design should a young person fall outside the referral criteria for evidence-based therapy programmes and interventions. In contrast to many other professionals, who may be trained in a specific therapeutic model, practitioner psychologists formulate from a broad-based knowledge of the science of psychology (rather than any one psychotherapeutic model or perspective), taking an integrated and multimodal perspective, which also locates personal meaning within its wider systemic, organisational and societal context (BPS 2011). This skill allows the delivery of individualised intervention based on an integration of models that may or may not have an existing evidence base, but nevertheless are likely to be of clinical value.

Benefits

The costs of interventions range significantly depending on the intensity and length of the service being offered. However, one of the major benefits of working systemically with young people and their families in the community is that of cost-effectiveness. It has been estimated that the annual cost for a young person being placed in a young offender's institute is £59,000 (Allen 2011b), £203,000 for a child looked after in a children's home and up to £211,000 for a child looked after in secure accommodation (YJB 2011). Whilst some of the evidence-based interventions are thought to be expensive in comparison to traditional interventions, these costs are far less than those of care or custody. The Munro Review of Child Protection (Munro 2011) also suggests that preventative services can do more to reduce abuse and neglect than reactive services.

A further benefit of systemic interventions is that many are multimodal or multidimensional. This means that the delivery of the treatment is varied and can be individualised to the needs that arise. The families are all likely to present with complex difficulties across a range of settings, thus it is important that interventions can target different problems simultaneously. Different therapeutic models may be used (from behavioural and cognitive to systemic approaches, such as strategic and structural family therapy). Although the parent/carer is seen as key to the success of a great number of the interventions, many of the evidence-based approaches also involve other parts of the system, including the young person, the school or the peer group. This also increases the psychological understanding of the wider systems.

Several of the systemic interventions offered provide a service out of the office, which means that the family does not have to travel to a clinic (thus reducing cost, childcare of other children and time for the caregiver). Parents frequently report these practical barriers as a reason for non-engagement in therapy (Garvey et al. 2006). Furthermore, the clinicians are better able to understand the environment within which the problems are occurring (and are often able to witness the issues live during sessions, such as how arguments might escalate). The interventions are, therefore, thought to be more ecologically valid. Some of the services highlighted operate outside of office hours (e.g. MST and MTFC), enabling parents who work to attend sessions with minimal disruption, and there are on-call support systems in place for evening and weekend contact during times of crisis. As such measures are more ecologically valid, the likelihood of change being sustained is thought to be increased. In reviewing the systemic interventions, those with good evidence are treatment models based on empirical knowledge of the family factors that predict antisocial behaviour, in particular poor parental supervision, lack of clear expectations and limits, inconsistent discipline and high levels of conflict (Datchi and Sexton 2013). There is also a high level of treatment fidelity. Successful systemic interventions appear to be driven by multifactorial formulations, are individualised to the needs of the young person and the context around them, they are flexible and they work with the wider systems.

Summary and conclusions

This chapter has highlighted the complexity of the psychological needs faced by young people within the criminal justice and looked after systems. FCAMHS have developed to assess and provide interventions for this vulnerable group. The psychological work undertaken within these services is diverse and challenging. Within the UK, there is a lack of a national framework for the service provision of FCAMHS, and hence they are all commissioned differently and deliver very diverse services, some based on diagnostic and traditional 'medical' models and others taking a more psychologically oriented approach. Thus, the provision across the country is inconsistent depending on area. In recent years, there has been an increase in evidence-based systemic interventions that have moved away from diagnostic labels to a more explanatory approach, working with the individual and their system in a more integrated, comprehensive approach, driven by multifactorial formulations. In the current climate of significant cuts to traditional CAMHS, the challenge to commissioners will be around reallocating resources, drawing on the evidence base as to what works and for whom, and looking at early intervention and preventative services that will enable young people and their families to steer a course away from looked after provision and custody.

References

Alexander, J.F., Pugh, C., Parsons, B.V., and Sexton, T.L. (2000) 'Functional Family Therapy', in D.S. Elliott (ed.), *Blueprints for Violence Prevention, Book 3*. 2nd edn. Boulder: University of Colorado, Institute of Behavioral Science, Centre for the Study and Prevention of Violence.

Allen, G. (2011a) *Early Intervention: The Next Steps*. London: HM Government.

Allen, G. (2011b) *Early Intervention: Smart Investment, Massive Savings*. London: HM Government.

Ardino, V. (2012) 'Offending behaviour: The role of trauma and PTSD', *European Journal of Psychotraumatology*, 3.

Baldwin, S.A., Christian, S., Berkeljon, A., Shadish, W.R., and Bean, R. (2012) 'The effects of family therapies for adolescent delinquency and substance abuse: A meta-analysis', *Journal of Marital and Family Therapy*, 38: 281–304.

Borduin, C.M. (1999) 'Multisystemic treatment of criminality and violence in adolescents', *Journal of the American Academy of Child and Adolescent Psychiatry*, 38: 242–249.

BPS (British Psychological Society) (2011) *Good Practice Guidelines on the Use of Psychological Formulation*. London: BPS.
Bridges, A. and Torchia, K. (2014) 'Overview of Forensic Services in the Community', in Z. Ashmore and R. Shuker (eds.), *Forensic Practice in the Community: Issues in Forensic Psychology*. London and New York: Routledge, 3–21.
Butler, S., Baruch, G., Hickey, N., and Fonagy, P. (2011) 'A randomized control trial of multisystemic therapy and a statutory therapeutic intervention for young offenders', *Journal of the American Academy of Child and Adolescent Psychiatry*, 50(12): 1220–1235.
Chamberlain, P., Leve, L.D., and DeGarmo, D.S. (2007) 'Multidimensional foster care for girls in the juvenile justice system: 2-year follow-up of a randomized clinical trial', *Journal of Consulting and Clinical Psychology*, 75(1): 187–193.
Chitsabesan, P., Kroll, L., Bailey, S., Kenning, C., Sneider, S., MacDonald, W., and Theodosiou, L. (2006) 'Mental health needs of young offenders in custody and in the community', *British Journal of Psychiatry*, 188: 534–540.
Datchi, C.C. and Sexton, T.L. (2013) 'Can family therapy have an effect on adult criminal conduct? Initial evaluation of functional family therapy', *Couple and Family Psychology*, 2(4): 278–293.
Davies, R.C., Williams, W.H., Hinder, D., Burgess, C.N., and Mounce, L.T. (2012) 'Self-reported traumatic brain injury and post-concussion symptoms in incarcerated youth', *Journal of Head Trauma Rehabilitation*, 27(3): 21–27.
Dent, M., Peto, L., Griffin, M., and Hindley, N. (2013) 'Community forensic child and adolescent mental health services (FCAMHS): A map of current national provision and a proposed model for future service', *An Interim Report for the Department of Health*. London: Solutions for Public Health.
DH (Department of Health) (2009) *Healthy Children, Safer Communities: A Strategy to Promote the Health and Well-Being of Children and Young People in Contact with the Youth Justice System*. London: Department of Health.
DH (Department of Health) (2011) *No Health without Mental Health: A Cross-Government Mental Health Outcomes Strategy for People of all Ages*. London: Department of Health.
Eddy, J.M., Whaley, R.B., and Chamberlain, P. (2004) 'The prevention of violent behavior by chronic and serious male juvenile offenders: A 2-year follow-up of a randomized clinical trial', *Journal of Emotional and Behavioral Disorders*, 12: 2–8.
Farrington, D.P., Lösel, F., Ttofi, M.M., and Theodorakis, N. (2012) *School Bullying, Depression and Offending Behavior Later in Life: An Updated Systematic Review of Longitudinal Studies*. Stockholm: National Council for Crime Prevention.
Fisher, P.A., Burraston, B., and Pears, K. (2005) 'The early intervention foster care program: Permanent placement outcomes from a randomised trial', *Child Maltreatment*, 10(1): 61–67.
Fonagy, P., Target, M., Cottrell, D., Phillips, J., and Kurtz, Z. (2002) *What Works for Whom? A Critical Review of Treatments for Children and Adolescents*. New York: Guilford Press.
Fox, S. and Ashmore, Z. (2011) 'An introduction to multisystemic therapy in England', *Forensic Update*, 103: 49–53.
Fox, S. and Ashmore, Z. (2014) 'The advantages and disadvantages of multisystemic therapy as an intervention to prevent young people entering the care system', *British Journal of Social Work*, 1–17.
Garvey, C., Julion, W., Fogg, L., Kratovil, A., and Gross, D. (2006) 'Measuring participation in a prevention trial with parents of young children', *Research in Nursing & Health*, 29: 212–222.
Hagell, A. (2002) *The Mental Health of Young Offenders. Bright Futures: Working with Vulnerable Young People*. London: Mental Health Foundation.

Harker, R. (2012) *Children in Care in England: Statistics*. Library: House of Commons.

Harrington, R., Bailey, S., Chitsabesan, P., Kroll, L., Macdonald, W., Sneider, S., Kenning, C., Taylor, G., Byford, S., and Barrett, B. (2005) *Mental Health Needs and Effectiveness of Provision for Young Offenders in Custody and in the Community*. London: Youth Justice Board.

Harvey, J. (2014) 'Assessment in Community Settings', in Z. Ashmore and R. Shuker (eds.), *Forensic Practice in the Community: Issues in Forensic Psychology*. London and New York: Routledge, 22–39.

Henggeler, S.W. and Borduin, C.M. (1990) *Family Therapy and Beyond: A Multisystemic Approach to Treating the Behavior Problems of Children and Adolescents*. Pacific Grove, CA: Brooks/Cole.

Henggeler, S.W., Schoenwald, S.K., Borduin, C.M., Rowland, M.D., and Cunningham, P.B. (1998) *Multisystemic Treatment of Antisocial Behaviour in Children and Adolescents: Treatment Manual for Practitioners*. New York: Guildford Press.

Henggeler, S.W., Schoenwald, S.K., Borduin, C.M., Rowland, M.D., and Cunningham, P.B. (2009) *Multisystemic Therapy for Children and Adolescents*, 2nd edn. New York: Guildford Press.

Jones, R., Everson-Hock, E.S., Papaioannou, D., Guillaume, L., Goyer, E., Chilcott, J., Cooke, J., Payne, N., Duenas, A., Sheppard, L.M., and Swann, C. (2011) 'Factors associated with outcomes for looked-after children and young people: a correlates review of the literature', *Child: Care, Health and Development*, 37(5): 613–622.

Kroll, L., Rothwell, I., Bradley, D., et al. (2002) 'Mental health needs of boys in secure care for serious or persistent offending: A prospective, longitudinal study', *Lancet*, 359, 1975–1979.

Lader, D., Singletone, N., and Meltzer, H. (2000) *Psychiatric Morbidity amongst Young Offenders in England and Wales*. London: Office for National Statistics.

Littell, J.H., Popa, M., and Forsythe, B. (2005) 'Multisystemic therapy for social, emotional, and behavioural problems in youth aged 10–17', *Cochrane Database of Systematic Reviews*, 4.

Meltzer, H., Gatward, R., Corbin, T., Goodman, G., and Ford, T. (2003) *The Mental Health Needs of Young People Looked after by Local Authorities in England: Summary Report*. London: Office for National Statistics on behalf of Department of Health.

Mental Health Foundation (1999) *Bright Futures: Promoting Children and Young People's Mental Health*. London: Mental Health Foundation.

Munro, E. (2011) *The Munro Review of Child Protection: Final Report – A Child-Centred System*. London: Department for Education.

NICE (National Institute for Health and Care Excellence) (2013) *Antisocial Behaviour and Conduct Disorders in Children and Young People: Recognition, Intervention and Management*, NICE Clinical Guideline 158.

NSPCC (National Society for the Prevention of Cruelty to Children) (2015) 'Statistics on looked after children', *NSPCC*. Available at: http://www.nspcc.org.uk/Inform/resourcesforprofessionals/lookedafterchildren/statistics_wda88009.html. Accessed 26 January 2015.

OFSTED (Office for Standards in Education, Children's Services and Skills) (2011) 'Children on the edge of care: Report of children's views by the Children's Rights Director for England', *OFSTED*. Available at: http://www.ofsted.gov.uk/resources/children-edge-of-care. Accessed 28 January 2015.

Ogden, T. and Hagen, K.A. (2006) 'Multisystemic therapy of serious behaviour problems in youth: Sustainability of therapy effectiveness two years after intake', *Journal of Child and Adolescent Mental Health*, 11: 142–149.

Roberts, R., Jones, H., and Scott, S. (2005) *Treatment Foster Care in England*. 2nd edn. Lyme Regis: Russell House Publishing.

Rogers, A., McMahon, J., and Law, D. (2011) 'Expanding therapy: Challenging the dominant discourse of individual therapy when working with vulnerable children and young people. A discussion paper', *Clinical Psychology Forum*, No. 222: 9–14.

Schaeffer, C.M. and Borduin, C.M. (2005) 'Long-term follow-up to a randomized clinical trial of multisystemic therapy with serious and violent juvenile offenders', *Consulting and Clinical Psychology*, 73(3): 69–91.

Sexton, T. and Turner, C.W. (2010) 'The effectiveness of functional family therapy for youth with behavioral problems in a community practice setting', *Journal of Family Psychology*, 24: 339–348.

Swenson, C.C., Penman, J., Hengeller, S.W., and Rowland, M.D. (2010) *Multisystemic Therapy for Child Abuse and Neglect*. Charleston, SC: Family Services Research Centre.

Van der Kolk, B. (2005) 'Developmental trauma disorder: Toward a rational diagnosis for children with complex trauma histories', *Psychiatric Annals*, 35(5): 401–408.

Westermark, P.K., Hansson, K., and Olsson, M. (2011) 'Multidimensional treatment foster care (MTFC): Results from an independent replication', *Journal of Family Therapy*, 33: 20–41.

Williamson, M. (2006) *Improving the Health and Social Outcomes of People Recently Released from Prisons in the UK: A Perspective from Primary Care*. London: Sainsbury Centre for Mental Health.

YJB (Youth Justice Board) (2000) *Asset*. London: Youth Justice Board.

YJB (Youth Justice Board) (2011) *Annual Report and Accounts 2010/11*. London: Youth Justice Board.

YJB (Youth Justice Board) (2014) Youth Justice Statistics 2012/13: England and Wales. Available at: https://www.gov.uk/government/uploads/system/uploads/attachment_data/file/278549/youth-justice-stats-2013.pdf. Accessed 29 January 2015.

4
Psychological Practice in Secure Settings

Clare Snodgrass and Jackie Preston

Introduction

Children and young people in secure settings present with a complex range of vulnerabilities, needs and risks. A significant number of them have been looked after in local authority care and have experienced trauma, neglect, loss and disruption (Bailey, Thornton and Weaver 1994; Casswell, French and Rogers 2012). These children and young people's early lives are reflected in behaviour that can be both risky to themselves and those around them. Across the range of secure settings, we will examine how young people present with similar levels of need and complexity and often have histories of trauma and deprivation. Young people may make transitions between secure settings, but psychological provision within these settings can provide consistency by helping the systems of care be psychologically informed to achieve the best possible outcomes.

Practitioners within secure settings need to adapt to work both directly with the young person and indirectly by supporting, enhancing and sometimes challenging the secure systems they are part of. This can be both the greatest obstacle and the greatest opportunity for change. In this chapter we will look at how psychology can be uniquely placed to bring a broad range of theories and models to bear on these most complex of issues, to develop a psychological framework through which meaning can be restored.

Overview of secure settings

It is estimated that there are over 2,200 young people held in secure settings in the UK at any one time and, over the course of a year, 9,900 young people will spend time in secure settings (Royal College of Paediatrics and Child Health 2013). The broader category of secure settings includes secure hospital provision, young offender institutions (YOIs), secure training centres (STCs)

Table 4.1 Overview of secure settings

	Young offender institutions	Secure training centre	Secure children's homes	Secure hospitals
Legal framework	Criminal justice	Criminal justice	Section 25 Children's Act 1989 Criminal justice	Mental Health Act Part 2/Part 3 Some Ministry of Justice restrictions
Age range	15–18	12–17	10–17	12–18 years
Number of beds	817 occupied (1)	290 271 occupied (1)	300 (2) 141 criminal justice beds (1)	100 medium secure No central record of low secure bed numbers
Gender	Male only	Male and female	Male and female	Three units all male All others male and female
Number of centres	6	4	16	Six medium secure Unknown low secure

Notes: (1) Ministry of Justice (2014).
(2) Department for Education (2012).

and secure children's homes (SCHs) (see Table 4.1 for an overview). Young people often move between these systems and the community, and experience transitions in, out and between settings.

In secure settings, young people are deprived of their liberty for the safety of others or themselves, and this requires a legal framework. The young people in hospital settings are detained under the Mental Health Act (1983), those in SCHs are secured under Section 25 of the Children's Act (1989) or under the Crime and Disorder Act (1998). In STCs and YOIs, young people are held under the Crime and Disorder Act (1998).

Psychological provision is a common feature of secure settings, but the position of practitioner psychologists can vary across settings from being integral members of the multidisciplinary team (MDT), to visiting in-reach workers as part of mental health in-reach teams, or providing sessional input as part of a separately commissioned service.

Young offender institutions and secure training centres

The largest population of young people in secure settings in England and Wales is to be found in YOIs. There are six YOIs in England and Wales, housing young men aged 15–18, and these operate under many of the same rules and policies as prisons for adult men and women. There are no longer any young women housed in YOIs. Statistics for 2012/13 showed that 74 per cent of the young people in secure settings are placed in YOIs. An additional 16 per cent of young people in secure settings in England and Wales are placed in STCs and 9 per cent are placed in SCHs (YJB 2014).

The number of children and young people in secure settings in England and Wales in 2012/13 was reported at around 1,544 under-18 year olds (YJB 2014). This figure does not include those placed in secure mental health hospitals and those placed in SCHs under a welfare order. While those in secure settings represent a declining group, clinical experience and anecdotal reports suggest they are an increasingly complex group. Since 2008/09 there have been 55 per cent fewer young people in the criminal justice system (CJS) in England and Wales (YJB 2014) and 36 per cent fewer young people held securely. The number of young people in custody on long-term sentences and remand has remained constant, whilst those on detention and training orders (DTOs) has fallen. Sentences predominantly comprise robbery (31 per cent), violence against the person (23 per cent) and burglary (17 per cent), and in 2012/13, 5 per cent of young people sentenced had 15 or more previous offences, a figure which has been steadily increasing (YJB 2014). Despite the falling numbers of young people in secure settings overall, proportionately, rates of self-harm and violence against staff and other young people is increasing, with a worrying rise of 45 per cent in the number of incidents of physical restraint and 22 per cent more assaults recorded between 2009/10 and 2012/13, and a 7 per cent increase in the rates of self-harm compared to the previous year (YJB 2014).

Secure children's homes

There are 16 individually managed SCHs in England and Wales, providing placements for 10–17-year-olds. The Department for Education has overall policy responsibility for SCHs in England and Wales, and the units are monitored and inspected by the Office for Standards in Education, Children's Services and Skills (OFSTED). There are two routes for young people into a SCH. One route is through a criminal conviction where a custodial sentence is deemed appropriate. In these cases, SCHs are used to place the most vulnerable young people, including those under the age of 12. The other route into a SCH is when a welfare order under Section 25 of the Children's Act (1989) has been made in order to keep the young person safe. For such an order to be granted, the local authority must be able to demonstrate that the young person:

- Has a history of absconding and is likely to abscond from any other descriptions of accommodation; *and*

- if they abscond they are likely to suffer significant harm; *or*
- if they are kept in any other description of accommodation they are likely to injure themselves or other persons.

There are approximately 300 beds for young people in SCHs, and currently approximately 141 are occupied by young people placed under the CJS (Ministry of Justice 2014).

Secure mental health hospitals

Young people in secure settings with the most serious and complex mental health problems can be transferred under the Mental Health Act 1983 (England and Wales) to inpatient units (DH 2011). NHS England commissions 100 medium secure adolescent inpatient beds across 6 sites in England, including 27 beds for young people with a learning disability. More detailed information about these units can be found on the NHS England website: http://www.england.nhs.uk/commissioning/spec-services/npc-crg/group-c/c11/ (2014). Similar provision based in Scotland, Wales and Northern Ireland is lacking. To be detained in a medium secure adolescent hospital young people must present a risk to others of direct violence liable to result in injury to people, sexually aggressive behaviour, or destructive and potentially life-threatening use of fire, or be in custodial care and in need of hospital treatment for mental disorder. There is additional low secure inpatient provision across the independent sector and the National Health Service (NHS), but there is no agreed co-ordination or central record of where these units are located and the number of beds available at any one time.

Young people in secure hospital settings may be detained under Section 2 or 3 of the Mental Health Act 1983 for assessment or treatment, they may be transferred from custodial settings to a secure hospital under Section 47 or 48 of the Mental Health Act 1983, or detained by the courts under Section 37 of the Act if the young person is deemed sufficiently unwell at the time of sentencing to require hospitalisation. A Section 37 may be given with or without a Section 41 restriction order, which imposes Ministry of Justice restrictions on leave, discharge and transfer between hospitals.

The secure systems for young people are highly complex and look after young people with both a high level of vulnerability or risk to themselves, and also behaviour that may pose a risk of harm to others. The units need to strike a balance between providing care that meets the developmental needs of young people, and providing a safe environment that attempts to minimise potential harm to them and others. They also need to effectively manage high-risk behaviours, whilst addressing the high levels of vulnerability and need, including mental health needs. Psychologically informed provision, by providing a holistic approach, can balance understanding and addressing the needs of young people, while comprehending the risks that they may pose.

Characteristics of the population

Over the last 20 years there has been a growing understanding of the complex needs and vulnerabilities of young people in secure settings. The outcomes for such young people are disturbingly poor. Young males in custodial settings are 18 times more likely than those in the general population to take their own lives (Fazell 2008) and, tragically, there have been 16 deaths of young people in secure care since 2000 (YJB 2014). The death rate for this group is higher than in equivalent age groups who have a diagnosis of schizophrenia or an eating disorder (Coffey et al. 2003). Mortality rates among young female offenders are 40 times higher than among young women in the general population, and drug use, suicide and non-intentional injury are the leading causes of death among young offenders (Coffey et al. 2003).

Children and young people in secure settings have experienced high rates of exposure to violence, abuse, neglect, loss and separation. One in 3 girls and 1 in 20 boys in custody have disclosed sexual abuse (Social Exclusion Unit 2002) and 90 per cent of young offenders have experienced at least one traumatic event, with over half being exposed 6 times or more (Abram et al. 2004). Three quarters of children and young people in custody have lived with someone other than a parent (YJB 2007). Eighty-four per cent of 12–18-year-olds in custody have problematic drug use (Galahad SMS Ltd. 2009), and 86 per cent of young men and 79 per cent of young women in the youth justice system (YJS) aged 15–18 years have been excluded from school (Parke 2009). Such high levels of adverse experiences also reflect a significant unmet need, with reports of over two-thirds of those having suffered abuse of a violent, sexual or emotional nature claiming not to have received any help (HM Inspectorate of Prisons 1997).

Mental health needs are three times more common among young people aged up to 18 in the YJS, than among their peers who do not offend (Hagell 2002). Studies of young people in custody indicate higher than average levels of depression (18 per cent), anxiety disorders (10 per cent) and psychotic-like symptoms (5 per cent) (Chitsabesan et al. 2006). Fazell (2008) reported that half of the sample of young people in custody met the criteria for a diagnosis of conduct disorder. In another study, almost nine out of ten young people aged 16–20 years in custody met the criteria for personality disorder diagnosis (Lader, Singleton and Meltzer 2000). Prevalence rates of attention deficit hyperactivity disorder (ADHD) diagnoses in young offenders have varied across studies, dependent on the methodology of the study. However, rates of ADHD diagnoses are significantly greater in both male and female young offenders in comparison with the general population, with rates between 11 and 16 per cent (Teplin et al. 2002; Fazell 2008). One study reported that almost all of the participants met criteria for a diagnosis of ADHD (Ståhlberg, Anckarster and Nilsson 2010).

Learning difficulties and communication problems are also significantly more common in young people in secure settings (Kroll et al. 2002; Ståhlberg, Anckarster and Nilsson 2010). The majority of young people with an identified intellectual disability (ID) have an impairment in the mild range, which may be overshadowed by their challenging behaviour. Nearly three quarters of young people in custody have been assessed as having some form of speech, language or communication need (Bryan, Freer and Furlong 2007). Initial studies looking at rates of traumatic brain injury in young offenders also suggest higher incidence in this population (Williams et al. 2010), although the use of self-report may affect the reliability of such findings.

Young women in custody are reported to have the highest rates of mental health difficulties, particularly depression, post-traumatic stress disorder (PTSD) and self-harm (Chitsabesan et al. 2006). One study found over a third of 17-year-old girls in YOIs had self-harmed in the previous month (Douglas and Plugge 2006). Young people from some black and minority ethnic (BME) communities (specifically black/black British young people and those of mixed heritage) are considerably overrepresented in the young people's secure estate and tend to receive longer sentences (House of Commons Home Affairs Committee 2007).

The picture that emerges from the clinical literature is of complex co-morbid emotional, behavioural and social problems. There are several disadvantages to the literature's use of a diagnostic approach to such complexity however. Diagnoses such as personality disorder, ADHD and conduct disorder have been found to be present at such high rates that this brings into question both their discriminatory ability and their clinical utility. In addition, significant co-morbidity has been highlighted in a number of studies. For example, Lader and colleagues found that eight out of ten of the young people had more than one mental health problem that met the criteria for a formal diagnosis (Lader, Singleton and Meltzer 2000), and, similarly, Ulzen and Hamilton (1998), using the Diagnostic Interview for Children and Adolescents – Revised (DICA-R), showed that over 85 per cent of young people in custody reached diagnostic criteria for at least one diagnosis. Other authors have suggested that theories of trauma and attachment may offer a more helpful framework for understanding the complex range of needs, difficulties and risks with which children and young people present (Casswell, French and Rogers 2012).

The findings described predominantly relate to young people in prison settings. There is little published research about the characteristics and mental health needs of young people in SCHs. The Secure Accommodation Network, which is the overarching body that represents SCHs in England and Wales, published a report in 2014: 'They helped me, they supported me: Achieving outcomes and value for money in secure children's homes' (Justice Studio 2014). The report suggested that a similar picture emerges for young people in SCHs, who have extremely complex needs, with backgrounds of sexual, physical or emotional abuse, neglect, domestic violence, family substance use and bereavements. Immediately prior to placement, young people are often looked after by the local authority, having experienced multiple placements and gaps in education. There is also a high proportion of young people involved in gangs or sexual exploitation, and they present with a range of complex and co-morbid mental health problems, difficulties forming relationships, aggression and deliberate self-harm (Justice Studio 2014).

There is a lack of published research about the characteristics of young people in adolescent inpatient units. Bailey and colleagues (1994) examined the clinical, individual and family background characteristics of the first 100 admissions to a secure psychiatric unit for adolescents. A third of adolescents presented with a risk to themselves and two-thirds had committed a recent serious offence. The background histories revealed high levels of disruption, disadvantage and need, with 80 per cent of young people having been in the care of local authorities at some stage in their lives, and most having had previous involvement with either mental health or special education provision. Forty-seven per cent moved on to a further secure establishment on discharge. Hill and colleagues (2014) examined the characteristics of 30 female patients admitted to an adolescent secure hospital. They noted the frequency and severity of problems reported on the Millon Adolescent Clinical Inventory (MACI) (Millon et al. 2006) and the fluctuating nature of the highly disturbed population. A relationship was found between disruption of early attachment relationships and trauma with the severity of presentation on the unit. Disruption in early attachment relationships, as reported by the Structured Assessment of Violence Risk in Youth (SAVRY) tool (Borum, Bartel and Forth 2003), and a history of childhood sexual abuse as measured by the MACI, correlated with the rates of aggressive and self-harm incidents.

Other studies have focused on analysing the type and frequency of incident rates, and note high incidence of violence to others, particularly nursing staff, and high levels of deliberate self-harm, particularly in young women. Hill and colleagues (2012) analysed all reported incidents involving 37 consecutively discharged young people from a mixed sex adolescent forensic hospital. Findings included a very high overall rate of incidents (2,388 incidents during a total of 6,161 cumulative occupied bed days). A small number of young women, meeting criteria for a diagnosis of emerging emotionally unstable personality disorder, accounted for the majority of violent incidents and other incidents. In an older evaluation, Kelsall, Dolan and Bailey (1995) found a slightly higher daily incident rate in the adolescent sample compared to studies of adult hospital environments. At least half of the population were involved in some form of violent episode over the 12-month period. Nursing staff were the most frequent targets of violence. In addition, young women displayed the highest rates of deliberate self-harm.

The psychosocial impact of the secure system

Psychological care for young people in secure settings takes place in a very specific context. Children and young people make a number of transitions from the community to custody, with associated stresses, losses and separations, including separation from family and friends, loss of role, of 'mortification of the self' (Goffman 1961), and the stress of the physical and psychological limbo of being 'between worlds with mastery of neither' (Gibbs 1982: 35). Harvey (2007) found that young people in a YOI often refused to accept the reality that their freedom and control had become limited, particularly if this was the first time they had come into a secure setting. Young people become fearful and preoccupied with safety, unsure about their new environment, its rules and challenges, with only the reputation of secure settings, or information from others to go on. For those young people on remand in Harvey's study, uncertainty about what would happen next added to the uncertainty they faced about how they would maintain relationships, how family and friends would manage without them, and what would happen on release. Heightened distress amongst young offenders in Harvey's (2007) study was associated with an external locus of control, a lower perception of adaptability to prison life and preoccupations with feeling unsafe.

There are few robust and comprehensive studies specifically exploring the impact of child custody on emotional well-being and mental health. The evidence that does exist is predominantly negative. For example, as outlined, we know that custodial units are a high-risk setting for some young people; young males in custodial settings are 18 times more likely to take their own life (Fazell 2008). Meltzer and Britain (1999) found that 20 per cent of male prisoners on remand aged 16–20 had attempted suicide. Suicidal behaviour and self-harm are particularly prevalent in the first month of custody, when young people face the greatest challenge in adapting to the secure environment. Harvey (2007) using Dear and colleagues' (2001) classification for self-harm in custody, identified four high-risk groups who self-harmed in custody. These were: young men who repetitively self-harmed for relief of tension; those who had mental health difficulties such as depression, hearing voices or symptoms of trauma; those who experienced particular difficulties adjusting to the early days of custody, including young people with physical withdrawal symptoms from drug or alcohol use; and, finally, young men who responded to a particular triggering event, such as problems in family relationships or conflict with peers.

Outcomes for young people in secure settings

There is little published about routine clinical outcomes for young people across different secure settings, although, in terms of the impact on offending, overall custody has been shown to have little effect on recidivism. Reoffending rates are high across the secure estate (over 70 per cent) for YOIs, STCs and SCHs (Ministry of Justice 2013).

Outcome research in generic (non-secure) adolescent inpatient care for young people has found that those admitted to inpatient units improve substantially during their stay and are generally satisfied with their care. Clinical outcomes are found to be affected by treatment climate and, specifically, by ward atmosphere (Tulloch et al. 2008).

Although there is not a routine collection of outcomes for young people in SCHs, indications are that they are able to provide a more positive impact for young people than other areas of the secure estate. The Youth Justice Board (YJB) and National Children's Bureau (2008) interviewed young people in SCHs, YOIs and STCs, and asked them to rate their perception of safety on a one to ten scale, and to make comparisons with other establishments they had resided in. Findings indicated that SCHs were experienced by young people as the safest in the secure estate. This is considered to be due to the smaller size and higher staffing ratios of SCHs, which make it easier for staff to get to know young people, and also the attitudes of staff who were experienced as more likely to treat them with respect, and to be more child-centred in their approach. There is tentative evidence that educational outcomes are also better in SCHs, with some qualitative evidence for increasing emotional well-being (Justice Studio 2014). SCHs' outcomes have been attributed to developing a sense of safety, pro-social modelling from highly motivated and trained staff, high staffing ratios that help the formation of relationships, an individualised approach to education and access to specific therapeutic work (Justice Studio 2014).

Mental health services for children and young people in secure settings

The last decade has seen a growing body of policy governing the health and social care of vulnerable children and young people and their families. These changes began with Every Child Matters (HM Government 2003), which aimed to reduce the differences in outcomes between children who do well and those who do not. Subsequent report recommendations have focused on improving access to services for all children, but especially for those who are most vulnerable, at risk of poor outcomes or perceived by services as hard to reach (Ministry of Justice 2008; Department for Schools, Children and Families, 2009 and the DH 2009; DH 2009a, 2009b). These recognise that every child and young person should have access to universal services; those with high-risk factors for poor outcomes may also need targeted support, and those with the most complex needs may need specialist input.

In 2001, Changing the Outlook (DH 2001) made the case for modernising the provision of mental health support for people in custody settings. It was argued that, rather than thinking about the equivalence of services in secure settings with what is provided outside, we should instead be thinking about what needs to happen to promote equivalence of outcomes for those in these settings. A focus on equivalence of outcomes therefore does not require the same pattern and level of services, but enhanced service provision in order to raise outcomes for those in secure settings to a level with those of children and young people in the wider community (Lines 2006). The Royal College of Paediatrics and Child Health have developed 'Healthcare Standards for Children and Young People in Secure Settings' (2013). These include standards for mental health and neurodisability care and intervention, and involve ensuring that all staff working with young people have access to consultation, advice and training from a CAMHS team, and that young people have access to dedicated CAMHS psychiatric and psychological input, and, through CAMHS, access to other multidisciplinary clinicians. In recognition of the poor health outcomes for young people in secure settings, there is a move to transfer commissioning responsibility for health services in SCHs and STCs in England to the NHS. The aim of this is to improve the health and well-being outcomes of children and young people detained in these units by providing care that is appropriate to their high level of need, and to improve continuity of care when they return to local communities (HM Government 2011).

A comprehensive CAMHS approach sees children and young people's mental health and emotional well-being as the responsibility of all workers in the secure estate, not just of specialist services, where 'a period in detention is currently a missed opportunity to detect, diagnose, and treat health problems in a population which is often hard to engage in the NHS' (Gould and Payne 2004: 550).

The role of psychology in secure settings

The role of the practitioner psychologist in secure settings has developed in recent years, from a focus on addressing offending and 'criminogenic' needs with a primary aim to reduce recidivism, to addressing broader mental health and psychological need and improving outcomes and well-being, not necessarily solely because there is a direct link between mental health and offending (Harvey and Smedley 2010). Practitioner psychologists in YOIs can form part of mental health in-reach teams or embedded integrated multidisciplinary mental health teams, or be organised within forensic psychology departments. Mental health provision in STCs and SCHs varies significantly. It is delivered by a range of providers, with local arrangements and disparity in levels of psychological and practitioner psychology input. The move to national commissioning, however, should enable a more unified approach to service delivery. In hospitals, practitioner psychology provision is an integral part of the MDT (Hill and Preston 2012).

Practitioner psychologists working with young people in secure settings need to have a systemic understanding of the context in which they are working (Harvey and Smedley 2010). In particular, it is essential that they are aware of the experience of being detained in that particular setting, that they be aware of the power imbalance and lack of trust that may exist in the relationship between the young person, care/custodial staff and the psychologist, and that they are aware of the dominant role of security (Figure 4.1).

Practitioner psychologists are uniquely placed in secure mental health services to use a broad-based approach to working both directly and indirectly with the young people in their care. By bringing together and integrating a range of psychological models and theories, including neurodevelopmental, behavioural, systemic, cognitive, trauma and attachment, psychologically informed services have an enhanced capacity to influence change.

The model in Figure 4.1 represents two interrelated dynamics: the mode of assessment and intervention informed by a psychological understanding, and its relationship to developmental psychological tasks or functions, underpinned by security of attachment relationships. There are four modes described:

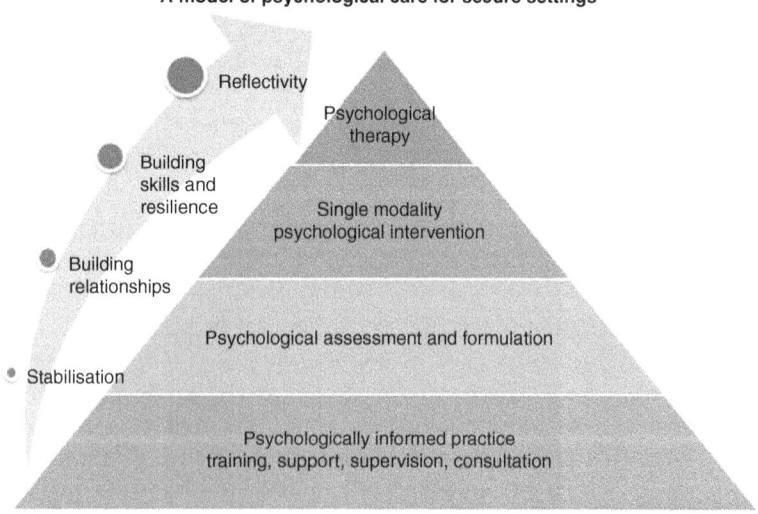

Figure 4.1 A model of psychological provision

psychologically informed practice, psychological assessment and formulation, single modality psychological intervention and psychological therapy. There are also four psychological tasks: stabilisation, building relationships, building skills and resilience, and reflectivity.

Achievement of each task is dependent on a foundation of dynamic individual, systemic, contextual and cultural factors, reflected in broad developmental models such as Bronfenbrenner's ecological model (Bronfenbrenner 1979), which emphasises the influence of the many layered ecologies, such as individual relationships, social networks, institutions, cultural and political spheres of which children are a part. The model also reflects attachment literature such as Golding's (2007) Pyramid of Need and trauma literature (Van der Kolk 2007), which suggest that the therapeutic needs of children are hierarchical, and need to begin with developing a sense of safety, developing relationships, and building resilience and skills.

For some young people, movement through different tasks reflects a developmental progression, others may move between tasks with front-line staff helping to promote stabilisation at times of crisis, whilst a small number may have the capacity and skills needed for reflection at an earlier stage in their journey. Rogers and Law (2010) stress the importance of working with the caregiving system when working therapeutically with young people in secure settings, and that the first priority is to develop safety and stability in the system and the young person. They propose three areas of intervention:

1. Psychoeducation for the young person and caregiving system.
2. Regulating distress and building coping resources for both the young person and the system.
3. Reprocessing trauma only when both the system is stable and the young person has sufficient skills in emotion regulation for this work to be carried out safely without retraumatising the young person.

The model is not prescriptive in what types of intervention may best meet a young person's needs. Different types of psychologically informed intervention may be undertaken by a range of staff, guided by a broad-based understanding of the young person's difficulties and needs. Creative approaches using stories, games, art and drama can be integral both to stabilisation and reflection, and, similarly, use of meaningful activity can be a medium to facilitate change across modes. What underpins all aspects of a psychologically informed approach is an overarching, cohesive, psychological formulation.

This model of psychological care for secure settings proposes that often the first task for the team working with young people in secure settings is to help the young people achieve a degree of stabilisation. The young person has moved to a new, often very unfamiliar environment, with a new team of adults in caregiving roles, as well as uncertainties over his/her peer group relationships. We can suppose that this transition may be highly anxiety provoking, and young people may use a range of strategies to attempt to manage this anxiety. They may present with high-risk behaviours or avoidant and isolative behaviours. Secure settings should provide a structure and routine, clear boundaries, certainty that basic needs will be met (regular meals and shelter), staff who are available consistently, and young people who are free from drugs and alcohol. As a result, the system itself can provide the foundations of stabilisation. The culture and ethos of the unit needs to manage the balance between providing care and nurturing, and control, consistency and boundary setting. We will describe the importance of a psychologically informed system of care, with a well-supported staff team who are equipped with knowledge of psychological theory and an understanding of the developmental needs of young people. This psychologically informed system of care enables a culture that can best support the young people to achieve a sense of safety and stabilisation.

The model proposes that, once a degree of stabilisation is achieved, the young person may be able to then build relationships with the professionals working with them; front-line staff in particular. Along with their histories of disrupted attachments and trauma, young people may have had difficult relationships with previous professionals, and may have dropped out of previous interventions in the community. As a result, it can be a significant challenge to form trusting relationships. The process of being in a secure unit means that the young people are separated from their most significant relationships in the community. The systems of care surrounding young people, which form the context for change, need to include reliable signals of care (Saxe, Ellis and Kaplow 2007) from front-line staff, who have a key caretaking role. As Saxe, Ellis and Kaplow (2007) describe, working with traumatised children and young people requires a 'critical mass' of signals of care communicating warmth, empathy and positive regard, sometimes where this has not been communicated before.

Practitioner psychologists have a role to play to help young people develop stabilisation, build relationships, develop new skills and develop reflexivity. Their role for most young people will be developing the system of care to provide psychologically informed practice through training, support, supervision and consultation, and through assessment and formulation. Psychological formulations, which are multifactorial, integrative and, therefore, by definition, not drawn from any single theoretical perspective, can help both the young person and those working with them make sense of complex interpersonal dynamics, so that both the system of care and signals of care are consistent and unified. A smaller number of young people may access single modality psychological interventions, where the key aim is to build skills and strengths in order to be able to access formal psychological therapy. Psychological therapy may draw from a number of psychological theories and approaches, and could include therapy directly addressing trauma, once it is felt that it is safe enough and young people are equipped with skills to regulate and manage their emotions and distress. For many young people this work is unlikely to occur in the secure setting (Box 4.1).

Box 4.1   Case example 1

A 17-year-old male in a YOI was presenting with self-harming and isolative behaviours. He was spending all of his time in his cell, refusing to mix with his peers, attend education or engage with other services. He had requested to be moved to another YOI. Prison staff investigated the possibility of bullying but found no evidence to support this. The psychologist hypothesised that he was dysregulated, anxious and hypervigilant, perceiving himself to be under threat. A request was made that he move to a specialist unit with smaller numbers and a higher staff ratio, where the formulation was shared with staff and a plan with the young person and staff developed in order to help him feel secure. Once stabilised, the young person engaged both with the regime and further psychological assessment and therapy, where one focus was core beliefs centred on being different to others.

Psychologically informed practice

There is increasing challenge to the idea that individual therapy is the most effective way to help young people who have experienced complex and traumatic attachment experiences and abuse (Rogers, McMahon and Law 2011). Therapeutic opportunities can happen through moment-by-moment everyday interactions between front-line carers and young people. Practitioner psychologists have an important role in working with the system of care to enable these therapeutic moments to be informed by sound clinical formulation and knowledge of psychological theory. These formulations can inform a collaborative identification of the therapeutic task and advice on the possible evidence-based ways of achieving the task. The intervention can be viewed as a systemic intervention, rather than necessarily being provided by a specialist therapist, who may meet with the young person for an hour a week.

Increasing emphasis is being placed on secure settings adopting a psychologically informed approach to service delivery, for example, the Secure Forensic Mental Health Service for Young People includes a psychologically informed model of care that forms part of the service specification (National

Commissioning Board 2013). The aim is for a psychological approach to underpin every aspect of care, therapy and security. Drawing from approaches to service delivery for homeless people known as psychologically informed environments (PIEs) (Johnson and Haigh 2010) and, in the CJS, known as psychologically informed planned environments (PIPEs), services run along these lines aim to help staff and services understand where emotional and behavioural problems, which can challenge mainstream service delivery, originate, and inform work with these service users. PIEs recognise that clients with challenging behaviour have particular support needs, often arising from earlier trauma and abuse. A theoretical psychological framework is developed from which staff and services develop clear and consistent responses to clients, and relationships and interactions are seen as central. PIPEs are psychologically led prison settings in the adult prison estate, where staff members have additional training to develop an increased psychological understanding of their work. There is a focus on the quality of relationships and interactions, with the ultimate aim of reducing risk behaviours, improving psychological well-being and encouraging prosocial living.

Whilst no such formal model exists as yet in the secure estate for young people, services have attempted to develop psychologically informed models of care, which take into account developmental perspective. The National Secure Mental Health Services for Young People have attempted to describe a psychologically informed model of care (National Commissioning Board 2013: 21), which aims for the therapeutic culture in the service to:

- Be delivered and maintained by staff who have a psychological understanding of their work and who are well supported and trained.
- Actively recognise the importance of the quality of relationships and interactions.
- Be informed by clinical formulation drawing from a range of theoretical perspectives.
- Be young-person and family centred, and to aim to maintain good links with the young person's wider support network.
- Promote well-being, the development of adaptive skills, the formation and maintenance of better relationships, and reduce problematic, challenging or risky behaviours.
- Promote positive risk taking using thorough risk assessment and risk management strategies.

The aim is to develop psychological mindedness within the system of care through training, clinical supervision and reflective practice, clinical and risk assessment, clinical formulation, psychologically informed interventions, and evaluation and measuring outcomes. Units may use an overarching framework of a model of care that provides a coherent structure and theoretical underpinning to the work of the unit, and provides structure and guidance for front-line staff to work in a psychologically informed manner (Box 4.2).

Box 4.2 Case example 2

Bluebird House, one of the national medium secure hospitals for young people, developed the Bluebird House Attachment and Trauma Model of Care. The model acknowledges the influence of the young persons' complex history in understanding the presenting needs, and provides guidance on how staff might meet these needs. It promotes interactions and relationships with front-line staff as primary facilitators of change. As part of the Model of Care, a two-day attachment and trauma training programme was developed by the unit psychologists and delivered to all clinical staff at Bluebird House.

Psychological assessment and formulation

Due to the round-the-clock care that secure settings provide, such settings enable a really comprehensive assessment of the young person and identification of their strengths and needs. A psychological assessment can contribute to the broader multidisciplinary assessment. Young people in secure settings have significantly greater, and often previously unidentified and unmet, mental and emotional health needs, and may not have received services before they were detained in a secure setting. Time in secure settings can be seen as a 'window of opportunity' to assess their needs (Royal College of Paediatrics and Child Health 2013). Assessments can consist of interviews with the young person, families and their wider system; observations in different settings including the unit, school, ward and community; psychometric assessments; and incorporating impressions and observations of front-line security, care, education and support staff. Psychologically informed assessments can be enhanced by using tools such as psychometric measures and structured clinical judgement approaches such as the SAVRY (Borum, Bartel and Forth 2003). Reviewing the case file can, in some cases, provide detailed information about a young person's early experiences, and, in other cases, highlight the lack of information and the gaps in this information that the system has accessed. It is important to connect the care pathway for young people so that information from any services with involvement prior to the young person being admitted to the secure setting is collated.

The assessments aim to provide an account of a young person's history, development and early experiences, patterns of relationships, mental health, behaviours and risk. It will also identify the strengths, values and goals of the young person, their family and wider system. Assessments can also provide a baseline from which change can be measured.

These assessments can then inform psychological formulations that draw from multiple theoretical perspectives and make sense of a young person's presentation in the context of their developmental history and experience. The formulations can be informed by the theoretical underpinnings of the overarching model of care. Psychological formulation can serve a range of purposes for teams, including generating new ways of thinking, achieving a consistent approach to intervention, helping to manage risk and raising staff morale (BPS 2011). Formulations have been found to improve team working, help with intervention planning and have a positive effect on staff perceptions of service users (Hollingworth and Johnstone 2014). One of the aims of sharing and developing formulations collaboratively with the staff team is to enable front-line staff to have increased empathy for young people, by helping them conceptualise young people's behaviours and patterns of interacting and relating to others as understandable, and even adaptive, given their early history. Clinical experience has found that developing clinical formulations with staff teams, when relationships with young people have become strained, has enabled improvements in relationships by helping staff gain a new perspective and clarity. The primary function of the formulation is to enable clarification of the therapeutic task at a particular point in the young person's journey, both for direct intervention and therapy, but also systemically by providing guidance to front-line staff. Presenting problems and challenging or high-risk behaviours can be conceptualised as having a function, such as emotion regulation, communication and so on, rather than being viewed as purely problematic behaviours, and the team's task can be to help the young person meet this need by developing alternative skills and positively reinforcing their use of these (Box 4.3).

Box 4.3   Case example 3

During routine group clinical supervision with nursing staff in a hospital setting, some staff identified that they were struggling to know how to work with a 15-year-old girl. She had developed strong attachments to a few members of staff, whom she could seek comfort from, but other staff did not feel that they had a role in working with her. A formulation meeting was held with nursing staff and the wider multidisciplinary team. The formulation was constructed collaboratively with the team and made links between the girl's early experiences of extreme neglect and her current difficulties communicating, forming relationships and managing her distress. The formulation highlighted three key therapeutic tasks that shaped the work of the team. The tasks were:

1. Communication and co-regulation: Hear and validate the meaning behind what she is trying to say; non-verbal art therapy; use of coloured balls to aid communication.
2. Play and identity: Allow opportunities for play and exploration; develop skills and hobbies.
3. Connect with system outside of hospital and promote relationships with stable attachment figures.

Single modality psychological interventions

Single modality psychological interventions are interventions that are rooted within one theoretical model, often addressing discrete problem areas, and encompass a broad range of individual and group-based approaches. They may be delivered by practitioners trained in this one theoretical model, and include manualised treatment packages. These are designed to enhance, support and develop cognitive, emotional, interpersonal, and adaptive skills and resources, so that children and young people can develop more adaptive, less damaging and risky ways of thinking, feeling and behaving. They are often present-moment focused, directive and goal oriented. The aim of these interventions is to help young people build skills in problem solving, emotion regulation, tolerating distress and managing relationships. They should always be informed by an understanding of the young person's developmental stage and levels of arousal (Perry 2013). This is important so as to ensure scarce resources are used to best effect (Saxe et al. 2005). Single modality interventions may be delivered by practitioner psychologists, or by a range of other professionals, usually under the governance structures of practitioner psychologists.

Group-based offending behaviour programmes, such as enhanced thinking skills programmes, from which juvenile enhanced thinking skills (JETS; Nichols and Mitchell 2004) was developed, would fit into the broad definition of single modality psychological interventions. They focus on cognitive skills deficits, are goal based and skills oriented, are directive in orientation, and are manualised rather than individualised, although, more recently, individual sessions have been incorporated into the group work approach (Clark 2010). Once again, the success of such programmes in terms of reducing reoffending has been found to depend on both individual and interpersonal factors, which are integral to developing an individualised understanding as part of a comprehensive psychological assessment and formulation. Clarke, Simmonds and Wydall (2004: 64) found that, in adult prisoners who had successfully completed a cognitive skills programme, change was attributed less to the programme itself, than to motivational and contextual factors, and concluded that:

> Motivation for programme participation and individual change are influenced by a complex combination of the individual's characteristics, the institutional context in which the programmes are delivered and how the individual engages with the programme.

Other examples of these kinds of interventions would include stage one dialectical behaviour therapy (DBT) targets for 'attaining basic capacities' such as decreasing life-threatening behaviours, decreasing therapy-interfering behaviours, decreasing quality-of-life-interfering behaviours and increasing behavioural skills (Miller, Rathus and Linehan 2007). Once again, having a psychologically informed system of care is needed to support such skills development, so that stress on caregivers does not replicate the type of invalidating environment (Linehan 1987) implicated in the development of difficulties regulating emotions. We will return to different secure settings and their capacity to validate young people's inner experiences later in the section 'Opportunity and challenges of secure settings'.

Whilst many single modality programmes and interventions focus on reducing problematic behaviour, our view is that emotion-focused interventions should not be overlooked. Frequently, clinical formulations suggest the function of behaviours as being a result of emotional dysregulation, or emotion overregulation, and, thus, helping young people to safely understand, express and tolerate emotions may be indicated.

Psychological therapy

Where the aim of single modality interventions is to support the development of discrete skills and build resilience, often focusing on the present, more formal therapeutic approaches are integrative, holistic, and incorporate past, present and future. It is likely that formal psychological therapy approaches will only be used with a small number of young people in these settings. Harvey and Smedley (2010) examine four psychological therapies used in prisons and secure settings (psychodynamic psychotherapy, cognitive analytic therapy (CAT), cognitive behaviour therapy (CBT) and systemic psychotherapy). The importance of using any intervention flexibly has been stressed (Smedley 2010). For example, a CBT approach, when used flexibly and collaboratively, can be tailored to an individual's needs. CBT can take a developmental perspective and help make sense of a young person's needs in the context of their early experiences; it can help understand how difficulties can be maintained on a day-to-day basis, or provide an explanation for a discrete symptom area.

Young people's early experiences, their cognitive functioning and their impulsivity can affect their ability to reflect on their early experiences and behaviours (Willis 2010). CAT has been used as a tool where the primary aim is to increase skills in recognition. Willis' audit of her practice suggested that young people reported that CAT had increased their understanding, but had less impact on revision of behaviours.

These therapeutic interventions can be tools to help a young person acquire skills to manage anxiety or low moods, which could provide sufficient foundations for future trauma work to safely be undertaken (Smedley 2010). However, there is an ethical dilemma as to whether secure settings provide a safe enough environment in which to engage in direct trauma reprocessing, and whether the young person's length of stay is sufficient to complete the work (Rogers and Law 2010).

Opportunities and challenges of secure settings

Developing relational security: Establishing a safe base

In forensic secure settings, the challenge is to balance security, and the restrictions that security can pose on a young person's liberty, choices and responsibility in order to manage risk, with a therapeutic culture that allows young people to understand themselves, take positive risks, and grow and develop. Questions arise as to whether the goals of developing a therapeutic culture and the security of a secure service are in conflict, and how this conflict can be reconciled. Security can be thought about in terms of procedural (policies, procedures and processes), physical (buildings and premises) and relational security. The ideal is that relational security is at the forefront of security, and procedural and physical security are robust and present, but in the background. Relational security is:

> The knowledge and understanding staff have of a patient and of the environment, and the translation of that information into appropriate responses and care... Safe and effective relationships between staff and patients must be professional, therapeutic and purposeful with understood limits.
>
> (DH 2010: 5)

Relational security aims to use therapeutic relationships to provide a sense of safety and containment that enables disturbed behaviour to be minimised in the least restrictive environment.

The safety and security that a secure setting provides can be an opportunity for young people and families to take therapeutic risks. The aim is to optimise choice, facilitating psychological functioning in a safe environment with the lowest level of external security possible, whilst still reducing risks. When relational security is at the forefront, risk assessments can be dynamic and can involve the young people. Making risk decisions within the context of boundaried therapeutic relationships allows positive risks to be taken to facilitate change.

Often, young people and families can be anxious about taking risks because these risks can lead to strong emotions. Historically, young people may have presented with violence, aggression and disturbed behaviour when emotionally dysregulated, and the security of a secure setting can allow families to practise having difficult conversations (Box 4.4).

Box 4.4   Case example 4

A parent used a family therapy session tell her daughter that the family pet had died. This was a conversation that previously would have been avoided due to the level of violence and aggression displayed by the young person when emotionally dysregulated. The mother was able to take the risk and use this as an opportunity to practise having difficult conversations, with confidence that the hospital setting could manage any resulting violence and aggression. As both the mother and her daughter became practised at managing difficult emotions, they were able to do this without the security of the setting, the young person was able to return home, and the family system felt more empowered to manage difficult emotions.

In general, it would appear from clinical experience that relational security is not at the forefront in a prison setting, where physical and procedural security predominate. However, the picture is more complex one than it first appears, with influences on the development of relational security at the institutional, political and cultural level. There is a lack of clarity about the aim and purposes of imprisonment within the wider CJS (House of Commons Justice Committee 2009), which has a less predictable influence on the development of relational security. This lack of cohesiveness was summed up by Professor Andrew Coyle in a report on the role of the prison officer, in which he stated that:

> In general terms we are fairly clear about the purpose of most of the large institutions in our society: the school for example, is there to educate young people, the hospital is there to heal people who are sick. There is no similar clarity about the role of the prison.
>
> (House of Commons Justice Committee 2009: 8)

This lack of clarity is influenced by a political debate, which is, in turn, influenced by powerful public perceptions about crime, loss of liberty and punishment. It has important implications for individual prison staff, for whom there is a potential clash between the perceived needs of security and discipline, and those of rehabilitation.

A further powerful institutional influence on the development of relational security is the lack of control in SCHs, STCs and YOIs when compared to hospital settings. Unlike a hospital, which can decide which young people to admit, YOIs, SCHs and STCs have to accept and manage whoever the courts sentence, and the YJB places with them. Dynamics such as lack of institutional clarity of purpose and aim, low levels of control and high levels of reactivity have significant influences at the microsystem level on developing stable, secure and consistent relationships between young people and front-line staff. Such dynamics need to be understood when developing individualised psychological formulations and intervention plans (Box 4.5).

Box 4.5   Case example 5

A 16-year-old in a YOI presented with disruptive and challenging behaviour: constantly ringing his cell bell, provoking other young people through name calling and challenging staff. As a consequence of his behaviour he lost privileges and entitlements, spending much of his time in his cell with little to occupy him. The mental health team hypothesised that he was emotionally dysregulated, and that his behaviours helped him to manage this, and the isolation and boredom. Although this formulation was shared with front-line staff with a view to increasing the amount of positive contact time he had with staff, many prison officers felt that his actions were designed to try and 'manipulate' them and most officers disengaged from him. The prison managed the demands he made on staff time through repeated discipline measures and moving him from wing to wing, destabilising him further and leading to an increase in his difficulties.

Creating dependency

For young people with complex histories of attachment, trauma and abuse, being in a custodial setting may be a source of threat. The young person will experience separation from family and other significant relationships. They may experience repetition of past experiences of neglect and separation, peer dynamics and bullying, and transitions and termination of relationships as staff members leave or change role (Harvey and Smedley 2010).

However, for others, institutions may in fact become a secure base. Secure settings can provide an opportunity for containment, clear consequences for behaviour, routine and meeting basic needs. Young people at risk to themselves can be managed with staff observations to prevent the most extreme self-harm, or to intervene in physical altercations between their peers. In STCs, young people reported that they mostly felt safe, that staff treated them with respect and that the education they had received would help them in the future, but they also often felt frightened and isolated (Elwood 2014). For at least some, then, there is a paradox of the environment being both a place of safety and security and also a place of threat (Haley 2010).

For many young people, community living is characterised by instability, insecurity, and low levels of support and care. This can create a risk of young people becoming reliant on institutions, the structure and routine, and, most importantly, relationships and attachments made with front-line staff (Box 4.6).

Box 4.6   Case example 6

A 17-year-old has returned to a secure setting for the fourth time, after breaching the conditions of his order. His previous convictions are for predominantly acquisitive offences. He was first placed in secure care aged 13, and has been in secure children's units, an STC and has served two sentences at a YOI, most recently in a specialist unit for vulnerable young people. He has professional support in the community, but has not had any contact with family for many years. In the community he struggles to manage day to day, having been placed in a hostel where he is expected to be able to budget and manage his time independently. When he returns to custody he tells staff that he is happy to be back as he considers the unit to be home.

Supporting front-line staff

The model of psychological provision proposed promotes the relationships and interactions of the young people and front-line staff as the key agents of change. Practitioner psychologists have important opportunities to work with the front-line staff to provide a supportive framework to enhance their interactions and relationships with young people. It is important that the front-line staff are sufficiently supported, trained and equipped to deal with the high levels of expressed emotion, challenging behaviour (including direct violence) and critical incidents, which they encounter as part of their day-to-day working lives.

The secure environments for young people are some of the most emotionally demanding environments to work in. High levels of burnout have been found for prison officers (Carlson and Thomas 2006), children's home staff (Heron and Chakrabarti 2003), and nursing staff in acute and forensic mental health inpatient settings (Jenkins and Elliott 2004; Dickinson and Wright 2008). Staff who experience burnout are likely to find it more difficult to be attuned to the needs of the young people, particularly because burnout is associated with depersonalisation, which can be defined as 'an unfeeling and impersonal response toward recipients of one's service, care treatment or instruction' (Maslach, Jackson and Leiter 1996: 4). There is, additionally, a potentially high level of PTSD and vicarious trauma experienced by staff working in these settings (Wright et al. 2006; Boudoukha et al. 2013).

Research has highlighted the importance of social support from co-workers within the prison (Harvey 2014) or hospital (Jenkins and Elliott 2004) in reducing emotional exhaustion; support from within the setting is more effective than from relationships outside of the work context. Practitioner psychologists can have a role to play in allowing staff time to talk together, and creating space within the demands of the day to do this. The importance of creating 'time to think' for staff to be able to hold in mind the young people has been stressed (Rose 2014).

Clinical supervision and reflective practice are commonplace methods used in health settings to provide support and thinking space for multidisciplinary staff (Hill and Preston 2012), but these approaches may be less familiar to other staff groups. To be successful, there needs to be an alignment between the supervision models and delivery and the aims and purpose of the units that is shared by all. The model needs to be embedded within the culture of the unit.

Keeping connected to systems outside of the secure setting

Young people in secure settings often have complex professional, family and carer systems. It can be important to keep the wider system of families and carers involved in the care and treatment of young people, but this can prove challenging when families may be geographically far away and the young people are being 'parented' by professionals. It has been suggested that treatment focused on the family can be more effective than focusing on the individual (Perkins-Dock 2001). Community treatments focusing on the whole system around the young person, specifically multisystemic therapy (MST), has been found to be one of the most effective treatments for young people in community settings, addressing both recidivism and mental health symptoms (Henggeler, Melton and Smith 1992; NICE 2013).

If the aim of the settings were to provide a stable base from which the young person can connect to the outside world, this could help translate skills learnt in a secure setting to the community context, and help the young person connect with significant relationships outside of the setting (Shelton 2010). Hospital settings may have more time, resources and dedicated family therapists to enable this connection to happen, and there is an expectation that families, carers and professionals will be involved in the planning of care. This is not as easy to achieve in other settings, due to the barriers and practical difficulties (Perkins-Dock 2001).

Practical and professional challenges of implementing a model of psychologically informed care across settings

Central to the model described in this chapter is the development of relational security so that young people can stabilise, building a safe base from which to develop and change. However, there are several practical challenges to developing relational security that need to be acknowledged.

Staffing levels, backgrounds and training vary widely across the secure estate. In hospitals, STCs and SCHs, where staffing ratios are higher, there is more opportunity to build and develop relationships between young people and front-line staff, leading to more individualised care. In YOIs, staffing levels are significantly lower, and staff are often moved between units to cover shortages, impacting on their ability to develop consistent, supportive relationships with the young people in their care. Although YOI staffing structures operate a personal officer system, where one member of staff is allocated to several young people as a source of support and guidance, it is our experience that this system rarely works well, as the dedication of scarce resources to ensuring the security and stability of the whole institution takes priority. As mentioned, hospitals, SCHs and STCs have higher staffing levels. However, high staff turnover and use of agency staff can impact on developing relational security. There is the risk, in secure environments, of the development of a vicious cycle of relational instability, leading to increased risk of harmful behaviours, leading to higher staff turnover, which, in turn, increases the risk of instability further.

Another important factor to consider in implementing psychologically informed interventions in secure settings is the clarity of purpose, aims and ethos of the setting. Whereas hospitals are more able to develop a sound framework around relational security as a clinical setting focused on care, the focus of other settings, even those with higher staff ratios and more resources, can be less clear. Physical and procedural security predominate in YOIs, where even some smaller units with higher staff ratios look to adapt the prison procedures, systems and policies of the parent setting.

Behaviour management in YOIs generally relies on coercive control through removal of privileges, and individualised, formulation-driven approaches are more difficult to attain. This contrasts with the individualised, collaborative approaches enabled by hospital settings, where shared decision-making with the young person is the norm. As the House of Commons review of the role of the prison officer concludes:

> Despite (the pedigree of the concept of 'dynamic security') and the potential benefits of engaging prisoners individually, it is evident to us that the current situation in the prison system mitigates against this approach.
> (House of Commons Justice Committee 2009: 59)

Nevertheless, there is some evidence that working to a psychologically informed model of care, where prison staff and mental health staff work in collaboration, has resulted in improvements in behavioural and social functioning of young people in one small YOI unit (Ryan and Mitchell 2011). This initial study suggests a promising future direction.

A further practical challenge for implementing the model in SCHs, STCs and YOIs is that duration of intervention is dictated not by clinical need, but by length of sentence. Practitioners need to be mindful of what can be achieved in the time frame available, which is often limited to several months, and which aspects of the intervention plan can be transferred to community settings, where resources are limited and thresholds for mental health referrals high. The opportunity secure settings offer to develop a comprehensive psychological formulation, which can be shared with community teams, and guide resettlement planning and management, should not, however, be underestimated.

Conclusion

Children and young people in secure settings have highly complex needs, often resulting from experiences of trauma, abuse and disrupted early attachments. As a consequence, they can display a complex range of behaviours (challenging behaviours, offending behaviour, mental health problems, drug and alcohol use, and poor educational achievement). This population is looked after in a range of settings governed by different bodies (Department of Education, NHS, Ministry of Justice), where the balance of relational, procedural and physical security may be differently weighted. Their needs, however, are more unified than this piecemeal approach to care would suggest. Recent practice and policy developments in delivering health care to this population, such as the Healthcare Standards (Royal College of Paediatrics and Child Health 2013), reflect an acknowledgement of the need for a coherent, equitable and unified approach across all secure settings.

The role of practitioner psychologists working in secure settings has many similar features, and the model described in this chapter reflects an overarching framework for embedding a psychologically informed approach. An essential element to the model is for the young person to achieve stability. Secure settings provide 24/7 care. This system of care, and the relationships formed between the professional caregivers and the young people, can be viewed as the key agents of change. This system can provide both opportunities and challenges, with some settings easier to align to an approach that requires building trusting and supportive relationships than others.

In the model, intervention is based on a comprehensive systemic psychological formulation, drawn from multiple theoretical perspectives, which enables an individualised understanding of needs and risk, and, in our view, is more useful than offering intervention based on diagnostic category, offence or social care need alone. Whilst there is a role for practitioner psychologists to engage in one-to-one therapy and group work with young people, a flexible approach is needed, and consideration of the system and the context in which the work is being carried out to ensure effectiveness and safety is paramount.

The challenges of implementing a psychological framework in secure settings may often lie beyond the influence of individual practitioners, being interwoven in complex systems of care, which differ in their capacity to embrace this kind of approach. For psychologically informed care to have meaningful impact, it requires collaboration with commissioners, managers and colleagues. In writing this chapter, it has become clear that, whilst implementation of psychologically informed care in secure hospital settings is well underway, progress is much slower and more piecemeal elsewhere. However, it is hoped that having a psychological framework and model, which can be shared, used to help communicate and influence, and from which evidence can begin to be generated, is a helpful start.

References

Abram, K.M., Teplin, L.A., Charles, D.R., Longworth, S.L., McClelland, G.M., and Duncan, M.K. (2004) 'Post-traumatic stress disorder and trauma in youth in juvenile detention', *Archives of General Psychiatry*, 61: 403–410.

Bailey, S.M., Thornton, L., and Weaver, A.B. (1994) 'The first 100 admissions to an adolescent secure unit', *Journal of Adolescence*, 17(3): 207–220.

Borum, R., Bartel, B., and Forth, A. (2003) *Structured Assessment of Violence Risk in Youth: Professional Manual*. Lutz, FL: Psychological Assessment Resources, Inc.

Boudoukha, A.H., Altintas, E., Rusinek, S., Fantini-Hauwel, C., and Hautekeete, M. (2013) 'Inmates-to-staff assaults, PTSD and burnout profiles of risk and vulnerability', *Journal of Interpersonal Violence*, 28(11): 2332–2350.

BPS (British Psychological Society) (2011) *Good Practice Guidelines on the Use of Psychological Formulation*. Leicester: British Psychological Society.

Bronfenbrenner, U. (1979) *The Ecology of Human Development: Experiments by Nature and Design*. Cambridge, MA: Harvard University Press.

Bryan, K., Freer, J., and Furlong, C. (2007) 'Language and communication difficulties in juvenile offenders', *International Journal of Language and Communication Disorders*, 42: 505–520.

Carlson, J.R. and Thomas, G. (2006) 'Burnout among prison caseworkers and corrections officers', *Journal of Offender Rehabilitation*, 43(3): 19–34.

Casswell, M., French, P., and Rogers, A. (2012) 'Distress, defiance or adaption? A review paper of at-risk mental health states in young offenders', *Early Intervention in Psychiatry*, 6: 219–226.

Chitsabesan, P., Kroll, L., Bailey, S., Kenning, C., Macdonald, W., and Theodosiou, L. (2006) 'Mental health needs of offenders in custody and in the community', *British Journal of Psychiatry*, 188: 534–540.

Clark, D. (2010) 'Therapy and Offending Behaviour Programmes', in J. Harvey and K. Smedley (eds.), *Psychological Therapy in Prisons and Other Secure Settings*. Abingdon: Willan Publishing, 234–251.

Clarke, A., Simmonds, R., and Wydall, S. (2004) 'Delivering cognitive skills programmes in prison: A qualitative study', *Home Office Findings*, 242. London: Home Office.

Coffey, C.F., Veit, F., Wolfe, R., Cini, E., and Patton, G.C. (2003) 'Mortality in young offenders: Retrospective cohort study', *British Medical Journal*, 326: 1064–1067.

Dear, G.E., Thomson, D.M., Howells, K., and Hall, G.J. (2001) 'Self-harm in Western Australian prison: Differences between prisoners who have self-harmed and those who have not', *Australian and New Zealand Journal of Criminology*, 34: 277–292.

Department for Education (2012) *Statistical First Release: Children Accommodated in Secure Children's Homes at 31 March 2012: England and Wales*. London: Department for Education.

Department for Schools, Children and Families (2009) *Think Family Toolkit: Improving Support for Families at Risk*. London: Department for Schools, Children and Families.

Department for Schools, Children and Families and the DH (Department of Health) (2009) *CAMHS Review: Children and Young People in Mind*. London: Crown Publications.

DH (Department of Health) (2001) *Changing the Outlook*. London: Department of Health.

DH (Department of Health) (2009a) *Healthy Children, Safer Communities*. London: Department of Health.

DH (Department of Health) (2009b) *New Horizons: A Shared Vision for Mental Health*. London: Department of Health.

DH (Department of Health) (2010) *See Think Act Relational Security Handbook*. London: Department of Health.

DH (Department of Health) (2011) *Procedure for the Transfer from Custody of Children and Young People to and from Hospital under the Mental Health Act 1983 in England*. London: Department of Health.

Dickinson, T. and Wright, K.M. (2008) 'Stress and burnout in forensic mental health nursing: A literature review', *British Journal of Nursing*, 17(2): 82–87.

Douglas, N. and Plugge, E. (2006) *A Health Needs Assessment for Young Women in the Secure Estate*. London: Youth Justice Board.

Elwood, C. (2014) *An Analysis of 12–18 Year Olds' Perceptions of Their Experience in Secure Training Centres*. HM Inspectorate of Prisons. Norwich: The Stationery Office.

Fazell, D. (2008) 'Mental disorders among adolescents in juvenile detention and correction facilities: A systematic review and metaregression analysis of 25 surveys', *Journal of the American Academy of Child and Adolescent Psychiatry*, 47(9): 1010–1019.

Galahad SMS Ltd. (2009) *Evaluation of the Substance Misuse Project in the Young Person's Secure Estate*. London: Youth Justice Board.

Gibbs, J. (1982) 'Disruption and Distress in Going from the Street to Jail', in N. Parisi (ed.), *Coping with Imprisonment*. London: Sage, 29–44.

Goffman, E. (1961/1991) *Asylums Essays on the Social Situations of Mental Patients and Other Inmates*. London: Penguin Press.

Golding, K.S. (2007) *Meeting the Therapeutic Needs of Looked after and Adopted Children*. Available at: http://www.cplaac.org.uk/downloads/files/Kims_Pyramid.doc. Accessed 7 July 2014.

Gould, J. and Payne, H. (2004) 'Health needs of children in prison', *Archives of Diseases in Childhood*, 89: 549–550.

Hagell, A. (2002) *The Mental Health of Young Offenders. Bright Futures: Working with Vulnerable Young People*. London: Mental Health Foundation.

Haley, M. (2010) 'Attachment-based Psychodynamic Psychotherapy', in J. Harvey and K. Smedley (eds.), *Psychological Therapy in Prisons and Other Settings*. Abingdon: Willan Publishing, 48–67.

Harvey, J. (2007) *Young Men in Prison: Surviving and Adapting to Life Inside*. Cullompton: Willan Publishing.

Harvey, J. (2014) 'Perceived physical health, psychological distress, and social support among prison officers', *The Prison Journal*, 94(2): 242–259.

Harvey, J. and Smedley, K. (2010) 'Introduction', in J. Harvey and K. Smedley (eds.), *Psychological Therapy in Prisons and Other Settings*. Abingdon: Willan Publishing, 1–18.

Henggeler, S.W., Melton, G.B., and Smith, L.A. (1992) 'Family preservation using multisystemic therapy: An effective alternative to incarcerating serious juvenile offenders', *Journal of Consulting and Clinical Psychology*, 60(6): 953.

Heron, G. and Chakrabarti, M. (2003) 'Exploring the perceptions of staff towards children and young people living in community-based children's homes', *Journal of Social Work*, 3(1): 81–98.

Hill, S.A. and Preston, J. (2012) 'The first three years of an inpatient adolescent forensic service', *Medicine, Science, and the Law*, 52(3): 156–161.

Hill, S.A., White, O., Lolley, J., Sidki-Gomez, A., and Williams, H. (2012) 'Incidents in an adolescent forensic secure inpatient service', *Medicine, Science and the Law*, 52(1): 27–31.

Hill, S.A., Brodrick, P., Doherty, A., Lolley, J., Wallington, F., and White, O. (2014) 'Characteristics of female patients admitted to an adolescent secure forensic psychiatric hospital', *Journal of Forensic Psychiatry & Psychology*, 25: 1–17.

HM Government (2003) *Every Child Matters*. Norwich: The Stationery Office.

HM Government (2011) 'Q&A on health services in secure children's homes (Youth Justice commissioned) and secure training centres in England'. London: Department of Health. Available at: https://www.gov.uk/government/publications/q-a-on-health-services-in-secure-children-s-homes-youth-justice-commissioned-and-secure-training-centres-in-england-august-2011. Accessed 7 September 2014.

HM Inspectorate of Prisons (1997) *Young Prisoners: A Thematic Review*. London: Home Office.

Hollingworth, P. and Johnstone, L. (2014) 'Team formulation: What are the staff views?' *Clinical Psychology Forum*, 257: 28–34.

House of Commons Home Affairs Committee (2007) *Young Black People and the Criminal Justice System. Second Report of Session 2006–2007: Volume 1*. London: The Stationery Office.

House of Commons Justice Committee (2009) *Role of the Prison Officer*. London: The Stationery Office.

Jenkins, R. and Elliott, P. (2004) 'Stressors, burnout and social support: Nurses in acute mental health settings', *Journal of Advanced Nursing*, 48(6): 622–631.

Johnson, R. and Haigh, R. (2010) 'Social psychiatry and social policy for the 21st century – new concepts for new needs: The "psychologically-informed environment"', *Mental Health and Social Inclusion*, 14(4): 30–35.

Justice Studio (2014) ' "They helped me, they supported me": Achieving outcomes and value for money in secure children's homes'. Available at: http://www.cypnow.co.uk/digital_assets/419/SAN_report_final.pdf. Accessed 7 July 2014.

Kelsall, M., Dolan, M., and Bailey, S. (1995) 'Violent incidents in an adolescent forensic unit', *Medicine Science and Law*, 35: 150–156.
Kroll, L., Rothwell, J., Bradley, D., Shah, P., Bailey, S., and Harrington, R.C. (2002) 'Mental health needs of boys in secure care for serious or persistent offending: A prospective, longitudinal study', *Lancet*, 359: 1975–1979.
Lader, D., Singleton, N., and Meltzer, H. (2000) *Psychiatric Morbidity among Young Offenders in England and Wales*. London: Office for National Statistics.
Linehan, M.M. (1987) 'Dialectical behavior therapy for borderline personality disorder: Theory and method', *Bulletin of the Menninger Clinic*, 51: 261–276.
Lines, R. (2006) 'From equivalence of standards to equivalence of objectives: The entitlement of prisoners to health care standards higher than those outside prisons', *International Journal of Prisoner Health*, 2(4): 269–280.
Maslach, C., Jackson, S.E., and Leiter, M. (1996) *Maslach Burnout Inventory: Manual*. 3rd edn. Palo Alto, CA: Consulting Psychologists Press.
Meltzer, H. and Britain, G. (1999) *Non-Fatal Suicidal Behaviour among Prisoners*. London: Office for National Statistics.
Miller, A.L., Rathus, J.H., and Linehan, M.M. (2007) *Dialectical Behaviour Therapy with Suicidal Adolescents*. New York: Guilford Press.
Millon, T., Millon, C., David, R., and Gossman, S. (2006) *Millon Adolescent Clinical Inventory: Professional Manual*. Minneapolis, MN: Pearson Assessments.
Ministry of Justice (2008) *Youth Crime Action Plan*. London: Ministry of Justice.
Ministry of Justice (2013) 'Transforming youth custody; putting education at the heart of detention', Consultation paper CP4/2013. The Stationery Office Limited.
Ministry of Justice (2014) 'Monthly statistics on the population in custody of children and young people within the secure estate', Youth Justice Report, November 2013.
National Commissioning Board (2013) '2013/14 NHS standard contract for Secure Forensic Mental Health Service for Young People: Particulars, schedule 2 – the services, a – service specification', *National Health Service*. Available at: http://www.england.nhs.uk/wp-content/uploads/2013/06/c11-sec-forensic-mh-young.pdf. Accessed 5 September 2014.
NICE (National Institute for Health and Clinical Excellence) (2013) 'Antisocial behaviour and conduct disorders in children and young people: Recognition, intervention and management', Clinical Guideline 158. Available at: http://www.nice.org.uk/CG158. Accessed 7 September 2014.
NHS England (2014) 'C11. Child & Adolescent Mental Health Service (CAMHS) Secure'. Available at: http://www.england.nhs.uk/commissioning/spec-services/npc-crg/group-c/c11/. Accessed 29 July 2014.
Nichols, C.E. and Mitchell, J. (2004) 'The JETS living skills programme: An integrated cognitive behavioural programme for juvenile offenders', Theory manual. HMPS Offending Behaviour Programmes Unit, Home Office.
Parke, S. (2009) *Children and Young People in Custody 2006–2008: An Analysis of the Experiences of 15–18 Year Olds in Prison*. London: HM Inspector of Prisons/Youth Justice Board.
Perkins-Dock, R.E. (2001) 'Family interventions with incarcerated youth: A review of the literature', *International Journal of Offender Therapy and Comparative Criminology*, 45(5): 606–625.
Perry, B.D. (2013) 'The Neurosequential Model of Therapeutics', in K. Brandt, B. Perry, S. Seligman and E. Tronick (eds.), *Infant and Early Childhood Mental Health: Core Concepts and Clinical Practice*. Arlington: American Psychiatric Publishing, 21–54.

Rogers, A. and Law, H. (2010) 'Working with Trauma in a Prison Setting', in J. Harvey and K. Smedley (eds.), *Psychological Therapy in Prisons and Other Settings*. Abingdon: Willan Publishing, 150–172.

Rogers, A., McMahon, J., and Law, D. (2011) 'Expanding therapy: Challenging the dominant discourse of individual therapy when working with vulnerable young people. A discussion paper', *Clinical Psychology Forum*, 222: 9–14.

Rose, J. (2014) *Working with Young People in Secure Accommodation: From Chaos to Culture*. Hove: Routledge.

Royal College of Paediatrics and Child Health (2013) *Healthcare Standards for Children and Young People in Secure Settings*. London: Royal College of Paediatrics and Child Health.

Ryan, T. and Mitchell, P. (2011) 'A collaborative approach to meeting the needs of adolescent offenders with complex needs in custodial settings: An 18-month cohort study', *Journal of Forensic Psychiatry & Psychology*, 22(3): 437–454.

Saxe, G.N., Ellis, B.H., and Kaplow, J.B. (2007) *Collaborative Treatment of Traumatized Children and Teens: The Trauma Systems Therapy Approach*. New York: Guildford Press.

Saxe, G.N., Ellis, B.H., Fogler, J., Hansen, S., and Sorkin, B. (2005) 'Comprehensive care for traumatized children', *Psychiatric Annals*, 35(5): 443–448.

Shelton, D. (2010) 'Systemic Psychotherapy in Prisons', in J. Harvey and K. Smedley (eds.), *Psychological Therapy in Prisons and Other Settings*. Abingdon: Willan Publishing, 130–146.

Smedley, K. (2010) 'Cognitive Behaviour Therapy with Adolescents in Secure Settings', in J. Harvey and K. Smedley (eds.), *Psychological Therapy in Prisons and Other Settings*. Abingdon: Willan Publishing, 71–97.

Social Exclusion Unit (2002) *Reducing Re-offending by Ex-prisoners*. London: Social Exclusion Unit.

Ståhlberg, O., Anckarster, H., and Nilsson, T. (2010) 'Mental health problems in youths committed to juvenile institutions: Prevalence and treatment needs', *European Journal of Child and Adolescent Psychiatry*, 19: 893–903.

Teplin, L.A., Abram, K.M., McClelland, G.M., Dulcan, M.K., and Mericle, A.A. (2002) 'Psychiatric disorders in youth in juvenile detention', *Archives of General Psychiatry*, 59(12): 1133–1143.

Tulloch, M.S., Lelliott, P., Bannister, D., Andiappan, M.M., O'Herlihy, M.A., Beecham, J., and Ayton, A. (2008) 'The costs, outcomes and satisfaction for inpatient child and adolescent psychiatric services (COSI-CAPS) study', *Report for the National Co-ordinating Centre for NHS Service Delivery and Organisation R&D*. London: HMSO.

Ulzen, T.P.M. and Hamilton, H. (1998) 'The nature and characteristics of psychiatric comorbidity in incarcerated adolescents', *Canadian Journal of Psychiatry*, 43: 57–63.

Van der Kolk, B.A. (2007) 'The Developmental Impact of Childhood Trauma', in L.J. Kirmayer, R., Lemelson, and M. Barad (eds.), *Understanding Trauma: Integrating Biological, Clinical, and Cultural Perspectives*. New York: Cambridge University Press, 224–241.

Williams, W.H., Cordan, G., Mewse, A., Tonks, J., and Burgess, C.N. (2010) 'Self-reported traumatic brain injury in male young offenders: A risk factor for re-offending, poor mental health and violence?' *Neuropsychological Rehabilitation*, 20(6): 801–812.

Willis, A. (2010) 'Cognitive Analytic Therapy with Young Adult Offenders', in J. Harvey and K. Smedley (eds.), *Psychological Therapy in Prisons and Other Secure Settings*. Abingdon: Willan Publishing, 102–126.

Wright, L., Borrill, J., Teers, R., and Cassidy, T. (2006) 'The mental health consequences of dealing with self-inflicted death in custody', *Counselling Psychology Quarterly*, 19(2): 165–180.

YJB (Youth Justice Board) (2007) *Accommodation Needs and Experiences of Young People Who Offend: Summary (B328)*. London: Youth Justice Board.

YJB (Youth Justice Board) (2014) *Youth Justice Statistics 2012/2013 England and Wales*. London: Youth Justice Board.

YJB (Youth Justice Board) and National Children's Bureau (2008) *A Review of Safeguarding in the Secure Estate: Summary of Findings and Action Plan*. London: Youth Justice Board.

5
Youth Violence Risk Assessment: A Framework for Practice

Lorraine Johnstone and Leanne Gregory

Introduction

The overarching aim of this chapter is to provide a framework for practitioners to aid their understanding and application of best practice principles in youth violence risk assessment. In order to achieve this goal, we set the scene by providing some statistics on youth violence, and detail the importance of robust risk assessments in supporting an overall management and support plan. Next, we highlight some of the key themes to emerge from the literature pertinent to understanding the phenomenon of youth violence. This is followed by a review of the different paradigms for assessing risk. Building on this, we take the view that the structured professional judgement (SPJ) paradigm provides the only feasible method of assessing violence risk, and we describe the available protocols that may be used to structure an evaluation for violent youth. However, we take the position that it is unacceptable to cease the assessment after merely identifying 'what' risk factors are present. A much deeper analysis must be achieved, addressing 'why' and 'how' risk manifests. We argue that a risk assessment is incomplete, and potentially misleading, in the absence of a risk formulation. Because the extant literature on clinical risk formulation is relatively scarce and, to our knowledge, no guidelines exist for understanding youth violence, we present a framework for practice that should assist evaluators. In the final substantive section, we acknowledge the still significant challenges that abound in youth violence risk assessment, and highlight key research and practice areas for development in the Conclusion.

Youth violence

The phenomenon of youth violence blights our communities and shapes the lives of many to come, whether they are victims or perpetrators. The statistics are astounding. Internationally, youth homicide accounts for 41 per cent of premature deaths (WHO 2011). Sexual violence (Vizard et al. 2007; Radford et al. 2011), cybercrime (Gerson and Rappaport 2011; Mishna et al. 2012), violent extremism (Home Office 2011), stalking and harassment (Brewster 2013), gang fighting (HM Government 2011; Madden 2013) and fire-setting (Mackay et al. 2014; Watt et al. 2014) by youths are also at worrying levels. In Scotland alone, with a population of only approximately 600,000 young people between the ages of 8 and 17 years, the data for 2012/13 revealed that 43,117 detected crimes were accounted for by this age group; and more than 1,300 of those were related to violence – murder, attempted murder, serious assault, robbery and assault with intent to rob, threats and extortion, cruelty to children, rape, assault with intent to rape, indecent assault and sexual offences against children (Scottish Government 2013). Similarly, in England and Wales, during 2011/12, 13.6 per cent (167,995) of all arrests were of people aged between 10 and 17 years of age; and in 2012/13 young people were primarily convicted of violent offences (over 19,000) and over 1,300 sexual offences (Ministry of Justice 2014). In the USA, between 15 and 20 per cent of all crime is committed by youth under the age of 18 years (Slobogin and Fondacaro 2011). Moreover, this data occurs in the context of a well-documented phenomenon that criminologists refer to as the 'dark figure of crime' – the number of offences that are underreported and/or undetected. Child-to-parent violence and inter-sibling violence – interpersonal or sexual – provide prime examples of behaviours where there will be significant barriers to reporting. Families will often go to great lengths to avoid involving statutory agencies for fear of 'criminalising' their children, or losing their children to the state or having unwelcome intrusions into their private family life.

When a child or adolescent perpetrates an act of serious harm, the state must consider how best to intervene. Across the international arena, there are varied responses. Whilst some jurisdictions adopt a punitive approach, others are more welfare orientated (see Johnstone 2011 for a discussion). Interventions can range from the innocuous and minimally intrusive, such as the offer of a befriender to facilitate socialisation and rehabilitation, all the way through to enacting legislation that allows for the deprivation of liberty and indeterminate state control. Indeed, in some jurisdictions, risk-assessment opinions have been used to justify the removal of a young person's liberty forever (see Amnesty International 2011). Irrespective of which philosophy dominates, those tasked with making decisions about a young person's future must have access to robust and reliable assessments about his/her risk. Key questions relate to whether a young person should be prosecuted, the nature of any legal intervention and disposal, where they should be placed, what level and type of secure placement is needed and for how long, what must be done in order to reduce the risk and optimise the young person's future, and how likely it is that any intervention will meet with success. With children and adolescents accounting for, and being at risk of, serious acts of violence, and the questions faced by policy makers, the Court, professionals and society at large about how to manage this, it is little wonder that assessing violence risk is a high priority for children's services. Nonetheless, the ability to identify or predict which child or adolescent will continue to engage in violent behaviour represents one of the most important challenges in the field of developmental criminology (Augimeri et al. 2010; Johnstone 2011). Whilst there exists a sizeable and informative research base, there remain significant challenges associated with the practice of risk assessment.

Understanding youth violence

Practitioners tasked with assessing youth should be aware of a myriad of pitfalls that could result in inaccurate conclusions about risk. It is beyond the scope of this chapter to discuss every relevant detail, but we can acknowledge key themes.

First, there is no single etiological theory of youth violence. A wide range of factors might be more or less relevant in any individual case. According to the literature, risk factors typically relate to individual-level variables (e.g. developmental problems, antisocial attitudes, coping ability, previous suicidality or self-harm, anger management problems), family-level variables (e.g. family stressors, parenting style, early caregiver disruption, parental criminality), peer-level variables (e.g. delinquent peers, peer rejection, socialisation problems), school factors (e.g. poor school attendance/attainment) and community-based factors (e.g. community disorganisation).

Second, many adolescents, including those with no prior history of conduct problems, engage in violent behaviour (Office of the Surgeon General 2001). Violent and delinquent behaviour is so common during this age period that it has been described as statistically normative (Moffitt 1993). By age 17, over 40 per cent of male youths engage in at least one serious assault, drug crime or theft (Bureau of Justice Statistics 2007, cited in Slobogin and Fondacaro 2011). Furthermore, only a small proportion will persist. Most do not become career criminals. This trend for a reduction in violent conduct in parallel with ageing and development highlights the potential for metamorphic change during childhood as part of a maturation process, which is an added layer of complexity in terms of assessing violence risk and considering the relevance of risk factors over time.

Third, children and young people that engage in serious violent behaviour are a vulnerable and marginalised group in many ways. Specifically, they often have complex presentations and multiple needs reflected in co-morbid neurodevelopmental and mental health needs, often underpinned by significant childhood maltreatment. This is well established across jurisdictions (Chitsabesan et al. 2006 (England and Wales); Rogers et al. 2006 (USA); Abram et al. 2007 (USA); Colins et al. 2009 (Belgium); Almond 2012 (England); Moore et al. 2013 (Australia); Kinner et al. 2013 (Australia); Dyer and Gregory 2014 (Scotland)). The challenge for assessors is to reliably conceptualise the relationship between co-morbid difficulties, and any potential link between mental health concerns and violence. This needs to be carefully considered on a case-by-case basis.

Fourth, much of our knowledge base derives from research concerned with the onset and development of delinquency (Loeber 1990; Lahey, Moffitt and Caspi 2003; Loeber, Farrington and Petechuk 2003; Siegel and Welsh 2008). This is problematic, as a young person exhibiting delinquent behaviour, such as alcohol consumption or vandalism, may not engage in any interpersonal violence. As such, the literature on delinquency may not be generalisable to, or inform, our thinking around violence per se.

Approaches to risk assessment

In its simplest terms, violence risk assessment is the process by which the extant literature is considered in relation to a particular person for the purposes of reaching an opinion about: (1) whether or not they will continue to engage in such behaviour; and (2) what intervention strategies should be implemented in order to mitigate the risk. Beyond this simple definition, when it comes to the topic of risk assessment, there is considerable variation on *what* constitutes a robust risk assessment. Casting an eye across the literature, there seem to be four prominent methodologies to risk assessment: (1) the unstructured clinical judgement (UCJ) approach; (2) the actuarial methodology; (3) checklists; and (4) the structured professional paradigm approach. It is a basic standard that any professional tasked with completing a violence risk assessment is aware of the whys and wherefores of the various methodologies. The pros and cons associated with these methodologies have been extensively discussed (see Otto and Douglas 2010; Hart and Logan 2011; Cooke and Michie 2013; Logan and Johnstone 2013) but, for the purposes of this chapter, we highlight the main issues below.

Option 1: The *Unstructured Clinical Judgement (UCJ)* approach. This paradigm was particularly prominent during the 1970s and 1980s when the emphasis with regard to the function of risk assessment was upon the clinical assessment and determination of dangerousness (McSherry 2013). The process of assessment is as follows. Drawing from one's own knowledge base, training and experience, the assessor may conduct one or more interviews with the young person and, after reflecting on the content of their responses, reach a view about their dangerousness and risk. There is no need to utilise any standardised assessment protocols or evaluations. The methodology and areas addressed are done so at the discretion of the assessing clinician. Some assessors may, whilst others may not, interview collaterals, read background reports and so on. The appeal of this approach is that it can be a highly individualised and person-centred one. It is also time- and cost-efficient. But this methodology has been highly criticised. From a violence risk assessment perspective, it is widely held that the UCJ approach fails to meet even the basic standards of forensic assessment. This stance has developed in the context of meta-analytic studies, which have demonstrated the superiority of structured risk assessments (Grove et al. 2000; Ægisdóttier et al. 2006). It is highly case-specific, lacks consistency, transparency and reliability, and, as experts have cautioned, is ultimately impeachable (Quinsey 1981; Douglas, Cox and Webster 1999; Hart et al. 2007). In addition, when the researchers examined the utility of the approach, they found no evidence to show any predictive validity. It has been suggested that the prevailing clinical stance was one of caution, and, as such, violence tended to be overpredicted (McAuley 1993). False positives were a common phenomenon (see *Dixon* v. *Attorney General* and *The People* v. *Baxtom*). It was suggested by Monahan (1981), following his review of risk assessments, that clinicians were accurate in their predictions in no more than one third of cases involving violence risk prediction. Experts in the field have argued that this approach should never be used to form a view about violence risk, and we would echo the points made by others that subjective clinical assessment has little, if any, relevance in professional and ethical risk assessment work with young people (DH 2002, 2007; Cooke and Michie 2013). Notwithstanding, among child and adolescent mental health services (CAMHS) clinicians, anecdotal evidence would suggest that this is exactly the type of approach that is used.

Option 2: The *Actuarial Risk Assessment (ARA)* approach. In the search for a more objective, empirically informed and scientific approach, a practitioner might be drawn to the ARA paradigm. Responding to the limitations of the UCJ, researchers turned their efforts to an entirely different approach. The ARA applies statistical methods, based on datasets of offender characteristics and retrospective data about reoffending behaviour (standardisation sample), to individual cases to make predictions about the likelihood of an individual reoffending. There are many examples of such protocols – the Stable and Acute 2007 (Hanson and Harris 2001), Risk Matrix 2000 (Thornton 2007), Violence Risk Appraisal Guide (Harris et al. 1993). These tools yield a percentage likelihood of reoffending within a certain time frame. Proponents of this approach argue that ARA is consistent and robust in terms of predictive validity, and that can be supplemented by using additional SPJ approaches (Burman et al. 2007).

However, the actuarial approach has been subjected to serious criticism. The list is long: a lack of sensitivity to change, failure to aid risk management and rigid in approach are among those criticisms listed by Douglas, Ogloff and Hart (2003). Perhaps fundamentally, a key limitation has been named as the fact that the predictions are about what an 'average' person will do, not what the individual will do. The issues have been discussed in depth elsewhere by Cooke and Michie (2013) and Hart, Michie and Cooke (2007), with specific reference to violence risk assessment. However, the problem is more widespread. Gigerenzer (2014), from the Max Planck Institute, showed how vulnerable many professions are to the uncritical acceptance of data and algorithms, only to provide highly misleading results to patients and peers, and concluded, 'Many doctors, financial advisers, and other risk experts themselves misunderstand risks or are unable to communicate them in an understandable way' (Gigerenzer 2014: 2). As such, experts have warned that a decision to utilise and rely on an ARA is likely to result in an inaccurate and indefensible opinion about risk (Hart, Michie and Cooke 2007; Cooke and Michie 2013).

Option 3: *The Risk Assessment Checklist*. Across many CAMHS and other children's services, practitioners may opt to use locally derived checklists designed by staff in the service. Services may attempt to capture or monitor risks by developing checklists, which, for instance, require a clinician to rate the presence or severity of certain behaviours, which relate to clinical risks. Such a checklist may be generated by a lone clinician or a small group, and thus reflect a highly subjective perspective in terms of the behaviours or items placed on it, and, as such, deemed to be reflective of risk. Consequently, the items used may not reflect unique or distinct constructs or risk factors. Nonetheless, anecdotal evidence suggests that acceptance of this approach is widespread, which is curious, especially in the face of the Royal College of Psychiatrists (RCP) position, which states that: 'reliance on locally developed, non-evidence based checklists' reflected an inadequate risk assessment process (RCP 2011).

Option 4: The *Structured Professional Judgement Paradigm (SPJ)*. The SPJ approach seeks to combine professional judgement and expertise about psychological theory and the individual in question, with information relating to empirical risk factors (both static and dynamic, and sometimes protective). The SPJ model involves several key steps. First, the assessor gathers a multimodal information set to enable a detailed analysis of the person's history and psychosocial functioning, including a detailed analysis of psychological disturbance, mental health and psychopathology. Next, after identifying the risks that exist, the assessor will select an evidence-based protocol to ensure that a minimum set of evidence-based risk factors are evaluated. In the adult field, there are many different protocols, including the Historical Clinical Risk-20, V2 (HCR-20 V2; Webster et al. 1997), Risk for Sexual Violence Protocol (RSVP; Hart et al. 2003), Sexual Violence Risk, 20 (SVR-20; Boer et al. 1997), Spousal Assault Risk Assessment (SARA; Kropp et al. 1995) and the Stalking Assessment Manual (SAM; Kropp, Hart and Lyon 2007). These have been developed to provide a narrative review of the literature, and include operationally defined risk factors and guidance on coding for both presence and relevance and both static and dynamic factors. Step three involves an exercise called scenario planning. Using catch-all terms such as 'high' or 'low' risk are meaningless. Scenario planning is a process by which assessors consider plausible futures, and it is a step in risk assessment that tolerates the uncertainty in the process. In the next step, all of the information is taken into account and considered in respect of risk management. After identifying what risks and risk factors are present, evaluators are required to articulate interventions such as treatment, monitoring, supervision and victim-safety planning.

The SPJ model is well established and a burgeoning literature attests to its utility in terms of its reliability, validity and clinical utility in adults (Douglas, Cox and Webster 1999). SPJ is considered a highly individualised and evidence-based process, with the advantage of creating tailored treatment targets and management strategies that can drive case management forward and generate the conditions necessary for change. Importantly, the SPJ framework allows for more than a cumulative risk model. Whilst there is a connection between the number of risk factors and level of risk (Webster and Hucker 2007), this is not a rule. The nature and configuration of risk factors is just as important to consider. For example, a single risk factor in adults – such as a diagnosis of paranoid psychosis – may be sufficient to drive high-risk behaviour (Johnstone 2013). However, we would add a note of caution, some protocols are promoted as SPJ approaches, but lack the requisite steps, and it is important for any assessor to be clear that the relevant stages are made explicit with a sound evidence, professional and practice base.

Risk protocols for assessing youth violence

Within the last two decades, several protocols have been put in place which purport to provide acceptable methods of youth violence risk assessment. We provide a brief snapshot of the most commonly utilised protocols falling into each of the approaches detailed in the section 'Approaches to risk assessment'. We reiterate the caution that not all of these tools incorporate what would be, in terms of forensic practice in risk assessment, the key steps in SPJ.

Asset (YJB 2000) is an actuarial tool, which contains both static and dynamic risk factors. It was developed at the Centre for Criminological Research, University of Oxford. It has been developed for use with children aged between 10 and 17 years of age, and is applied routinely in youth justice settings, especially in England and Wales. It is used to plan the allocation of resources and inform sentencing in that context. Young people are rated across 12 domains on a scale of 0 to 4, and scores are summed to yield a total Asset score, which is designed to be indicative of the level of risk. A revised version of the Asset, 'AssetPlus' is currently in development.

The Assessment, Intervention and Moving-On project (AIM) (Print, Morrison and Henniker 2002) was designed by services in Manchester and is geared towards the assessment of children and young people aged between 10 and 17 who display harmful sexualised behaviours. It contains a number of factors relating to both risks and strengths, and has been designed for use among multi-agency colleagues in order to facilitate communication and shared language and approach.

Internet-Assessment, Intervention and Moving-On (I-AIM) is a manual designed primarily for social workers to facilitate the assessment of adolescents between the ages of 12 and 18 who have engaged in harmful sexual behaviour through their usage of the Internet. It is designed to supplement the AIM.

The Youth Level of Service/Case Management Inventory (YLS-CMI) (Hoge and Andrews 2002) is an actuarial tool, which assesses the risk of general recidivism. It was developed in Canada and is designed for use with young people aged between 12 and 18 years. It has been described as a fourth-generation tool, which aims to emphasise effective treatment and to facilitate clinical supervision (Andrews, Bonta and Wormith 2006).

The Early Assessment Risk List for Boys (EARL-20B) (Augimeri et al. 2001) and the Early Assessment Risk List for Girls (EARL-20G) (Levene et al. 2001) are SPJ guides for evaluating known risk factors for antisocial behaviour in children under the age of 12 years. The EARLS reflect the first systematic attempts to provide practitioners with a framework for organising their assessments, in terms of method and coverage, when assessing pre-adolescent children.

The Structured Assessment of Violence Risk in Youth (SAVRY) (Borum, Bartel and Forth 2002, 2006), also a SPJ model, was devised to assist clinicians in the evaluation of risk for violence, including sexual assault, in male and female adolescents aged between 12 and 18 years.

The Short-Term Assessment of Risk and Treatability: Adolescent Version (START: AV) (Nicholls et al. 2010) is a SPJ tool that was developed in order to capture a range of clinical risk in youth, including violence risk. It has some unique features in that it is largely composed of dynamic risk items, which are rated in terms of both strengths and vulnerabilities for each item.

The Multiplex Empirically Guided Inventory of Ecological Aggregates for Assessing Sexually Abusive Adolescents and Children (MEGA) (Miccio-Fonseca 2006; Miccio-Fonseca and Rasmussen 2006) was developed to assess sexual violence risk in children aged 19 and younger. It is a 75-item tool designed for use by clinicians and non-clinicians.

The Estimate of Risk of Adolescent Sexual Offence Recidivism Version 2.0 (ERASOR) (Worling and Curwen 2001) was developed to assess the short-term risk of sexual recidivism in juveniles aged 12–18 years who have previously committed a sexual assault. It is a 25-item tool. Items are evaluated using qualitative ratings, and evaluators are required to make a structured clinical assessment regarding the level of risk that is present.

The Juvenile Sex Offender Assessment Protocol (J-SOAP-II) (Prentky and Righthand 2003) was developed for assessing sexual violence risk in adolescents aged between 12 and 18 years. The first version was designed as an actuarial instrument, but the most recent version is described as a structured decision-making tool.

The Sexually Harmful Adolescent Risk Protocol (SHARP) (Richardson 2009) is a SPJ protocol that assesses 50 factors across 12 domains that might be relevant to understanding sexually harmful behaviour in children.

FACE – Child and Adolescent Risk Assessment Suite (FACE-CARAS) (FACE Measurement and Recording Systems) was developed at the University of Durham, and it is described by its developers as a 'systematic and structured approach to assess the relevant static and dynamic risk factors. This supports clinicians by identifying key risk factors that are used to formulate and implement risk management plans.' It contains nine schedules (e.g. relating to aggression, sexual harm or learning disability), which are administered differentially, and dependent on responses to an initial set of screening questions.

Utility of the tools

We argue that the utility of any tool can be adjudged by its performance across a range of criteria, such as its methodological, conceptual, empirical properties, as well as, in the case of youth, developmental properties. Of course, other practical concerns such as assessment time, competencies required, the clinical benefits of its outputs and so on are also relevant in real-life settings, where demand is high and resource is low. Considering the protocols mentioned, we draw attention to the following.

In relation to the ASSET (Baker et al. 2002; 2005), AIM (Griffin and Beech 2004) and YLS-CMI (Jung and Rawana 1999; Schmidt et al. 2005; Schwalbe 2007; Olver, Stockdale and Wormith 2009), broadly speaking, the extant literature suggests moderate performances in terms of psychometric properties and predictive validity. However, this does not negate the problems associated with applying them at the individual level and, given that, interpreted in another way, these statistics reveal that, a certain percentage of young people who resemble high-risk youth do not recidivate – this is a precarious way to reach a view. Considering the FACE-CARAS, key steps in the SPJ are omitted and little, if any, guidance given on how assessors move from risk factors to formulation to scenarios to risk management. In addition, the rationale for risk factors included is not clear, and there is arguably a potential lack of specificity and sensitivity in the risk factors included.

Considering the SPJ paradigm, when examined for predictive validity and reliability, again speaking in broad terms, the data suggests similar and at times better performance when compared with other types of assessment methodology (Welsh et al. 2008; Olver, Stockdale and Wormith 2009; Schmidt, Campbell and Houlding 2011; Childs et al. 2014). However, both the ARA and SPJ paradigms are characterised by other conceptual and developmental difficulties. These have been discussed in detail elsewhere (see Johnstone 2011), but suffice to say that the protocols are limited due to: (1) their narrow conceptualisation of the SPJ model and an emphasis on cumulative risk models; (2) poor risk specificity and failure to consider co-morbidity in risk; (3) absence of compelling psychometric properties; (4) overreliance on delinquency and criminogenic models; and (5) absence of developmental sensitivity in relation to the failure to account for heterogeneity and homogeneity, equifinality and multi-finality, issues of change and stability and transient developmental phenomena, and the direction of effects in risk processes.

Henceforth, with these challenges exposed, practitioners must take a careful and cautious approach to their risk evaluations. Drawing on the practice of formulation, we propose that this is a fundamental stage in violence risk assessment and a viable approach to tolerating and working with uncertainty for the purposes of producing a reliable opinion.

Using formulation and risk formulation to enhance the SPJ paradigm

As Johnstone (2013) and others (Johnstone and Dallos 2006) have observed, formulation is not a new or novel concept. It is a process that is used by practitioner psychologists and psychotherapists to bridge the gap between assessment and therapy in each of the main models of treatment – behavioural, cognitive-behavioural, cognitive-analytical therapy, dialectical behavioural treatments, psychodynamic, systemic and integrative. Irrespective of approach, clinical case formulation shares the same core elements.

Formulation moves beyond a simple listing of events or experiences. It is a narrative: an individualised explanation of the past and the present. It provides a summary of the person's main problems. Formulation is theory driven and therefore enables an inferential and evidence-based stance. It incorporates the research and practice base. It is ampliative and informative. It results in a deeper understanding and enables the generation of testable hypotheses. It is the building blocks of change. Formulation is a core component of practitioner psychological practice and is considered to provide a more useful intervention than the categorical approach of psychiatric diagnosis.

A 'risk formulation' shares all the core components of a formulation but can be considered as reflecting a specific focus on risk of harm. Building on the concept of clinical case formulation, it is concerned with those variables that are most relevant to understanding why and how a person has made a choice to commit harm in the past, and why and how they might commit harm again in the future. In the last few years, it has been recognised that it is a critical stage in the risk assessment process (Hart et al. 2011; Cooke and Michie 2013; Johnstone 2013; Logan and Johnstone 2013). It is no longer acceptable to merely provide a list of risk factors. Formulation is key to elucidating treatment targets and modalities.

Formulation provides a framework for structuring and organising complex information. As detailed, in order to understand youth violence, the assessor must consider literatures from across a broad range, as far and wide as those pertaining to temperament, attachment, parenting, abuse and trauma, and mental disorder, as well as those more commonly associated with criminological literatures. The assessor must also be able to disentangle common presentations from unusual and more concerning presentations. Furthermore, as indicated, any cross-sectional analysis of an adolescent population might fail to reveal those features that set the persisters apart from desisters. Thus, considering the need to integrate multi-theoretical and multi-level biopsychosocial theories, it is essential to use a framework capable of synthesising and making sense of the data. Indeed, we would go as far as to say that risk assessment should be viewed as incomplete in the absence of a risk formulation. That said, because the extant literature on clinical risk formulation is relatively scarce and, to our knowledge, there does not exist any specific guidelines on youth violence risk formulation, we present a framework for practice that should assist evaluators.

Given the complex mix of variables that can act, react and interact with each other to result in risk, formulation needs to be pragmatically grounded. In other words, unlike a model-specific approach, such as cognitive behavioural therapy, which links early experiences, core schema and distorted thinking, feelings and behaviour, risk formulation should be broader in its scope and draw from an eclectic and integrated framework. This is essential where no definitive theory exists to explain the occurrence of a particular phenomenon. That is not to exclude model-specific formulation, as this may well be what is recommended in risk management, but the risk formulation should be seen as a step before. It has been argued elsewhere that Weerasekera's (1996) four Ps model is an appropriate framework to organise data pertaining to risk. Applying this to the assessment of children and adolescents, Carr (1999) explained that formulation is a process which distinguishes between factors which *predispose* a child to developing a problem, such as personal predisposing factors like genetic vulnerabilities, pre- and perinatal complications and so on, and contextual risk factors, such as poor attachment, poor parenting, parental alcohol and substance use, parental criminality, stress such as abuse, loss and so on, from factors that *precipitate* the onset or marked exacerbation of the difficulties, such as acute life stress, abuse, transition, loss, trauma and so on, and maintaining factors which perpetuate the problems once they have begun. These can include personal factors such as biological features including emotional dysregulation,

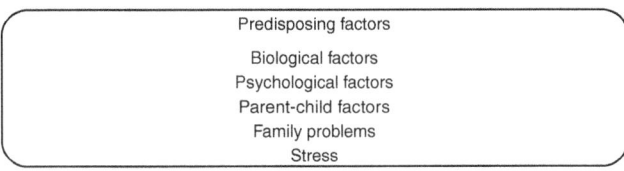

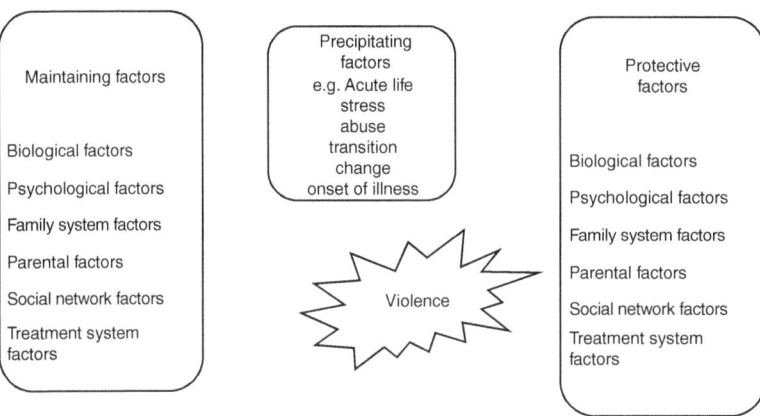

Figure 5.1 Formulation of risk of violence
Source: Adapted from Carr (1999).

family system factors, parental factors, social network factors and treatment system factors. Protective factors – the fourth P – prevent further deterioration and have implications for prognosis. Similarly, these can also be categorised according to whether they are biological, psychological or contextual in the family and/or social network. Drawing from Carr's framework for producing a formulation, Figure 5.1, shows the first stage and how risk factors can be organised into these different systems to provide the building blocks of an in-depth understanding. By organising them in this manner, the diachronic nature of the variables can be revealed, as can the relevant areas.

After organising variables in this manner, it is necessary to move to the next phase relating to the narrative. Figure 5.2 shows the process by which formulation makes a key link between the information and the outcome.

In developing a narrative risk formulation, a key task for the clinician is to articulate hypotheses about the likely multifactorial mechanisms of risk. This is done by moving beyond a simple listing of relevant factors, as per

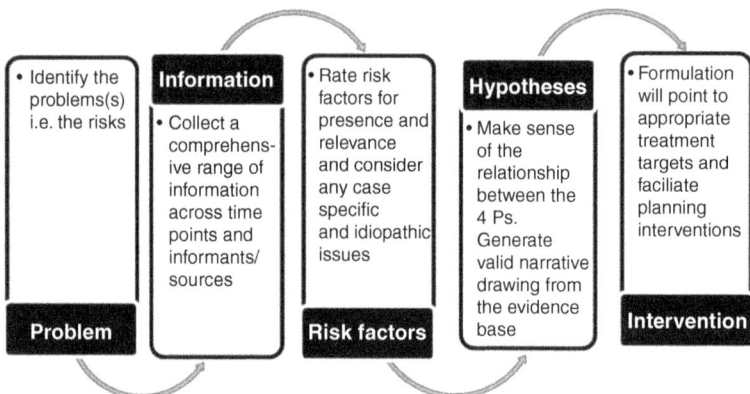

Figure 5.2 The process of risk formulation

the four Ps model, and detailing what impact a certain event or phenomenon has had on the development of a young person and/or their current state or behaviour. An example, using the common predisposing factor of childhood maltreatment, can be used to illustrate this process. The narrative can combine case-specific information with clinical wisdom and theoretical knowledge to outline how the experience of maltreatment likely impacted upon the young person, and how that relates to risk. There may be a number of distinct or overlapping mechanisms, reflecting the multifarious routes to similar outcomes. For instance, in one scenario an individual may experience physical abuse in childhood as a form of punishment and boundary setting by one parent in an environment where their other physical and emotional needs are met. This experience may model violence, as per social learning theory, as an acceptable means of problem solving, and be relevant to later instrumental violence perpetrated by the young person. Alternatively, another individual may experience maltreatment in the form of chronic emotional abuse and emotional neglect, and consequently fail to develop protective emotional regulation skills, as per attachment theory, which may laterally make them vulnerable to reactive interpersonal violence at times of distress. A third scenario may involve a child who experiences sexual abuse and associated powerlessness and shame, as per psychodynamic thinking, in the longer term this child may develop a violent and domineering interpersonal style in order to avoid experiencing intolerable powerlessness again.

Despite the obvious qualitative differences between each of the case vignettes outlined briefly here, when rated on a risk tool, all would score highly in relation to maltreatment. Thus, a risk-factor rating in the absence of an individualised case formulation may neglect or obscure vital idiosyncratic information which is relevant to risk. One of the key benefits of formulation is that the process yields treatment needs and, as such, facilitates risk management.

As discussed, principles of clinical case formulation and forensic case formulation have been proposed and discussed in the literature. It is suggested that, when formulating violence, or any clinical risk, with children and young people in mind, that formulations should *additionally* be:

Developmentally informed. When formulating violence risk with a young person it is vital that both chronological and developmental age and stage are considered. This relates to a number of domains of functioning, including cognitive, social, emotional, physical and moral development. Much of the literature, and especially the forensic literature, has developed based on what we know about adult populations. It is imperative that we adjust our expectations and thinking when it comes to high-risk youth. As such, knowledge of normative child development and abnormal psychology are key and can facilitate a balanced view on risk. Linked to this, we would also take the view that to formulate risk in the absence of understanding attachment is pointless. These very early building blocks of development deserve unreserved attention, analysis and understanding.

Systems informed. Children and young people are embedded in family, school and community systems over which they have little control. They lack the resources, autonomy or often the understanding to recognise or change these external factors. It follows then that a child cannot be best understood in a vacuum, and when formulating risk the perpetuating influence of systemic factors, whether they be parenting influences, family stressors, bullying or school issues, cannot be underestimated. It is critical to adopt a whole systems approach to assessment.

Trauma informed. The links between childhood trauma of all forms and poor outcomes, including violent conduct, later in life are becoming increasingly recognised. Locally, for instance, a small sample of recent Scottish data relating to a youth justice population suggested that over three quarters of high-risk youth had been exposed to domestic violence, and almost 90 per cent had experienced, largely multiple types of, childhood maltreatment (Dyer and Gregory 2014). It is suggested that, traditionally, the impact of trauma on development has been poorly understood or responded to, and, as such, has not translated into practice or service models. Furthermore, it is argued that the complex, and co-occurring difficulties commonly apparent in high-risk youth are often best captured by a complex trauma conceptualisation rather than multiple diagnostic labels. It is our view that a trauma-informed stance will most often enhance conceptualisation and increase the potential for appropriate interventions.

Vulnerability informed. It is well established that the population of young people considered to be high risk in terms of violent conduct are a marginalised and vulnerable group. This pertains not just to experiences of childhood adversity and poor outcomes in terms of mental health, but is also relevant in terms of most other vulnerabilities, including global and specific learning difficulties, social communication problems, acquired brain injuries, substance misuse (SM) difficulties and physical health problems, to name just a few. As such, to successfully conceptualise violence risk for this group, clinicians need to be able to either differentiate between these varying difficulties, or, more likely in our experience, understand the complex interaction between multiple difficulties.

An illustrated case study

In the case study that follows, we present a complex case with co-morbid risks to illustrate how the SPJ approach, including formulation, contributed to a better understanding of how the risk developed, what could trigger harm and what the key targets should be for treatment.

The referral

As the multidisciplinary team (MDT) convenes for its usual Tuesday morning clinical team meeting, the chair alerts her colleagues to a very concerning referral – Eric. He is a 16-year-old boy. He has been living in a residential children's home for the last four months. He was taken there after he assaulted his mother, broke her jaw and fractured four ribs when she removed his Xbox from his bedroom as a punishment for truanting. He has been referred by social work colleagues for a 'specialist risk assessment' to aid decisions about his ongoing placement and treatment. Consideration is being given to moving Eric to a secure school. Eric has been described as being 'out of control for some time', and his most recent assault on his mother occurs in the context of a history of gang-fighting, fire-setting and an allegation of sodomy against his younger cousin. He has also admitted to having viewed extreme child pornography and is unusually candid in his beliefs that this should be viewed as a right and claims that paedophilia is a sexual preference that merits the same respect as homosexuality. He has also been self-injuring. Apparently, this is a long-standing concern. When he was younger, he would cause himself friction burns by rubbing particular materials across his arms. Of late, he has been engaging in highly concerning risk-taking behaviours, and it is believed that he was prostituting himself for money for new psychoactive substances. Attempts to support him have met with ridicule and rejection.

The risk assessment
Step 1: Background information.

Given that reliable risk assessment requires an in-depth understanding of an individual, a broad scope was taken in terms of gathering information. Various data sources were utilised, and information relating to experience and functioning across differing time points was sought. This included clinical interviews with Eric and his parents, along with some standardised assessments; interviews were also conducted with Eric's social worker and care staff; and educational, health and social work records were reviewed. The information gleaned was then synthesised and reported under organised headings including: family composition and history; developmental history; educational functioning; social functioning; mental health; physical health; psychosexual development; substance/alcohol misuse; offending behaviour; interests/hobbies; future plans.

Step 2: Risks and risk-factor ratings.

Based on the information obtained, it is clear that Eric presents with complex and co-morbid risks. In order to ensure a thorough analysis, several protocols were selected to inform the assessment: the SAVRY (Borum, Bartel and Forth 2006), the RSVP (Hart et al. 2003) and the Northgate Firesetter Risk Assessment (Taylor and Thorne 2005). The risk factors rated as present and relevant are emboldened in Table 5.1.

Step 3: Risk formulation.

A narrative formulation was developed, using the four Ps framework, and with cognisance of the principles outlined previously in the section 'Using formulation and risk formulation to enhance the SPJ paradigm'. Excerpts from same are italicised as follows:

> *The available information suggests that there are a number of vulnerability factors, which interact to predispose Eric to his current difficulties and presentation. Of central importance is the presence of an autistic spectrum disorder (ASD), which has resulted in Eric having significant difficulties coping with the demands of life due to ASD-associated challenges in relation to adaptive social, cognitive, behavioural, communication and interpersonal functioning. It would appear that he has a very low frustration tolerance, is prone to perceiving threat, lacks impulse control and is unable to regulate his emotions effectively. He has been volatile from an early age and it is possible that his constitutional difficulties have been compounded by environmental and social learning experiences whereby aggression has become reinforced for him – he has been able to have his needs met via this method of behaviour. Furthermore, the experience of physical discipline at the hands of his father earlier in life likely modelled the use of violence and aggression as a means of social problem solving and communication. It is also possible that inconsistent schooling, parenting and educational experiences have further compounded these problems, resulting in unpredictability and destabilising experiences for Eric. He seems to have been unable or unwilling to engage in the more prosocial aspects of his life and has withdrawn from (or been rejected by) age-appropriate peers and*

Table 5.1 Summary of risk factors for Eric

SAVRY (Borum et al. 2006)	RSVP (Hart et al. 2003)	Northgate (Taylor and Thorne 2005)
H1. History of Violence	1. Chronicity of Sexual Violence	H1. History of childhood (pre-16) fire-setting
H2. History of Non-Violent Offending	2. Diversity of Sexual Violence	H2. Previous incidents of fire-setting as an adult
H3. Early Initiation of Violence	3. Escalation of Sexual Violence	H3. Previous incidents of targeted fire-setting
H4. Past Supervision/Intervention Failures	4. Physical Coercion in Sexual Violence	H4. Previous hoax calls to emergency services
H5. History of Self-Harm or Suicide Attempts	5. Psychological Coercion in Sexual Violence	H5. Previous self-harm/suicidal gestures
H6. Exposure to Violence in the Home	6. Extreme Minimisation or Denial of Sexual Violence	C1. Recent build-up of depression or stress
H7. Childhood History of Maltreatment	7. Attitudes that Support or Condone Sexual Violence	C2. High levels of anger
H8. Parental/Caregiver Criminality	8. Problems with Self-Awareness	C3. Poor interpersonal conflict resolution skills
H9. Early Caregiver Disruption	9. Problems with Stress or Coping	C4. Impulsivity
H10. Poor School Achievement	10. Problems Resulting from Child Abuse	C5. Current or recent signs of major mental illness (using DSM/ICD criteria)
SC11. Peer Delinquency	11. Sexual Deviance	C6. Low social attention
SC12. Peer Rejection	12. Psychopathic Personality Disorder	OTHER CASE SPECIFIC Autistic Spectrum Disorder
SC13. Stress and Poor Coping	13. Major Mental Illness	
SC14. Poor Parental Management	14. Problems with Substance Use	
SC15. Lack of Personal/Social Support	15. Violent or Suicidal Ideation	
SC16. Community Disorganisation	16. Problems with Intimate Relationships	
I17. Negative Attitudes	17. Problems with Non-Intimate Relationships	
I18. Risk Taking/Impulsivity	18. Problems with Employment	
I19. Substance Use Difficulties	19. Non-Sexual Criminality	
I20. Anger Management Problems	20. Problems with Planning	
I21. Low Empathy/Remorse	21. Problems with Treatment	
I22. Attention Deficit/Hyperactivity Difficulties	22. Problems with Supervision	
I23. Poor Compliance		
I24. Low Interest/Commitment to School		
P1. Prosocial Involvement		
P2. Strong Social Support		
P3. Strong Attachment and Bonds		
P4. Positive Attitude Towards Intervention and Authority		
P5. Strong Commitment to School		
P6. Resilient Personality Traits		

other prosocial outlets. Parent accounts indicated that throughout childhood and early adolescence, Eric was more at ease socially with younger peers, likely secondary to his social problems with peers in school and the community. This process of emotional of social congruence with younger children is likely relevant to his sexualized conduct.

With precipitating factors or triggers in mind, again, there are a number of apparent factors – both inter and intrapersonal. Certain internal states appear to serve as triggers for violent and aggressive conduct, strong emotions such as stress, frustration, or sadness tend to precede violent conduct and indicate the difficulty that Eric has with regulating his emotions. As such, significant life events or stressors are especially difficult for Eric to manage; this has been especially apparent in recent months in relation to the deterioration in Eric's presentation secondary to his being received into care. Less apparently significant events, such as not getting his needs met or experiencing social misunderstanding have also proven difficult for Eric to cope with. Whilst Eric's violent and aggressive conduct have been relevant in one form or another in the longer term, his delinquent conduct (SM, vandalism, firesetting) has developed more recently in the context of finding his first experience of peer acceptance with an antisocial peer group in the community. As such, peer influence and the need to fit in socially are also relevant precipitants. With sexualized behaviour in mind, the available information suggests that the beginning of puberty and, in parallel, ownership of a personal laptop precipitated the onset of sexualized activity online, sexualized comments towards peers at school, and ultimately sexual behavior perpetrated against his cousin.

With regard to maintenance factors there are a number of hypothesized factors that perpetuate Eric's difficulties. A negative view of self and others secondary to long-term interpersonal problems underpin negative emotional states and negative predictions about other people's intentions. Poor social skill, limited emotional regulation skills, and sensory difficulties likely perpetuate ongoing deliberate self-harm, and interpersonal problems; with the latter likely particularly pertinent to Eric's preference for younger peers, and inappropriate use of the internet for acceptance, intimacy, and control. Rigid and concrete thinking styles in general, and some specific and concerning beliefs (e.g. men and dominance in the household; sexual interest in children as normal and benign; and females as particularly weak), along with empathy deficits associated with the absence of theory of mind, are all thought to maintain risk. Simultaneous peer rejection at school, and acceptance by antisocial peers in the community, reinforce delinquent conduct. Whilst poor social understanding of risks and sexual relationships and perceived benefits of SM (in Eric's case relaxing and euphoric states) drive risky sexualized conduct in relation to prostitution.

There were a number of strengths that serve as a means of potential protection against further risky behavior. For instance, Eric is intelligent and has some goals and aspirations for the future. He is particularly interested in science and engineering, despite his recent disinterest in formal education. Eric's parents remain loving and committed to him and are motivated to engage with supports.

Step 4: Scenario planning.

Scenario planning is a technique used to assist in planning and preparation for future events. Applied to the field of risk management, this technique can assist in the identification of an individual's risk in plausible, yet speculative, environmental and situational contexts – this is not about prediction of a future event, rather a method of planning to minimise risk. With Eric in mind, a number of scenarios were articulated in relation to: violent conduct, sexualised conduct, delinquent behaviour and risks to self. Comments were made upon hypothesised antecedents to, nature of, and likelihood, imminence and severity of particular types of risky behaviour.

Step 5: Risk management.

In order to manage Eric's diverse and co-morbid risks it was recommended that multi-agency and multimodal interventions were necessary. In particular, detailed and concrete suggestions based on both empirical and professional knowledge and organised under the headings of further assessment, intervention, monitoring and supervision were made. In other words, professionals knew what to do, when, why and ultimately by whom.

Reflections and recommendations

We have already emphasised that, when undertaking risk assessment, the overarching challenge is understanding who will desist and who will persist in terms of offending behaviour. The purpose of the risk assessment is to identify persisters, along with a sense of what offending behaviour might look like, and in what context it is likely to occur. To achieve this end, there are various risk assessment paradigms and tools available to practitioners, which have been summarised in the **Approaches to risk assessment and Risk protocols for assessing youth violence** sections As highlighted, there are strengths and weaknesses to all approaches, and even the most robust available methodology, which in our view is SPJ, has its limitations. Thus, it is in an imperfect context that practitioners are asked to form a view on risk, in essence attempting to speculate with some certainty about future events, which, some might argue, is a next to impossible task. As such, the weight of the task at hand, the absence of an infallible methodology and the significant implications of an opinion on risk can be viewed as challenges in themselves by virtue of the anxiety-provoking nature of the task. In practice, there are many further challenges for risk assessors, for instance, the common tension that arises when assessors also have a therapeutic relationship with a service user; working within legal frameworks; or access to a breadth of reliable and relevant background information or collateral informants, to name just a few. These and other general issues and conflicts around risk assessment are well documented in the literature. Here, we are specifically interested in those unique challenges pertaining to risk assessment practice in terms of youth violence.

Building upon what has already been highlighted in terms of potential pitfalls and complexities when risk-assessing violent youth – for instance, the need to be informed about developmental stage, be systems focused, and understand the role of trauma and/or complex psychopathology – there are several other key issues. Of significance is the need to balance the often-competing agendas of two strong drivers: child welfare and public protection. The multi-agency ethos that underpins best practice in risk assessment and management compels public servants from many backgrounds to work together: social work and care, police, health, education, state prosecution services and so forth. As such, the highest level of successful multi-agency communication, liaison and joint working is called for in terms of working towards shared goals. Arriving at a shared understanding is a vital part of this work, with risk assessment often being the vehicle with which to conceptualise that understanding. However, each agency or professional has a potentially different attitude or brief and, as such, there may be divergent opinions and concerns regarding any one young person. For instance, some views may be weighted towards the vulnerability of the child associated with unmet needs, and others informed more by the seriousness of offending behaviour and concerns about future risk and public protection. This issue becomes even more complex when the dynamic nature of childhood is taken into account. Thus, not only are there questions regarding the balance of need and risk at any one point in time, but also other uncertainties to be tolerated regarding how a child will mature or change in the short to medium term, and what this means in terms of their risks and needs. Experience has taught us that even in the most hopeless or worrying of cases there is the potential for risk to lessen significantly, even within short time frames. For example, change of placement or protection from abuse can result in almost immediate changes, whereas high-intensity and expertly delivered psychological therapies can move cases within several months.

Despite the numerous challenges, violence risk assessment has become an integral part of the state response to offending behaviour, and can be viewed as key in ensuring an appropriate and measured response, especially where case presentations are complex and risks severe. In order that assessors have the best possible chance of succeeding in their task, and that young people have access to the most robust and reliable opinions, it is suggested that risk assessment practice continues to evolve and improve.

Here, we have proposed that risk formulation is a vital and useful adaptation to supplement practice. Whilst formulation is well described in the clinical literature, it is not well evaluated as a methodology or intervention in either clinical or forensic evidence bases. Research testing the validity and utility of risk formulations would be a welcome addition. The content and purpose of formulation is to consider the mechanisms of risk. Understanding risk mechanisms is vital to prevention and intervention. As such, developing our understanding of how an event (risk factor) influences our behaviour (risk) and what factors mediate or moderate this process is of immense value. There is a paucity of research in general in relation to violence and youth. This has led to practice being largely informed by the adult forensic literature, which has significant limitations. The gaps in the literature are too numerous to list here, suffice it to say that the empirical evidence for forensic practice with children and young people needs significant expansion in broad terms.

1In terms of practice development, it is suggested that models of working that tolerate co-morbidity in terms of both differing mental health and risk presentations are required. Practice that artificially separates different aspects of a person's functioning, or fails to account for aspects of how they present, increases the potential for false negatives, and limits the potential success of subsequent risk management efforts or intervention. It is clear that violent youth are among the most vulnerable in terms of their mental health needs. Despite this, access to mental health services for violent youth, particularly psychologically informed provision and formulation for either the purposes of risk assessment or mental health intervention, varies. Clear pathways and access to services are needed in order to ensure mental health and psychologically informed assessments and complex formulation are available. Where services are accessible, it is vital that evidence-based risk assessment methodologies are adopted and the use of the UCJ approach eliminated. Whilst best practice gets bedded in, it is resource heavy in terms of clinician time and training needs. As such, improving practice has significant implications in this regard. Violence risk assessment is inherent in the role of youth justice social workers, who represent the front line in terms of working with high-risk youth. Highlighting again what we know about the complex neurodevelopmental, trauma and other mental health needs of this group, it is suggested that there is a significant role for mental health services and psychologically informed provision in supplementing and supporting this work. Such a service can be provided based on need, consultation or formulation being the least intense intervention, followed by specialist assessments, or psychological or medical interventions at the highest intensity.

Conclusion

Recent decades have seen important strides in the development of risk assessment practice. That said, the phenomenon of youth violence has garnered less attention, from an assessment perspective, than is required to ensure the best possible responses and outcomes. Here, we have proposed the practice of risk formulation, along with several principles, as an integral and necessary development in terms of violence risk assessment in youth, given its highly individualised stance and the inherent capacity to inform risk management and intervention. It is our view that risk formulation, or understanding the mechanisms of risk, is a practice that holds great promise and utility as an element of risk assessment. This hypothesis is open to testing, and is only one aspect of many that still require to be understood in terms of managing and supporting young people who present with high risk.

References

Abram, K.M., Washburn, J.J., Teplin, L.A. et al. (2007) 'Posttraumatic stress disorder and psychiatric comorbidity among detained youths', *Psychiatric Services*, 58(10): 1311–1316.

Ægisdóttier, S., White, M.J., Spengler, P.M., Maugherrnan, A.S., Anderson, L.A., Cook, R.S., Nichols, C.S., Lampropolous, G.K., Walker, B.S., Cohen, G. and Rush, J.D. (2006) 'The metaanalysis of clinical judgment project: Fifty-six years of accumulated research on clinical versus statistical prediction', *The Counseling Psychologist*, 34: 341–82.

Almond, T. (2012) 'The provision of mental health care and services in young offenders institutions', *Social Work in Action*, 24(3): 189–200.

Amnesty International (2011) *This Is Where I'm Going to Be When I Die: Children Facing Life Imprisonment without the Possibility of Release in the USA*. London: Amnesty International Ltd.

Andrews, D., Bonta, J., and Wormith, S. (2006) 'The recent past and near future of risk and/or need assessment', *Crime and Delinquency*, 52: 7–27.

Augimeri, L.K., Enebrink, P., Walsh, M., and Jiang, D. (2010) 'Gender-Specific Childhood Risk Assessment Tools: Early Assessment Risk Lists for Boys (EARL-20B) and Girls (EARL-21G)', in R.K. Otto and K.S. Douglas (eds.), *Handbook of Violence Risk Assessment*. Oxford: Routledge, Taylor & Francis, 43–62.

Augimeri, L.K., Koegl, C.J., Webster, C.D., and Levene, K. (2001) *Early Assessment Risk List for Boys: EARL-20B, Version 2*. Toronto: Earlscourt Child and Family Centre (now called Child Development Institute).

Baker, K., Jones, S., Merrington, S., and Roberts, C. (2005) *Further Development of Asset*. London: Youth Justice Board.

Baker, K., Jones, S., Roberts, C., and Merrington, S. (2002) *Validity and Reliability of ASSET*. London: Youth Justice Board.

Boer, D.P., Hart, S.D., Kropp, P.R., and Webster, C.D. (1997) *Manual for the Sexual Violence Risk – 20: Professional Guidelines for Assessing Risk of Sexual Violence*. Vancouver: The Mental Health, Law, and Policy Institute.

Borum, R., Bartel, P., and Forth, A. (2002) *Manual for the Structured Assessment of Violence Risk in Youth (SAVRY)*. Tampa, FL: Mental Health Institute.

Borum, R., Bartel, P., and Forth, A. (2006) *Structured Assessment for Violence Risk in Youth (SAVRY)*. Tampa, FL: Mental Health Institute.

Brewster, M.P. (2013) 'Children and stalking', *Family and Intimate Partner Violence Quarterly*, 5(3): 247–270.

Burman, M., Armstrong, S., Batchelor, S., McNeill, F., and Nicholson, J. (2007) 'Research and practice in risk assessment and risk management of children and young people engaging in offending behaviours: A literature review', *Risk Management Authority*. Available at: http://www.rmascotland.gov.uk/files/1612/7263/5799/Research%20and%20Practice%20in%20Risk%20Assessment%20and%20Risk%20Management%20of%20Children%20and%20Young%20People%20Engaging%20in%20Offending%20Behaviours%20-%20A%20Literature%20Review.pdf. Accessed 29 October 2014.

Carr, A. (1999) *Handbook of Clinical Child and Adolescent Psychology: A Contextual Approach*. London: Routledge.

Childs, K., Frick, P.J., Ryals, J.S., Lingonblad, A., and Villio, M.J. (2014) 'A comparison of empirically based and structured professional judgment estimation of risk using the structured assessment of violence risk in youth', *Youth Violence and Juvenile Justice*, 12(1): 40–57.

Chitsabesan, P., Kroll, L., Bailey, S., Kenning, C., Macdonald, W., and Theodosiou, L. (2006) 'Mental health needs of offenders in custody and in the community', *British Journal of Psychiatry*, 188: 534–540.

Colins, O., Vermeiren, R., Schuyten, G., and Broekaert, E. (2009) 'Psychiatric disorders in property, violent and versatile offending detained male adolescents', *American Journal of Orthopsychiatry*, 79(1): 31–38.

Cooke, D.J. and Michie, C. (2013) 'Violence Risk Assessment: From Prediction to Understanding – or from What? to Why?', in C. Logan and L. Johnstone (eds.), *Managing Clinical Risk: A Guide to Effective Practice*. Abingdon: Routledge, 3–25.

DH (Department of Health) (2002) *Mental Health Policy Implementation Guide: Adult Acute Inpatient Care Provision*. London: Department of Health.

DH (Department of Health) (2007) *Best Practice in Managing Risk: Principles and Evidence for Best Practice in the Assessment and Management of Risk to Self and Others in Mental Health Services*. London: Department of Health.

Dixon v. Attorney General of Commonwealth of PA. (1971) Available at: http://www.leagle.com/decision/19711291325FSupp966_11107.xml/DIXON%20v.%20ATTORNEY%20GENERAL%20OF%20COMMONWEALTH%20OF%20PA. Accessed 18 January 2015.

Douglas, K.S., Cox, D.N., and Webster, C.D. (1999) 'Violence risk assessment: Science and practice', *Legal and Criminological Psychology*, 4: 149–184.

Douglas, K.S., Ogloff, J.R.P., and Hart, S.D. (2003) 'Evaluation of a model of violence risk assessment among forensic psychiatric patients', *Psychiatric Services*, 54: 1372–1379.

Dyer, F. and Gregory, L. (2014) 'Mental health difficulties in the youth justice population: Learning from the first six months of the IVY project', *CYCJ Briefing Paper No. 5*. Available at: http://www.cycj.org.uk/wp-content/uploads/2014/04/Briefing-Paper-5-final.pdf. Accessed 29 October 2014.

FACE-CARAS (FACE – Child and Adolescent Risk Assessment Suite) (n.d.) *Face Recording and Measurement Systems*. Available at: http://www.face.eu.com/solutions/assessment-tools/caras. Accessed 17 January 2015.

Gerson, R. and Rappaport, N. (2011) 'Cyber cruelty: Understanding and preventing the new bullying', *Adolescent Psychiatry*, 1(1): 67–71.

Gigerenzer, G. (2014) *Risk Savvy: How to Make Good Decisions*. United States of America: Penguin Group.

Griffin, H. and Beech, A. (2004) 'Evaluation of the AIM framework for the assessment of adolescents who display sexually harmful behaviour', *Youth Justice Board*. Available at: http://yjbpublications.justice.gov.uk/Resources/Downloads/AIM%20Full%20Report.pdf. Accessed 18 January 2015.

Grove, W.M., Zald, D.H., Lebow, B.S., Snitz, B.E., and Nelson, C. (2000) 'Clinical versus mechanical prediction: A meta-analysis', *Psychological Assessment*, 12: 19–30.

Hanson, R.K. and Harris, A.J. (2001) 'A structured approach to evaluating change among sexual offenders', *Sex Abuse*, 13: 105–122.

Harris, G.T., Rice, M.E., and Quinsey, V.L. (1993) 'Violent recidivism of mentally disordered offenders: The development of a statistical prediction instrument', *Criminal Justice and Behavior*, 20, 315–335.

Harris, G.T., Rice, M.E., Quinsey, V.L., Lalumière, M.L., Boer, D.P., and Lang, C. (2003) 'A multisite comparison of actuarial risk instruments for sex offenders', *Psychological Assessment*, 15: 413–425.

Hart, J., O'Toole, S., Price-Sharps, J., and Shaffer, T. (2007) 'The risk and protective factors of violent juvenile offending: An examination of gender differences', *Youth Violence and Juvenile Justice*, 5: 367–384.

Hart, S.D., Michie, C. and Cooke, D. (2007) 'Precision of actuarial risk assessment instruments: Evaluating the "margins of error" of group v. individual predictions of violence', *British Journal of Psychiatry*, 190(49): s60–s65.

Hart, S.D, Sturmey, P., Logan, C. and McMurran, M. (2011) 'Forensic case formulation', *International Journal of Forensic Mental Health*, 10: 118–128.

Hart, S.D., Kropp, P.R., Laws, D.R., Klaver, J., Logan, C., and Watt, K.A. (2003) *The Risk for Sexual Violence Protocol (RSVP): Structured Professional Guidelines for Assessing Risk of Sexual Violence*. Burnaby: Mental Health, Law, and Policy Institute, Simon Fraser University.

Hart, S.D. and Logan, C. (2011) 'Formulation of violence risk using evidence-based assessments: The structured professional judgement approach', in P. Sturmey & M. McMurran, (eds.). *Forensic Case Formulation*. Chichester, UK: Wiley Blackwell, 83–106.

HM Government (2011) *Ending Gang and Youth Violence: A Cross-Government Report Including Further Evidence and Good Practice Case Studies*, November 2011.

Hoge, R. and Andrews, D. (2002) *Youth Level of Service/Case Management Inventory*. Toronto: Multi-Health Systems.

Home Office (2011) *'Prevent' strategy*, *Home Office*. Available at: https://www.gov.uk/government/uploads/system/uploads/attachment_data/file/97976/prevent-strategy-review.pdf. Accessed 1 September 2014.

I-AIM (Internet-Assessment, Intervention and Moving-On) (n.d.). Available at: http://aimproject.org.uk/?page_id=83. Accessed 18 January 2015.

Johnstone, L. (2011) 'Assessing and Managing Violent Youth: Implications for Sentencing', in B. McSherry and P. Keyzer (eds.), *Dangerous People: Policy, Prediction, and Practice*. New York: Taylor & Francis Group, 123–146.

Johnstone, L. (2013) 'Mental Disorder and Violence', in C. Logan and L. Johnstone (eds.), *Managing Clinical Risk: A Guide to Effective Practice*. Abingdon: Routledge, 56–87.

Johnstone, L. and Dallos, R. (eds.) (2006) *Formulation in Psychology and Psychotherapy: Making Sense of People's Problems*. London and New York: Routledge.

Jung, S. and Rawana, E. (1999) 'Risk and need assessment of juvenile offenders', *Criminal Justice and Behaviour*, 26: 69–89.

Kinner, S.A., Degenhardt, L., Coffey, C., Sawyer, S., and Hearps, S. (2013) 'Complex health needs in the youth justice system: A survey of community-based and custodial offenders', *Journal of Adolescent Health*, 54(5): 521–526.

Kropp, P.R., Hart, S.D., and Lyon, D.R. (2007) *Stalking Assessment and Management*. Vancouver: Proactive Resolutions.

Kropp, P.R., Hart, S.D., Webster, C.D., and Eaves, D. (1995) *Manual for the Spousal Assault Risk Assessment Guide*, 2nd edn. Vancouver: British Columbia Institute of Family Violence.

Lahey, B., Moffitt, T.E., and Caspi, A. (2003) *The Causes of Conduct Disorder and Serious Juvenile Delinquency*. New York: Guilford Press.

Levene, K., Augimeri, L. Pepler, D., Walsh, M., Webster, C., and Koegl, C. (2001) *Earl 21-G: Early Assessment Risk List for Girls*. Toronto: Earlscourt Child and Family Centre.

Loeber, R. (1990) 'Development and risk factors of juvenile antisocial behavior and delinquency', *Clinical Psychology Review*, 10: 1–41.

Loeber, R., Farrington, D.P., and Petechuk, D. (2003) *Child Delinquency: Early Intervention and Prevention*, Bulletin. Washington, DC: US Department of Justice, Office of Justice Programs, Office of Juvenile Justice and Delinquency Prevention.

Logan, C. and Johnstone, L. (2013) 'Future Directions in Clinical Risk Assessment and Management', in C. Logan and L. Johnstone (eds.), *Managing Clinical Risk: A Guide to Effective Practice*. Abingdon: Routledge, 313–318.

McAuley, F. (1993) *Insanity, Psychiatry and Criminal Responsibility*. Dublin: Round Hall Press.

Mackay, S., Feldberg, A., Ward, A.K., and Marton, P. (2014) 'Firesetting', *Encyclopedia of Adolescence*, 1036–1048.

McSherry, B. (2013) *Managing Fear: The Law and Ethics of Preventative Detention and Risk Assessment*. New York: Routledge Taylor Francis Group.

Madden, V. (2013) 'Understanding the mental health needs of young people involved in gangs'. A Tri-borough Public Health Report produced on behalf of the Westminster Joint Health and Wellbeing Board.

Miccio-Fonseca, L.C. (2006) *Implementing MEGA: A New Tool for Assessing Risk and Concern for Sexually Abusive Behaviour in Youth Ages 19 and under: An Empirically Guided Paradigm for Risk Assessment, Revised Version*. San Diego, CA: Author.

Miccio-Fonseca, L.C. and Rasmussen, L.A. (2006) *Multiplex Empirically Guided Inventory of Ecological Aggregates for Assessing Sexually Abusive Children and Adolescents (Ages 19 and under) – MEGA: Professional Manual*. San Diego, CA: Author.

Ministry of Justice (2014) 'Youth justice statistics 2012/2013 England and Wales', *Ministry of Justice*. Available at: https://www.gov.uk/government/uploads/system/uploads/attachment_data/file/276098/youth-justice-stats-exec_summary.pdf. Accessed 18 January 2015.

Mishna, F., Khoury-Kassabri, M., Gadalla, T., and Daciuk, J. (2012) 'Risk factors for involvement in cyber bullying: Victims, bullies and bully-victims', *Children and Youth Services Review*, 34: 63–70.

Moffitt, T.E. (1993) 'Adolescence limited and life-course persistent antisocial behavior: A developmental taxonomy', *Psychological Review*, 100: 674–701.

Monahan, J. (1981) *Predicting Violent Behavior: An Assessment of Clinical Techniques*. Beverly Hills, LA: Sage.

Moore, E., Gaskin, C., and Indig, D. (2013) 'Childhood maltreatment and post-traumatic stress disorder among incarcerated young offenders', *Child Abuse and Neglect*, 37(10): 861–870.

Nicholls, T.L., Viljoen, J.L., Cruise, K.R., Desmarais, S.L., and Webster, C.D. (2010) *Short-Term Assessment of Risk and Treatability: Adolescent Version (START: AV)* (Abbreviated Manual). Coquitlam: BC Mental Health and Addiction Services.

Office of the Surgeon General (US, 2001) *Youth Violence: A Report of the Surgeon General*. Department of Health and Human Services.

Olver, M., Stockdale, K., and Wormith, S. (2009) 'Risk assessment with young offenders: A meta-analysis of three assessment measures', *Criminal Justice and Behaviour*, 36: 329–353.

Otto, R.K. and Douglas, K.S. (eds.) (2010) *Handbook of Violence Risk Assessment*. New York: Routledge, Taylor & Francis Group.
The People v. *Baxton* (1957) *Justia*. Available at: http://law.justia.com/cases/illinois/supreme-court/1957/34115-5.html. Accessed 18 January 2015.
Prentky, R. and Righthand, S. (2003) *Juvenile Sex Offender Assessment Protocol-II (J-SOAP-II)*. Available at:https://www.ncjrs.gov/pdffiles1/ojjdp/202316.pdf. Accessed 14 January 2015.
Print, B., Morrison, T., and Henniker, J. (2002) *Working with Young People Who Display Sexually Inappropriate and Abusive Behaviour*. Manchester: AIM Project.
Quinsey, V.L. (1981) 'The Long-Term Management of the Mentally Disordered Offender', in S.J. Hucker, C.D. Webster and M. Ben-Aron (eds.), *Mental Disorder and Criminal Responsibility*. Toronto: Butterworths, 137–155.
Quinsey, V.L., Harris, G.T., Rice, M.E., and Cormier, C. (2006) *Violent Offenders: Appraising and Managing Risk*. 2nd edn. Washington, DC: American Psychological Association.
Radford, L., Corral, S., Bradley, C., Fisher, H., Bassett, C., Howat, N., and Collishaw, S. (2011) *Child Abuse and Neglect in the UK Today*. London: NSPCC.
RCP (Royal College of Psychiatrists) (2011) 'Response to: Consultation on preventing suicide in England: A cross-government outcomes strategy to save lives', *Royal College of Psychiatrists*. Available at: http://www.rcpsych.ac.uk/pdf/Final%20response%20to%20the%20Suicide%20Strategy.pdf. Accessed 18 January 2015.
Richardson, G. (2009) 'Sharp Practice: The Sexually Harmful Adolescent Risk Protocol', in M.C. Calder (ed.), *Sexual Abuse Assessments: Using and Developing Frameworks for Practice*. Lyme Regis: Russell House Publishing, 108–147.
Rogers, K.M., Pumariega, M.D., Atkins, D.L., and Cuffe, S.P. (2006) 'Conditions associated with identification of mentally ill youths in juvenile detention', *Community Mental Health Journal*, 42(1): 25–40.
Schmidt, F., Campbell, M.A., and Houlding, C. (2011) 'Comparative analyses of the YLS/CMI, SAVRY, and PCL:YV in adolescent offenders: A 10-year follow-up into adulthood', *Youth Violence and Juvenile Justice*, 9: 23–42.
Schmidt, F., Hoge, R., and Gomes, L. (2005) 'Reliability and validity analyses of the Youth Level of Service/Case Management Inventory', *Criminal Justice and Behaviour*, 32: 329–344.
Schwalbe, C. (2007) 'Risk assessment for juvenile justice: A meta-analysis', *Law and Human Behavior*, 31: 449–462.
Scottish Government (2013) 'Scottish policing performance framework, 2012–13', *Edinburgh: Scottish Government*. Available at: http://www.scotland.gov.uk/Publications/2013/11/6914. Accessed 22 October 2014.
Siegel, L.J. and Welsh, B.C. (2008) *Juvenile Delinquency: The Core*. 3rd edn. Belmont: Thomson Wadsworth.
Slobogin, C. and Fondacaro, M.R. (2011) *Juveniles at Risk: A Plea for Preventative Justice*. New York: Oxford University Press.
Taylor, J.L. and Thorne, I. (2005) 'Northgate Firesetter Risk Assessment', unpublished manual. Northgate and Prudhoe NHS Trust.
Thornton, D. (2007) 'Scoring guide for the Risk Matrix 2000.9/SVC', *Birmingham University*. Available at: http://www.birmingham.ac.uk/Documents/college-les/psych/RM2000scoringinstructions.pdf. Accessed 18 January 2015.
Vizard, E., Hickey, N., French, L., and McCrory, E. (2007) 'Children and adolescents who present with sexually abusive behaviour: A UK descriptive study', *Journal of Forensic Psychiatry and Psychology*, 18(1): 59–73.

Watt, B.D., Geritz, K., Hasan, T., Harden, S., and Doley, R. (2014) 'Prevalence and correlates of firesetting behaviours among offending and non-offending youth', *Legal and Criminological Psychology*, 21(1): 19–36.

Webster, C.D. and Hucker, S.J. (2007) *Violence Risk Assessment and Management*. Chichester: John Wiley & Sons.

Webster, C.D., Douglas, K.S., Eaves, D., and Hart, S.D. (1997) *HCR-20: Assessing Risk for Violence, Version 2*. Burnaby: Simon Fraser University.

Weerasekera, P. (1996) 'A Formulation of the Case of Antoinette: A Multiperspective Approach', in P. Sturmey (ed.), *Clinical Case Formulation: A Variety of Approaches*. Oxford: Wiley Blackwell, 145–156.

Welsh, J., Schmidt, F., McKinnon, L., Chattha, H., and Meyers, J. (2008) 'A comparative study of adolescent risk assessment instruments: Predictive and incremental validity', *Assessment*, 15(1): 104–115.

WHO (World Health Organization) (2011) 'Youth violence: Factsheet no. 356', *World Health Organization*. Available at: http://www.who.int/mediacentre/factsheets/fs356/en. Accessed 24 October 2014.

Worling, J.R. and Curwen, T. (2001) 'Estimate of Risk of Adolescent Sexual Offense Recidivism (Version 2.0: The "ERASOR")', in M.C. Calder (ed.), *Juveniles and Children Who Sexually Abuse: Frameworks for Assessment*. Lyme Regis: Russell House Publishing, 372–397.

YJB (Youth Justice Board) (2000) *Asset*. London: Youth Justice Board.

6
Whole Systems Approaches

Brigitte Squire, Tom Jefford and Cindy Cupit Swenson

Introduction

Aggression and antisocial behaviours are the most common mental health and behavioural difficulties experienced by children and young people aged 5 to 16 years (ONS, 2005). These behaviours significantly impact functioning and quality of life during childhood and adolescence, and are associated with an increased rate of mental health need during adulthood (NICE 2013). Children and youth who display antisocial behaviours are more likely to perform poorly in school, abuse substances, have contacts with the criminal justice system (CJS) and experience social isolation during adolescence.

Whilst many antisocial acts are common (and even normative during adolescence), the duration, frequency or severity of antisocial behaviours may be so concerning that specialist support is warranted. In fact, the youth's behaviours can be so serious that placement out of the home for intensive treatment is a possibility. As young people are assessed for treatment, their behaviour and presentations may attract a variety of diagnoses, such as conduct disorder or attention deficit hyperactivity disorder (ADHD), for example. Regardless of the diagnosis, to effect meaningful change, intervention and support must focus on target behaviours that are in need of change; such behaviours may be multiple (e.g. aggression, low mood, family conflict) and complex. Moreover, multiple agencies and providers may be involved in the care and treatment of these children and young people. For example, children and young people may require the support of different agencies to manage school problems, substance abuse, mental health difficulties and broader family needs. Multi-agency involvement creates a challenge in the effective co-ordination of care across agencies. In the UK, the National Institute for Health and Clinical Excellence (NICE) and the Social Care Institute of Excellence (SCIE) have developed guidelines for recognition, intervention and management of the difficulties associated with antisocial behaviour. The guidance (NICE 2013) acknowledges that identifying which interventions and agencies are most appropriate is challenging, and the most appropriate agency depends on whether they operate on a preventative level or are treating more complex presentations. A care pathway is presented in the guidance, based on research into effective interventions. The pathway distinguishes between preventative interventions for children aged 3 to 14 with, or at high risk of developing, a 'conduct disorder', and promotes group, and, if necessary, individual parent and foster training programmes alongside some child-focused treatments, such as group social and cognitive problem-solving programmes. For adolescents aged 11–17, who may attract a diagnosis of conduct disorder, multimodal interventions are considered to be needed. Somewhat unsurprisingly, pharmacological interventions are contraindicated for the routine management of behavioural problems and those attracting a diagnosis of conduct disorder, although, in the experience of the authors, due to the lack of psychologically oriented practitioners within services and a predominance of a medical model of understanding behaviour, this guidance is not necessarily followed widely. There are recommendations for the sparing use of pharmacological interventions, such as for managing severe aggressive behaviour or for managing young people with a diagnosis of coexisting ADHD, but these are not recommended for use in isolation from psychological interventions. There remains considerable debate as to the effectiveness of medication in the long run for such young people.

There is a significant body of research on the effectiveness of parenting programmes as primary interventions for the prevention of complex conduct difficulties (Scott 2010; Gardner 2011). In 2007, the National Academy for Parenting Practitioners was set up in England to deliver the training and dissemination of evidence-based parenting programmes, such as Triple-P (Sanders 2008; Sanders, Prinz and Shapiro 2012) and Incredible Years (Webster-Stratton, Rinaldi and Jamila 2011), and many UK local authorities now offer a range of parenting interventions (Scott 2010). However, Scott's research into the implementation of these programmes revealed that a high proportion of parents did not engage (one third did not attend), or dropped out prematurely (mean of 7 of the 18 sessions), and that the skill set of practitioners was paramount for good outcomes. He also noted that staff tended to navigate to 'easy', non-evidenced-based programmes with no effect on child outcomes. Prevention programmes also do not reach families with the highest needs and who have multiple risk factors that contribute to poor child outcomes (Scott et al. 2010). There is a need for more specialist services that are multimodal and are able to engage these families.

Utting, Monteiro and Ghate (2007), commissioned by the UK Department of Health (DH), and the Prime Minister's Strategy Unit in 2006, conducted a selective review of interventions with children and young people with conduct problems and their families. The review explored interventions that evidence effectiveness in reducing antisocial and behavioural difficulties displayed by children and adolescents, including substance abuse and/or a reduction in reoffending and reconviction rates for young offenders. Utting concluded that the selected home visiting programmes – Nurse-Family Partnership Home Visiting Programme (Olds 2006); multisystemic therapy (MST; Henggeler et al. 2009), multidimensional treatment foster care (MTFC; Chamberlain 2003) and functional family therapy (FFT; Alexander et al. 2013) – shared a number of general principles of effective implementation and overall effectiveness. These included: a strong, coherent and clearly articulated theoretical basis; professional, qualified and trained staff to deliver the interventions; high programme fidelity assisted by manuals and training programmes; flexibility within the programme to assess and meet the needs of the clients (individually tailored); high degree of face-to-face work with parents and children; partnership (collaboration) with families; programme delivery in the community and natural environment of the young people; multimodal/multidimensional approaches to tackle multiple risks and problems simultaneously; a tiered approach so that support can be ratcheted up to the next level; and a relatively sustained treatment period (Utting, Monteiro and Ghate 2007).

In this chapter we will focus on the multisystemic or multimodal approaches that are usually employed with older youth (age 12+) who exhibit serious antisocial behaviours. As such, these youth are considered at high risk of placement and the interventions necessary for behaviour change are intensive.

Evidence-based multi-systemic approaches for young people with severe antisocial behaviour

In recent years, demands have increased for delivery of research-supported treatments for young offenders and young people who display antisocial behaviour. Numerous organisations internationally (e.g. Blueprints for Violence Prevention in the US; Elliott 1998; NICE in the UK) have developed criteria to determine if a treatment is evidence-based to guide practice. In order for a programme to be accepted on to the published lists of model programmes, such as the US Office of Juvenile Justice and Delinquency Prevention list (OJJDP; http://www.ojjdp.gov/mpg) or the Blueprints list (developed by the University of Colorado; http://www.blueprintsprograms.com), it has to reach standards set by the list holders.

Blueprints programmes are classed as either 'promising programmes' or, for the higher standard, a 'model' programme. To achieve the 'Promising' listing there is an independent expert review of the intervention specificity, intervention impact and dissemination readiness, which includes the requirement that a treatment manual be published. There is also an assessment of the quality of evaluation, which requires published trials to produce valid and reliable findings with a minimum of one 'high quality randomised control trial or two quasi-experimental evaluations' (Mihalic and Irwin 2003; http://blueprintsprograms.com).

For the 'model' programme classification, there are two additional standards to meet, with a minimum of either two 'high quality randomised control trials or one high quality randomised controlled trial plus one high quality quasi-experimental evaluation' (Mihalic and Irwin 2003; http://blueprintsprograms.com). There is also a requirement that positive intervention impact is sustained for a minimum of 12 months after the end of the intervention. It is interesting to note at this point the stress placed on the Blueprints website for the additional qualification of a randomised control trial (RCT) as being required to be of a 'high quality'.

Largely, the identified 'model' evidence-based treatments for young people who exhibit severe antisocial behaviour are family and ecologically based. The development of such treatments rose out of cross-sectional and longitudinal studies showing that youth antisocial behaviour is determined by multiple risk factors across multiple systems, including individual youth, family, peer, school and neighbourhood (e.g. Howell 2008; Loeber, Burke and Pardini 2009). Examples of individual youth risk factors include beliefs such as favourable attitudes towards antisocial behaviour and attributing hostile intent to others, reduced verbal skills and 'psychiatric symptoms'. Family factors that increase risk include limited monitoring, ineffective discipline, low warmth, high conflict, and parental problems such as substance misuse (SM) or diagnosis of a 'psychiatric disorder' (Liberman 2008). Young people that associate with negative peers and have limited exposure to, or have been rejected by, prosocial peers, are at higher risk of antisocial behaviour (Elliott, Huizinga and Ageton 1985). With regard to school factors, antisocial youth exhibit low achievement and a lack of commitment to education, with behavioural problems and suspensions. Family and school factors are predictive of antisocial behaviour because they predict association with negative peers (Tighe et al. 2012). Finally, antisocial youth tend to receive low support from resources in the community, and their communities are often characterised by high disorganisation and psychosocial stress, availability of weapons and drugs, and a high mobility among members (Swenson et al. 2009).

The literature on the aetiology of antisocial behaviour noted earlier in this section supports the overriding conclusion that comprehensive multifactorial interventions (e.g. parenting, community support, school-based and peer) are needed to address the multiple risk factors that lead youth to engage in antisocial behaviour. A multifactor or multisystemic conceptualisation (Henggeler et al. 2009) is consistent with Bronfenbrenner's (1979) theory of social ecology, which suggests that young people are embedded in multiple systems and behaviour is a function of individuals' interactions within and between these systems. As such, to be effective, interventions must be tailored to the primarily individualised multifactorial or multisystems formulation of needs.

Clinical assessments, formulation of need and interventions, therefore, must take into account a wide variety of possible contributors to behavioural problems, both within and between systems, and they have to be ecologically valid. Assessments and interventions need to be conducted within the natural environment and context of the young person. Emphasis will be placed on sequences of behaviour and the reciprocal nature of influences and interactions that shape certain behaviours. Considering the empirical research on protective and risk factors of severe antisocial behaviour, the most effective treatments will have the capacity to address a comprehensive array of risk factors and concomitantly build protective factors (Henggeler et al. 2009).

The intervention programmes that have been listed as 'model' programmes for this client group are FFT (Alexander et al. 2013), MST (Henggeler et al. 2009) and MTFC (Chamberlain 2003), which we will describe in the following three sections.

Functional family therapy

Developed by Alexander and colleagues in the 1970s (Alexander and Parsons 1973, 1982), FFT is a widely disseminated evidence-based treatment, whose participants range from status offenders to young people presenting serious antisocial behaviour. FFT views the young person's presenting problems as being symptoms of dysfunctional family relations. Interventions focus on establishing and maintaining new patterns of family behaviour. They aim to reduce defensive communication patterns, increase supportive interactions, and promote supervision and effective discipline (Brosnan and Carr 2000). FFT is typically delivered by therapists who work in teams of 3 to 8 and carry caseloads of 12–15 families each. The treatment comprises three phases of intervention, with each phase having clear goals and assessment objectives, addressing different risk and protective factors (Sexton and Alexander 1999). In the first engagement and motivation phase, the therapist addresses and challenges maladaptive perceptions, beliefs and emotions, to increase the belief that change is possible and to shift the family's focus to developing positive family relationships. Next, behavioural, cognitive-behavioural and family systems approaches are used to highlight dysfunctional patterns of family behaviour and encourage interactions that foster positive functioning among all family members. The therapist's role is to provide concrete behavioural interventions that guide and support specific behavioural changes. This may include suggested parenting techniques, as well as communication and conflict management strategies. The final stage of treatment involves sustaining treatment gains and generalising change to the social ecology, such as school and community. The whole intervention consists of 8 to 12 hours of direct service, extending to 26–30 hours for more serious cases, and is delivered over a 3- to 4-month period in the home or in clinic settings as an outpatient therapy (Lane et al. 2004).

FFT has been evaluated across multiple efficacy and effectiveness trials. In the initial randomised efficacy trial (Alexander and Parsons 1973), young people whose families participated in FFT had better improvements in family interactions and decreases in recidivism for status offences, but not criminal offences. In subsequent quasi-experimental studies (Gordon et al. 1988) FFT evidenced an 84 per cent reduction in recidivism and, 32 months later, showed fewer arrests compared to youth in a comparison condition (Gordon, Graves and Arbuthnot 1995). Regarding effectiveness research, Friedman (1989) conducted a randomised trial comparing FFT to a parent group intervention for young people who abuse substances and who were in 'outpatient' treatment programmes. Despite higher rates of family engagement, FFT was not more effective than the comparison intervention in decreasing young people's externalising behaviour problems or SM. In a large-scale randomised trial in 14 different countries, comparing FFT to probation, 12 months post treatment rearrest rates were comparable for both conditions, but the lack of differences may have been due to low adherence (Sexton and Turner 2010).

In the UK there are currently nine sites (England – six; Northern Ireland – one; Scotland – two) implementing FFT (see http://www.fftllc.com), with one site in England involved in RCT evaluation.

Multisystemic therapy

MST (Henggeler et al. 2009) is a treatment model for young people aged 12 to 17 with very serious behavioural problems and their families. Based on Bronfenbrenner's theory and the aetiology of antisocial behaviour, treatment addresses risk factors across each of the systems and differs from individual to individual. As such, the specific interventions are bespoke to each family. The major goal of MST is to prevent out-of-home placement and to improve family relations through an intensive home-based treatment administered by a team of a half-time MST supervisor and three to four therapists working with four to six families. The focus of assessment is on determining the factors (across multiple systems) that drive the target referral behaviours. The therapist and family develop collaborative goals for treatment based on the desired outcomes of the members of the ecology. Therapists visit the family three or more times a week and treatment requires daily effort from the family members to reach the collaborative goals. Progress against these goals is reviewed weekly, and barriers to progress are addressed on the way. The family has access to a 24-hour on-call system to assist and support them whilst addressing the problems. Treatment lasts an average of three to five months and sessions are conducted in places and at times convenient to families. Doing so overcomes the barriers to office-based appointments, which fit into a standard time frame but may not be possible for families who work during those hours or do not have transport. MST is used most efficiently as an alternative to out-of-home placement. Considerable attention is devoted to the role of extra-familial systems (e.g. peers, school, neighbourhood, family network) in determining or maintaining identified problems. MST interventions are drawn from existing evidence-based techniques, such as behaviour therapies, cognitive-behavioural therapies, pragmatic family therapy approaches and, in some cases, pharmacological treatments (e.g. for ADHD). An intensive quality assurance system surrounds the implementation of the service and involves initial orientation training, weekly group supervision, weekly consultation with an MST expert, ongoing training, and feedback about treatment fidelity that is gathered from the parent or carer on a monthly basis. MST is a licensed programme with Multisystemic Therapy Services in Charleston, South Carolina (http://mstservices.com), which oversees the implementation of the model and secures the quality assurance.

Over 30 years of rigorous research supports the efficacy and effectiveness of MST for the specific group of young people for whom it is intended. In efficacy trials conducted out of a university setting, Borduin and colleagues (see Schaeffer and Borduin 2005) have demonstrated the capacity of MST to improve family relations, reduce youth and parent mental health difficulties, and decrease rearrest and incarceration among youth by more than 50 per cent through a 14-year follow-up. Multiple randomised clinical trials conducted through community-based agencies have demonstrated the effectiveness of MST at improving family and peer relationships and decreasing recidivism and out-of-home placements (Henggeler, Melton and Smith 1992; Henggeler et al. 1993). A key aspect of dissemination of MST has been the quality assurance programme that supports the fidelity of the model. That is, when the model is followed with fidelity, favourable clinical outcomes are more likely to be achieved (Henggeler et al. 1997).

MST currently operates more than 500 teams across 15 countries, serving more than 23,000 youth annually (http://mstservices.com). The Departments of Health and Education have supported the dissemination of MST in the UK and there are, at the time of writing, 46 teams in the UK (Northern Ireland – 4; England – 37; Scotland – 5) with a UK-based MST Expert Network Partnership to guide and support the sites.

In recent years, RCTs have been conducted to adapt MST to youth populations with specific needs. MST for youth with problem sexual behaviour (MST-PSB) is an intervention to support young people who engage in criminal sexual behaviour such as the sexual assault, rape and molestation of younger children. MST-PSB is built on the foundation of standard MST and attempts to address the many factors that influence problem sexual behaviour (PSB). MST-PSB has been shown in RCTs to be effective for reducing recidivism of young people who display sexually harmful behaviour. In a small initial study (Borduin et al. 1990), compared to individual counselling, MST-PSB reduced sexual offending by 93 per cent at a 3-year follow-up. In a larger randomised efficacy study, families that were supported by MST-PSB (compared to usual community services) showed significant reductions in recidivism for sexual offences, rearrest for other crimes and days incarcerated at a nine-year follow-up (Borduin, Schaeffer and Heiblum 2009).

MST-substance abuse (MST-SA, also known as MST-CM for MST enhanced with contingency management protocols; Henggeler et al. 2012) supports youth who are abusing drugs and alcohol. In addition to standard MST, MST-SA is the only other adaptation that has proven to be effective with this population. Whilst its foundation is MST, in which therapists work with only a few families at a time to give parents and caregivers guidance, MST-SA is highly focused on drug and alcohol use. For example, at every session the therapist determines whether the adolescent is currently using drugs and drinking alcohol. If the answer is yes, the underlying reasons for the substance abuse (peer pressure and boredom, for example) are sought, and an intervention is built. If the answer is no, the factors that led to the youth stopping are leveraged to influence future behaviour.

MST-SA has been evaluated across two randomised clinical trials. In the first (Henggeler, Pickrel and Brondino 1999), MST produced decreased drug use post-intervention and decreased days in out-of-home placements. At a four-year follow-up (Henggeler et al. 2002), young adults receiving MST evidenced decreased violent crime and increased marijuana abstinence. The second study integrated MST into juvenile drug courts (Henggeler et al. 2006) and showed that MST enhanced substance use outcomes for alcohol and marijuana.

In the case example that follows we will illustrate how MST approaches severe antisocial behaviour during adolescence.

Case example

Colin is 13 years old and lives with his mother, Marilyn and his older brother, James, who is 18 years old. His father died a year ago from lung cancer and, since the death, Colin's mother has shown signs of depression and has had difficulty leaving the home.

Colin has not attended school in the past year, is mixing with antisocial peers at night who are known for vandalising buildings and cars, and sleeps most of the day or plays video games. He has been arrested when riding in a stolen car with one of the youths and was sentenced to a referral order. His mother suspects that he is using drugs, as his behaviour has changed and he is more irritable and restless at home. Although James can see that his mother is not strict enough with Colin, he doesn't want to upset her by criticising her. Colin's grandmother lives nearby and is supporting Colin's mother and keeping her company in the evening.

At the start of treatment, the MST worker obtains the desired outcomes of all significant people (personal and professional) in the young person's life and assesses how they can be a resource in obtaining the desired outcomes. Based on the concerns at referral and the desired outcomes of the significant people and the young person himself, the following collaborative overachieving goals were agreed: (1) Colin is to attend school full-time as evidenced by school reports; (2) Colin is not to commit any further offences as evidenced by police and youth officer's reports; (3) Colin's mother will increase her parental authority and her monitoring of Colin as evidenced by age-appropriate rules and boundaries and clear expectations of his whereabouts; and (4) Colin will stop using drugs as evidenced by clear drug screens.

To plan the interventions, the MST worker needs to have a good understanding (conceptualisation) of all the factors in the different systems contributing to and perpetuating the presenting problems (risk factors). To this end, s/he will talk to all involved to hear their views as to why this behaviour is occurring. At the same time, the worker will look for strengths (protective factors) in each of the systems (individual, family, school, peers and community) the young person is embedded in and use these as a leverage for change.

The following reasons (fit factors) for Colin not going to school were identified: there were no consequences at home for not going; he was not getting up in time due to late nights out; anxiety of not being able to catch up having missed so many lessons; anxiety and worry about his mother being sad and trying to protect her by not leaving her alone at home; unresolved grief due to the sudden death of his father; involvement with older antisocial peers who don't attend school either; Mum not having a direct link with school.

Additional factors related to the other goals were: Mum's depression; not using the social support systems (grandmother and James) in an efficient way; boredom and lack of structure; no clear rules and expectations with appropriate consequences and rewards; lack of monitoring; access to pocket money to be able to buy drugs; lack of involvement in prosocial activities in the community; Mum feeling sorry for him being at home all day.

Several interventions were designed to address these factors in a step-by-step approach, reviewing the advances and barriers in trying to achieve the agreed intervention steps in weekly supervision and consultation meetings.

To get Colin back in school, the MST worker planned the following interventions: a behavioural plan with rewards and consequences was drawn up with Marilyn to encourage Colin to attend school. This included removal of all electronics during school time and limiting access to them after school attendance. A curfew and bedtime rule were put in place to help Colin wake up in time. Pocket money was directly related to him attending school, and increased access to his video games was an earned reward. James and Grandma were informed of the plan and asked to support Marilyn in removing the electronics and to assist her in sticking to the plan. A school meeting with Marilyn was set up to agree a staged return back, with the support of an assistant teacher to help Colin catch up. A communication link via a daily diary was agreed to address any barriers as they came up. Family sessions were arranged to work on the grief over the loss of Dad and to deal with feelings of guilt and responsibility, so that Colin did not feel he had to stay home with his mother at all times.

In relation to his offending behaviour and drug use, the worker re-engaged Colin in the local football team whilst his mother monitored his whereabouts and made it very clear with whom she didn't want him to mix. She discovered the places where he would meet with antisocial peers and would call and inform the police if necessary to make such meetings more challenging for him. Colin would not receive money, but the rewards he would earn would be agreed goods that Mum would purchase until he demonstrated that he was not using any drugs. Colin and his mother were offered a contingency management programme where Marilyn was drug screening Colin, who could earn a significant amount of rewards as a contingency for clean screens.

Marilyn was encouraged to see her GP for her depression and the worker supported her to take better care of herself so that she felt energetic enough to deal with Colin's problems. The worker also managed to connect Marilyn with the local community learning centre, where she embarked on an IT course. The worker addressed some of Marilyn's negative cognitions related to her guilty feelings and also in relation to her views about the importance of education.

The process of reaching the overarching goals had a difficult start as Colin was not happy with his curfew and having to get up on time. It was also difficult for Marilyn not to get persuaded by him to allow him out or to have access to his electronics, as she could easily get emotionally involved and feel sorry for him. James was a major help in supporting Marilyn to stay strong and also in encouraging Colin to go to school and join the football team. He removed all electronics from the house until Colin attended school. There was a clear ritual in the morning to get Colin up and Marilyn joined him on the bus on several days to get him to school. The assistant teacher did a brilliant job in getting him back on track and he managed to sit some exams with satisfactory results.

Marilyn had to call the police on one occasion when he had left the house at night and didn't return home. She could give the address of the place he was staying and they collected him from there. His friends didn't like this police involvement and were less keen to have him round any longer. His full-time attendance at school and his involvement in local community activities, together with the rewards he earned, made him less interested in using drugs.

Through family sessions, grief over the loss of his father was addressed and the family came up with ways to remember him. They began to talk openly and easily about him and the memories they had of him.

After finishing her IT course, Marilyn did a volunteer job in the local hospital and really enjoyed being out and being helpful to others.

Although MST has a well-supported research base for its efficacy and effectiveness, it is targeting a specific client group and has well-defined referral criteria, which eliminates certain adolescents or younger children with a similar presentation. Local pathways for referral to MST differ between agencies, and therefore some guidelines to provide multi-model evidence-informed practice to adolescents and their families with complex presentations who cannot access MST is needed. These guidelines would need to include multifactorial formulations and interventions that have shown to be effective to address some of the identified problems. An interesting development that confronts this issue is the work of Chorpita and Daleiden (2009), who distilled the practice elements of over 600 evidence-based interventions in the child mental health field and developed the modular approach to therapy for children (MATCH) protocols for the treatment of common mental health problems (Chorpita and Weisz 2009). Their suggested interventions are delivered in a modular form based on consensus studies of best practice, and their system gives guidance on how to meet the changing complex needs of children and families.

Multidimensional treatment foster care

For youth who require placement out of the home, MTFC (Chamberlain 2003) is an evidence-based community alternative to institutional care. MTFC provides extremely high-quality foster care placements for youth presenting serious antisocial behaviour, and a team of treatment staff (e.g. case manager, family therapist, individual therapist and other resource staff) surrounds each individual. The chief goal of MTFC is to reunite young people with their family, so interventions focus, alongside the foster placement, on the family of origin and pertinent extra-familial systems. MTFC is based on social learning theory and, as such, the interventions are drawn from behavioural or cognitive behavioural approaches. Young people take part in a structured behavioural management programme in their foster home. The MTFC team work with no more than ten young people at any one time and the team is led by a full-time Master's-level programme supervisor, with competencies in the delivery of psychological intervention. Only one young person is placed with a particular foster family for a 6- to 9-month period. Intervention typically continues post-reunification. If reunification (with the primary family) is not possible, the focus will be on securing a lasting permanent placement by reducing the problem behaviours.

MTFC has been evaluated across three hybrid efficacy–effectiveness studies (i.e. real-world providers, but managed from a research centre). The most rigorous research, a randomised clinical trial, showed greater reductions in criminal charges one-year post-discharge, and 60 per cent fewer days incarcerated for young people receiving MTFC versus those receiving group care (Chamberlain and Reid 1998). A two-year follow-up study supported the sustainability of these treatment effects (Eddy, Whaley and Chamberlain 2004). Research identified more rapid improvements in children's behaviour, decreased levels of aggression and/or delinquent behaviour, good levels of subsequent residency in more lenient and less restrictive settings, and increased placement stability.

In 2005, the Department of Education and Skills supported setting up some MTFC schemes in the UK, and a national treatment foster care team based at the Maudsley Hospital in London was established to provide support, training and consultation to the new sites. They support three different versions of MTFC designed for pre-school, 6–11-year-olds and adolescents.

Implementation of evidence-based interventions

An emerging body of work is being published and peer reviewed on implementation research, which is becoming known as 'implementation science'. This is the study of implementation as a distinct set of processes, and is closely allied to the nascent evidence-based practice movement. As evidence-based practice seeks to define itself, so researchers are working to define a new taxonomy for implementation research as meta-analyses, such as those demonstrated by Fixsen and colleagues (2005). Researchers are creating multiple definitions of concepts and processes, as it is argued that 'the lack of such a framework inhibits the shared understanding of the exact nature of specific implementation strategies' (Mazza et al. 2013: 2).

Mihalic and Irwin (2003) outline the history of evidence-based practice from the 'nothing works' pessimism of the 1970s in criminal justice interventions, when few, if any, of the methodologies and systems in place were having any discernible effect on crime and delinquency. This led to renewed efforts in research, which created the 'what works' movement that emerged in the 1990s (Davies, Nutley and Smith 2000). Mihalic and Irwin (2003) point out that what was largely being routinely ignored was the relationship between the process and the product and, specifically, implementation as a distinct entity to be considered. Practitioners were left:

> [W]ith a list of model or best-practice programmes that produced favourable outcomes during research trials, but very little information available about how to implement these programmes. In other words, we now have some knowledge about what to implement, but we know very little about how.
>
> (Mihalic and Irwin 2003: 308)

Biglan and Ogden (2008) record similar sentiments in their review of emerging evidence-based practice in Norway, stating that, from 30 years of research, 'we know far more about how to affect young people than we know about how to influence the social systems that will have to adopt evidence-based practices if the fruits of recent discoveries are going to be realized' (Biglan and Ogden 2008: 81). Therefore, the question has moved from 'does this evidence-based programme work?' to 'can this evidence-based programme work in this particular setting?'

This stresses the importance of implementation as a process, and the readiness, or not, of both professional practice *and* of organisational systems to adapt to new ways of working in order to adopt the innovations of evidence-based practice. These ideas were extensively reviewed by Greenhalgh and colleagues (2004), whose systematic review considered the diffusion of innovations in services within the health system in the UK. Greenhalgh's work is a logical starting point for thinking about implementation research, drawing as it does on constructs from social psychology, organisational behaviour theories and management theory. She concluded that the research prior to her review lacked robustness and specificity, tending to confuse the diffusion of knowledge, implementation and change management. Greenhalgh set new questions for future implementation researchers, to find out 'by what processes are particular innovations in health service delivery and organisations implemented and sustained (or not) in particular contexts and settings, and can these processes be enhanced?' (Greenhalgh et al. 2004: 620). This highlights the need to pay closer attention to both the setting and the system in which an innovative practice is implemented.

A systematic review of implementation research by Fixsen and colleagues (2005) at the National Implementation Research Network in North Carolina, USA, helpfully develops understanding of how the preparation of the team, service, professional disciplines, wider stakeholders and community are central to successful implementation. According to the schematic framework proposed by Fixsen, it can be demonstrated how deficits in any of these domains will tend to lead to reduced outcomes for the evidence-based programme being implemented.

Continuing attempts to develop a general theory of implementation and conceptual frameworks abound (e.g. Grol et al. 2007; Feldstein and Glasgow 2008). May and colleagues (2009) have taken a broadly sociological perspective to expand understanding of the processes by which new ways of working are embedded into practice. This has become known as normalisation process theory. In more recent work, May (2013) has continued to refine his model by integrating additional constructs to create a general implementation theory, which develops and expands the reach of his original work with four interrelated core constructs – capability, capacity, potential and contribution. For May, as a sociologist, the important core element is the notion of human agency in shaping and modifying the social system and the social processes that then result.

Kitson and colleagues (2008) have started to refine a conceptual framework, developed in 2002, called the Promoting Action on Research Implementation in Health Services (PARiHS) framework. Like others before, it seeks to define a clear typology and to describe the core component elements that are relevant to implementation. This research reflects upon the almost infinite number of potential interactions between these components, and invites others to test out parts of the framework to begin to give it validity.

Based upon a wide-ranging systematic review, Damschroder and colleagues (2009) set out the Consolidated Framework for Implementation Research (CFIR), identifying five major domains: intervention characteristics, outer setting, inner setting, characteristics of the individuals concerned and implementation process. Each domain has further constructs within, which are further defined, making 37 constructs in all. Damschroder adds in the domain of the individual to the PARiHS framework. The contextual nature of the approach and the reach of the framework are comprehensive. In terms of research methodology, the CFIR sets out how the evaluation of qualitative information can use standardised coding to test out and describe the various implementation constructs. This allows future research to build upon the model. The visual representation of the CFIR is designed to demonstrate the dynamic relationship between the domains in complicated ways, recognising both individual actors as well as organisational influences. The model acknowledges the adaptive nature and process of implementation, and the jigsaw shape of the model leads one to consider how components have to adapt to create a fit or risk disconnection. Unlike the PARiHS framework, the CFIR explicitly recognises the temporal nature of implementation as a stage in a process which will adapt over time.

In the first testing of the CFIR and as a demonstration model, Damschroder and Lowery (2013) evaluated a large-scale weight management programme for military veterans called 'MOVE!' using the CFIR constructs and then started the process of refining their model. It was found to offer a good fit for many of the variables tested and that, 'of the 31 CFIR constructs assessed, 10 constructs strongly distinguished between facilities with low versus high MOVE implementation effectiveness' (Damschroder and Lowery 2013: 1). There were mixed results for a further 16 constructs, with insufficient data to assess the remainder, with the individual domain not tested in this research. Damschroder and Lowery (2013) has now established a model with the explicit ambition of setting a template for future research, and has established an online collaborative system by way of an open source research wiki to encourage the widespread testing of CFIR and the reporting of results (which can be found at http://cfirguide.org/).

Challenges in the implementation of evidenced-based interventions

Having implemented MST in several settings, the CFIR resonates with the experience of implementation as a multilayered and time-phased process. Seeking to embed MST within a complex system, such as a children's service of a local authority, requires cultural, organisational, practical and managerial change that must take place at a team, first line manager and strategic management level. Deficits in any strata can permeate across to create blocks and obstacles. Finding the means to overcoming these issues may not be immediately obvious, especially when disguised compliance may mask deep-seated antipathy towards practice, which challenges working practices in fundamental ways.

MST services have, over time, paid more attention to those multilayered factors that are important for effective outcomes. In some RCTs of MST where there were less favourable outcomes (Leschied and Cunningham 2002; Ogden and Halliday-Boykins 2004), a major contributor to this was the team's lack of treatment fidelity. Alongside an in-depth site assessment where agencies have to demonstrate their commitment to the full implementation of MST, they developed an intensive quality assurance system to secure ongoing fidelity to the model. Despite this framework, ongoing attention is needed to change agency and team factors, and some modification and adaptation is necessary without losing treatment fidelity.

Feedback-informed services

Although implementation research is contributing to making dissemination of evidence-based practices more efficient, leading to better outcomes for clients, there is also a growing body of research that shows that a core group of general therapeutic factors are responsible for successful outcomes regardless of the approach or model (Lambert, Shapiro and Bergin 1986; Lambert 1992; Hubble, Duncan and Miller 1999). There are client and extra-therapeutic factors that are independent of treatment, and that refer to what the client brings to therapy, their circumstances and events in their life. In addition to these client and extra-therapeutic factors are therapist effects: some clinicians are more effective than others (Wampold and Brown 2005); alliance effects: the quality and strength of the collaborative relationship between client and therapist is the largest contributor to outcome (Norcross 2011); the expectancy and allegiance effect: the client's and therapist's expectations and beliefs of potential effects of therapy; and the model and technique effects: they provide structure and focus in treatment and engage and inspire participants (Lambert and Bergin 1994).

To improve outcomes in treatment it is important to seek and obtain valid and reliable feedback from clients regarding the therapeutic alliance and ongoing outcome progress, to adjust treatment as needed. Miller (2011) summarised the impact of routinely monitoring and using outcome and alliance data from

13 RCTs involving 12,374 consumers, and demonstrated that it doubles the effect size, decreases dropout rates by half and decreases deterioration by 33 per cent. As the alliance between client and therapist impacts most strongly on treatment outcomes, monitoring this alliance by using client feedback allows clinicians to identify and correct problems with engagement and reduce early dropout or risk of negative outcome. The fact that MST does whatever it takes to secure client engagement and alliance might be one of the contributing factors to its success.

Agencies that adopt session-by-session feedback can improve their services, evaluate all treatments that take place in their agency and make the real-time treatment more effective. This practice-based evidence approach can supplement the evidence-based programmes that cannot reach all clients in need of treatment.

Conclusion

As severe antisocial behaviour in adolescents is a major and growing problem in mental health, it is important to have interventions that have a proven record of effectiveness. We have discussed some multi-model interventions that are ecologically valid and that address the multiple risk factors associated with this complex presentation. These interventions are often embedded in intense quality assurance systems, to secure treatment fidelity to the model in order to protect effective outcomes. We discussed the fact that, despite this treatment adherence to the model, practitioners need to be aware of the necessary local conditions, to make the treatment work within a certain setting, agency and culture, and that there are continuous changing circumstances that need a flexible model adaptation without losing treatment fidelity. We highlighted the fact that these treatment models have a clear target client group, and that local services also need a system to evaluate the effectiveness of other treatments for complex behavioural problems by, for example, using client session-by-session feedback measures to improve practice.

References

Alexander, J.F. and Parsons, B.V. (1973) 'Short-term behavioral intervention with delinquent families: Impact on family process and recidivism', *Journal of Abnormal Psychology*, 81(3): 219–225.

Alexander, J.F. and Parsons, B.V. (1982) *Functional Family Therapy: Principles and Procedures*. Carmel, CA: Brooks/Cole.

Alexander, J.F., Waldron, H.B., Robbins, M.S., and Neeb, A.A. (2013) *Functional Family Therapy for Adolescent Behavior Problems*. Washington, DC: American Psychological Association.

Biglan, A. and Ogden, T. (2008) 'The evolution of evidence-based practices', *European Journal of Behavior Analysis*, 9(1): 81–95.

Borduin, C.M., Schaeffer, C.M., and Heiblum, N. (2009) 'A randomized clinical trial of multisystemic therapy with juvenile sexual offenders: Effects on youth social ecology and criminal activity', *Journal of Consulting and Clinical Psychology*, 77(1): 26–37.

Borduin, C.M., Henggeler, S.W., Blaske, D.M., and Stein, R.J. (1990) 'Multisystemic treatment of adolescent sexual offenders', *International Journal of Offender Therapy and Comparative Criminology*, 34(2): 105–113.

Bronfenbrenner, U. (1979) *The Ecology of Human Development: Experiments by Design and Nature*. Cambridge, MA: Harvard University Press.

Brosnan, R. and Carr, A. (2000) 'Adolescent Conduct Problems', in A. Carr (ed.) *What Works with Children and Adolescents? A Critical Review of Psychological Interventions with Children, Adolescents and their Families*. Florence, KY: Taylor & Francis/Routledge, 131–154.

Chamberlain, P. (2003) *Treating Chronic Juvenile Offenders: Advances Made through the Oregon Multidimensional Treatment Foster Care Model*. Washington, DC: American Psychological Association.

Chamberlain, P. and Reid, J.B. (1998) 'Comparison of two community alternatives to incarceration for chronic juvenile offenders', *Journal of Consulting and Clinical Psychology*, 66(4): 624–633.

Chorpita, B. and Daleiden, E. (2009) 'Mapping evidence-based treatments for children and adolescents: Application of the distillation and matching model to 615 treatments from 322 randomised trials', *Journal of Consulting and Clinical Psychology*, 77: 566–579.

Chorpita, B. and Weisz, J. (2009) *MATCH-ADTC: Modular Approach to Therapy for Children with Anxiety, Depression, Trauma or Conduct Disorder*. Satellite Beach, FL: PractiseWise, LLC.

Damschroder, L.J. and Lowery, J.C. (2013) 'Evaluation of a large-scale weight management program using the consolidated framework for implementation research (CFIR)', *Implementation Science*, 8(1): 51.

Damschroder, L.J., Aron, D.C., Keith, R.E., Kirsh, S.R., Alexander, J.A., and Lowery, J.C. (2009) 'Fostering implementation of health services research findings into practice: A consolidated framework for advancing implementation science', *Implementation Science*, 4(1): 50.

Davies, H.T.O., Nutley, S.M., and Smith, P.C. (2000) *What Works? Evidenced-Based Policy and Practice in Public Services*. Bristol: Policy Press.

Eddy, J.M., Whaley, R.B., and Chamberlain, P. (2004) 'The prevention of violent behavior by chronic and serious male juvenile offenders: A 2-year follow-up of a randomized clinical trial', *Journal of Emotional and Behavioral Disorders*, 12(1): 2–8.

Elliott, D.S. (1998) *Blueprints for Violence Prevention*, series edn, University of Colorado, Center for the Study and Prevention of Violence. Boulder, CO: Blueprints.

Elliott, D.S., Huizinga, D., and Ageton, S.S. (1985) *Explaining Delinquency and Drug Use*. Beverley Hills, CA: Sage.

Feldstein, A.C. and Glasgow, R.E. (2008) 'A practical, robust implementation and sustainability model (PRISM)', *Joint Commission Journal on Quality and Patient Safety*, 34(4): 228–243.

Fixsen, D.L., Naoom, S.F., Blase, K.A., Friedman, R.M., and Wallace, F. (2005) *Implementation Research: A Synthesis of the Literature*. Tampa, FL: The National Implementation Research Network, Louis de la Parte Florida Mental Health Institute, University of Florida.

Friedman, A.S. (1989) 'Family therapy vs. parent groups: Effects on adolescent drug abusers', *American Journal of Family Therapy*, 17(4): 335–347.

Gardner, F. (2011) 'Preventing Mental Health Problems through Very Early Intervention', Presentation at the 2011 Emanuel Miller Lecture and Day Conference, London.

Gordon, D.A., Graves, K., and Arbuthnot, J. (1995) 'The effect of functional family therapy for delinquents on adult criminal behavior', *Criminal Justice and Behavior*, 22(1): 60–73.

Gordon, D.A., Arbuthnot, J., Gustafson, K.E., and McGreen, P. (1988) 'Home-based behavioral-systems family therapy with disadvantaged juvenile delinquents', *American Journal of Family Therapy*, 16(3): 243–255.

Greenhalgh, T., Robert, G., Macfarlane, F., Bate, P., and Kyriakidou, O. (2004) 'Diffusion of innovations in service organizations: Systematic review and recommendations', *Milbank Quarterly*, 82(4): 581–629.

Grol, R.P., Bosch, M.C., Hulscher, M.E., Eccles, M.P., and Wensing, M. (2007) 'Planning and studying improvement in patient care: The use of theoretical perspectives', *Milbank Quarterly*, 85(1): 93–138.

Henggeler, S.W., Melton, G.B., and Smith, L.A. (1992) 'Family preservation using multisystemic therapy: An effective alternative to incarcerating serious juvenile offenders', *Journal of Consulting and Clinical Psychology*, 60(6): 953–961.

Henggeler, S.W., Pickrel, S.G., and Brondino, M.J. (1999) 'Multisystemic treatment of substance abusing and dependent delinquents: Outcomes, treatment fidelity, and transportability', *Mental Health Services Research*, 1(3): 171–184.

Henggeler, S.W., Clingempeel, W.G., Brondino, M.J., and Pickrel, S.G. (2002) 'Four-year follow-up of multisystemic therapy with substance-abusing and substance-dependent juvenile offenders', *Journal of the American Academy of Child and Adolescent Psychiatry*, 41(7): 868–874.

Henggeler, S.W., Melton, G.B., Brondino, M.J., Scherer, D.G., and Hanley, J.H. (1997) 'Multisystemic therapy with violent and chronic juvenile offenders and their families: The role of treatment fidelity in successful dissemination', *Journal of Consulting and Clinical Psychology*, 65(5): 821–833.

Henggeler, S.W., Melton, G.B., Smith, L.A., Schoenwald, S.K., and Hanley, J.H. (1993) 'Family preservation using multisystemic treatment: Long-term follow-up to a clinical trial with serious juvenile offenders', *Journal of Child and Family Studies*, 2(4): 283–293.

Henggeler, S.W., Schoenwald, S.K., Borduin, C.M., Rowland, M.D., and Cunningham, P.B. (2009) *Multisystemic Therapy for Antisocial Behavior in Children and Adolescents*. London: Guilford Press.

Henggeler, S.W., Halliday-Boykins, C.A., Cunningham, P.B., Randall, J., Shapiro, S.B., and Chapman, J.E. (2006) 'Juvenile drug court: Enhancing outcomes by integrating evidence-based treatments', *Journal of Consulting and Clinical Psychology*, 74(1): 42–54.

Henggeler, S.W., Cunningham, P.B., Rowland, M.D., Schoenwald, S. K., Swenson, C.C., Sheidow, A.J., McCart, M.R., Donohue, B., Navas-Murphy, L.A., and Randall, J. (2012) *Contingency Management for Adolescent Substance Abuse: A Practitioner's Guide*. New York: Guilford Press.

Howell, J.C. (2008) *Preventing and Reducing Juvenile Delinquency: A Comprehensive Framework*. Portland, OR: Sage.

Hubble, M., Duncan, B., and Miller, S. (eds.) (1999) *The Heart and Soul of Change: What Works in Therapy*. Washington, DC: American Psychological Association.

Kitson, A.L., Rycroft-Malone, J., Harvey, G., McCormack, B., Seers, K., and Titchen, A. (2008) 'Evaluating the successful implementation of evidence into practice using the PARiHS framework: Theoretical and practical challenges', *Implementation Science*, 3(1): 1.

Lambert, M. (1992) 'Implications of Outcome Research for Psychotherapy Integration', in J.C. Norcross and M.R. Goldfried (eds.), *Handbook of Psychotherapy Integration*. New York: Basic Books, 94–129.

Lambert, M. and Bergin, A. (1994) 'The Effectiveness of Psychotherapy', in A. Bergin and S. Garfield (eds.), *Handbook of Psychotherapy and Behavior Change*. 4th edn. New York: Wiley, 143–189.

Lambert, M., Shapiro, D., and Bergin, A. (1986) 'The Effectiveness of Psychotherapy', in S. Garfield and A. Bergin (eds.), *Handbook of Psychotherapy and Behavior Change*. 3rd edn. New York: Wiley, 157–211.

Lane, E., Gardner, F., Hutchings, J., and Jacobs, B. (2004) 'Nine to thirteen: Risk and protective factors; Effective interventions', in C. Sutton, D. Utting, and D.P. Farrington (eds.), *Support from the Start: Working with Young Children and Their Families to Reduce the Risks of Crime and Antisocial Behaviour*. London: Department of Education and Skills, 57–68.

Leschied, A.W. and Cunningham, A. (2002) *Seeking Effective Interventions for Young Offenders: Interim Results of a Four-Year Randomized Study of Multisystemic Therapy in Ontario, Canada*. London, ON: Centre for Children and Families in the Justice System.

Liberman, A.M. (ed.) (2008) *The Long View of Crime: A Synthesis of Longitudinal Research*. New York: Springer.

Loeber, R., Burke, J.D., and Pardini, D.A. (2009) 'Development and etiology of disruptive and delinquent behavior', *Annual Review of Clinical Psychology*, 5: 291–310.

May, C. (2013) 'Towards a general theory of implementation', *Implementation Science*, 8(18): 1–14.

May, C.R., Mair, F., Finch, T., MacFarlane, A., Dowrick, C., Treweek, S., Rapley, T., Ballini, L., Ong, B., Rogers, A., Murray, E., Elwyn, G., Legare, F., Funn, J., and Montori, V.M. (2009) 'Development of a theory of implementation and integration: Normalization process theory', *Implementation Science*, 4: 29–37.

Office for National Statistics (2005) Mental Health of Children and Young People in Great Britain. Hampshire: Palgrave Macmillan.

Mazza, D., Bairstow, P., Buchan, H., Chakraborty, S.P., Van Hecke, O., Grech, C., and Kunnamo, I. (2013) 'Refining a taxonomy for guideline implementation: Results of an exercise in abstract classification', *Implementation Science*, 8(1): 32.

Mihalic, S.F. and Irwin, K. (2003) 'Blueprints for violence prevention from research to real-world settings: Factors influencing the successful replication of model programs', *Youth Violence and Juvenile Justice*, 1(4): 307–329.

Miller, S. (2011) *Psychometrics of the ORS and SRS: Results from RCTs and Meta-Analyses of Routine Outcome Monitoring and Feedback: The Available Evidence*. Chicago, IL: ICCE.

NICE (National Institute for Health and Clinical Excellence) (2013) *Conduct Disorders and Antisocial Behaviour in Children and Young People: Recognition, Intervention and Management (CG158)*. London: British Psychological Society and Royal College of Psychiatrists. Available at: http://guidance.nice.org.uk/CG158/. Accessed 1 May 2015.

Norcross, J. (ed.) (2011) *Psychotherapy Relationships that Work: Evidence-Based Responsiveness*. 2nd edn. New York: Oxford University Press.

Ogden, T. and Halliday-Boykins, C.A. (2004) 'Multisystemic treatment of antisocial adolescents in Norway: Replication of clinical outcomes outside of the US', *Child and Adolescent Mental Health*, 9(2): 77–83.

OJJDP (Office of Juvenile Justice and Delinquency Prevention) (n.d.) OJJDP: Model Programs Guide. Available at: http://www.ojjdp.gov/mpg. Accessed 26 January 2015.

Olds, D.L. (2006) 'The nurse–family partnership: An evidence-based preventive intervention', *Infant Mental Health Journal*, 27(1): 5–25.

Sanders, M.R. (2008) 'The triple P-positive parenting program as a public health approach to strengthening parenting', *Journal of Family Psychology*, 22(4): 506–517.

Sanders, M.R., Prinz, R.J., and Shapiro, C. (2012) 'Parenting and Child Maltreatment as Public Health Issues: Implications from the Triple P System of Intervention', in A. Rubin (ed.), *Clinician's Guide to Evidence-Based Practice: Programs and Interventions for Maltreated Children and Families at Risk*. Hoboken, NJ: John Wiley & Sons, Inc., 297–312.

Schaeffer, C.M. and Borduin, C.M. (2005) 'Long-term follow-up to a randomized clinical trial of multisystemic therapy with serious and violent juvenile offenders', *Journal of Consulting and Clinical Psychology*, 73(3): 445–453.

Scott, S. (2010) 'National dissemination of effective parenting programmes to improve child outcomes', *British Journal of Psychiatry*, 196: 1–3.

Scott, S., O'Connor, T., Futh, A., Matias, C., Price, J., and Doolan, M. (2010) 'Impact of a parenting program in a high-risk, multi-ethnic community: The PALS trial', *Journal of Child Psychology and Psychiatry*, 51(12): 1331–1341.

Sexton, T. and Alexander, J. (1999) *Functional Family Therapy: Principles of Clinical Assessment and Implementation*. Henderson, NV: RCH Enterprises.

Sexton, T. and Turner, C.W. (2010) 'The effectiveness of functional family therapy for youth with behavioral problems in a community practice setting', *Journal of Family Psychology*, 24(3): 339–348.

Swenson, C.C., Henggeler, S.W., Taylor, I.S., and Addison, O. (2009) *Multisystemic Therapy and Neighborhood Partnerships: Reducing Adolescent Violence and Substance Abuse*. New York: Guilford Press.

Tighe, A., Pistrang, N., Casdagli, L., Baruch, G., and Butler, S. (2012) 'Multisystemic therapy for young offenders: Families' experiences of therapeutic processes and outcomes', *Journal of Family Psychology*, 26(2): 187–197.

Utting, D., Monteiro, H., and Ghate, D. (2007) *Interventions for Children at Risk of Developing Antisocial Personality Disorder*. Report to the Department of Health and Prime Minister's Strategy Unit, Policy Research Bureau.

Wampold, B. and Brown, G. (2005) 'Estimating variability in outcomes attributable to therapists: A naturalistic study of outcomes in managed care', *Journal of Consulting and Clinical Psychology*, 73(5): 914–923.

Webster-Stratton, C., Rinaldi, J., and Reid, J.M. (2011) 'Long-term outcomes of incredible years parenting program: Predictors of adolescent adjustment', *Child and Adolescent Mental Health*, 16(1): 38–46.

7
Violence among Young People: A Framework for Assessment and Intervention

Wendy Morgan

Introduction

Violence among young people has significant personal, emotional and financial costs (David-Ferdon and Simon 2014). Official crime statistics from both the USA (Hockenberry and Puzzanchera 2014) and the UK (MoJ 2014) show that approximately 20 per cent of all recorded crime committed by young people is of a violent nature. Given the scope and scale of this issue, it is unsurprising that a considerable amount of clinical and political attention has been directed towards understanding and reducing violence perpetrated by young people. This has resulted in a large body of published work about risk assessment processes, intervention strategies and specific programmes. However, rather than assisting the practitioner, this multitude of advice can be contradictory, overwhelming, biased, context specific or simply out of date.

The picture is complicated by shifting public and political narratives. For example, behaviour that, 30 years ago, would have been treated by discretionary welfare initiatives, is now dealt with through punitive criminal justice sanctions (Muncie 2008). Individuals who work with young people are therefore increasingly being asked to work within a formalised framework of violence risk assessment, risk reduction and risk intervention. As a result, the focus sometimes shifts away from a holistic assessment of the young person (e.g. their strengths, interests and aspirations, as well as areas of concern), and solely considers their problematic antisocial behaviour.

This chapter presents a holistic framework which integrates a wide range of scientific and ethical principles into work with young people who have committed violence. The Framework for the Assessment and Intervention with Violence (FAIV) is not a prescriptive approach. It is a set of best practice guidelines that consider the young person, their behaviour and the clinician all to be essential elements which need to be integrated to effectively assess and reduce violent behaviour.

Defining violence

Clarifying what constitutes violent behaviour is not a simple task. Definitions differ across jurisdictions (Hazel 2008), time periods (Muncie 2008), clinicians and researchers (Howells, Daffern and Day 2008). When considering violent behaviour in young people, intent is useful to have at the core of a definition, because it allows for the developmental process to be considered explicitly. A 2-year-old who, when angry, throws objects and lashes out, does not have a primary motivation to harm others; their behaviour is reflective of immature emotional control. In contrast, *most* 12-year-olds will have the capacity to decide upon different courses of action when frustrated. Even if their decision-making is poor, and adversely affected, there is still an element of choice in their response (Borum and Verhaagen 2006).[1]

Whilst most psychologists agree that motivation and insight are essential to defining violence, there is less consensus over the type and severity of harm that should be included. When working with young people, there are advantages to adopting a narrow definition of violence. It ensures problematic behaviour (such as making verbal threats) is not pathologised, individuals are not pejoratively labelled and those most clearly in need of help are accurately identified. However, there are also advantages to including a wider range of behaviours. For example, *credible* threats of harm that create fear or distress in others may be useful when assessing risk of harm towards a specific individual (such as a parent, authority figure or dating partner) (Stader 2011; Leen et al. 2013; Holt 2013). Within this chapter, violence is defined as acts that are *intended* to cause fear, distress or physical harm to another individual. It is recognised that sexually harmful behaviour may also fit within this definition of violence. Whilst there are some overlaps between risk factors for adolescent sexual and violent behaviour, there are also some distinct differences (Seto and Lalumiere 2010). The risk factors included within the FAIV are specifically drawn from non-sexual violent offending studies. Whilst many of the variables and good practice suggestions are highly applicable to work with young people who engage in sexually harmful behaviour, this chapter has not been designed with this population in mind.[2]

Framework for the Assessment and Intervention of Violence (FAIV)

There exists a large body of work in relation to assessment and intervention of violent behaviour. Psychiatrists, social workers, criminologists, psychologists and treatment providers have all made valuable contributions to work in this field. However, there has been relatively little cross-fertilisation across these different disciplines and approaches. This chapter has drawn together best practice principles from across a range of theoretical and practitioner perspectives to help practitioners within a range of settings and client groups. The result is FAIV. The framework is not intended to be a detailed prescriptive approach. It is recognised that different individuals, practitioners and settings will require variations in practice. However, there are some ethical, theoretical and clinical concerns which are core to work with young people who have engaged in violent behaviour; it is these that the FAIV attempts to articulate.

The FAIV is illustrated in Figure 7.1. Client-related variables are presented first. These capture essential elements of the young person's functioning and well-being. Factors that relate to practitioner well-being and skills are at the base of the model. These act as a foundation to clinical work with young people. The client and the practitioner factors inform, and are informed by, risk assessment and intervention activity, and these are placed in the centre of the model. Assessment and intervention are presented as explicitly linked (see Tharinger, Gentry and Finn 2013), with psychological formulation a process extending across both elements (see Rich 2011). Because FAIV focuses on core principles, it is applicable within different settings and policy frameworks. Moreover, current good practice guidance on risk assessment, as well as new developments, can be incorporated.

Client factors

In clinical practice it is impossible to parcel out client-related factors from the wider issues of assessment and intervention. Likewise, there is necessarily an

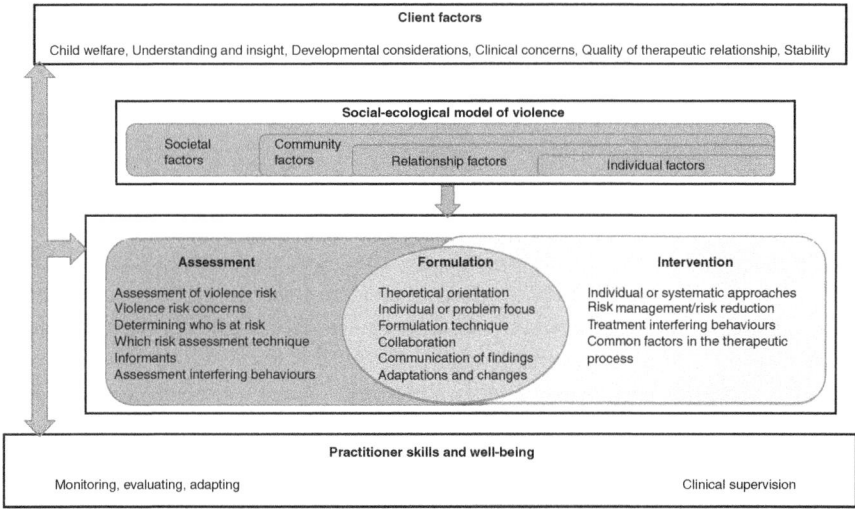

Figure 7.1 Framework for the assessment and intervention with violence (FAIV)

interaction between the client and the clinician. However, it is important to consider those aspects which relate to general aspects of the young person's functioning or well-being, and the way these impact upon the assessment and intervention process.

Child welfare

When a young person presents a risk of harm to others, there is a danger *their* vulnerability or welfare concerns can be underemphasised (Bailey 2002). It is beyond the scope of this chapter to address all the issues which may be of relevance. The Child Welfare Information Gateway (https://www.childwelfare.gov), the Social Care Institute for Excellence (http://www.scie.org.uk) and the National Society for the Prevention of Cruelty to Children (http://www.nspcc.org.uk) all contain excellent resources which cover assessment of a range of welfare concerns (e.g. risk of physical, psychological or sexual harm). However, other concerns are subtler in nature and are less frequently discussed. One such issue is that of diagnosis, sometimes referred to as the double-edged sword (Dell 2011). Diagnosis can allow for clear identification of concerns and access to appropriate treatment. However, it can also result in stigmatisation, prevention of access to mainstream treatments and the pathologisation of otherwise normal behaviour (Dell 2011). When deciding upon whether a diagnosis should, or should not, be provided, there is no unambiguously clear answer. Personal and professional obligations and preferences, the characteristics of the client, provision of available treatment and relevant policy requirements all need to be reflected upon and balanced in coming to the final decision.

Understanding and insight

Intentionality is at the core of the definition of violence used within the FAIV. However, the extent of an individual's insight and understanding (and hence the extent to which they intended to harm another) is complex to assess. Even when acts are intentional, the meaning to the young person, their assessment of risk and their appreciation of the consequences, need to be considered. For example, becoming involved in rioting or gang violence may reflect the young person's lack of expectations for the future, or their need to express their identity (Baker and Kelly 2011) and not primarily their desire to harm others.

Experience of maltreatment or poor attachment to caregivers also has a direct impact upon insight (Fonagy 2003). Youths with a history of trauma tend to process emotional and neutral faces differently from those without aversive childhoods, to have a lower IQ and be less able to effectively discriminate emotions (Hart and Rubia 2012). These deficits lead to a number of social and behavioural concerns and difficulties that create problems for the young person and those around them. For example, violent outbursts within residential care may, for some young people, reflect an interaction between their cognitive and emotional deficits and a sense of powerlessness triggered by their location (Baker and Kelly 2011).

In addition, young people who have been traumatised may respond violently to situations when they feel fearful (Nader 2011) or encounter situations which remind them of the trauma (either directly or at an unconscious level (van der Kolk 1989)). In other instances, violent behaviour may reflect an unconscious desire to re-enact the trauma situations (which may include harm to self or violence towards others (van der Kolk 1989)). All of these factors should be considered when considering the extent to which a young person is able to access his or her internal states (van der Kolk 2005).

Developmental considerations

Developmental considerations are essential to informing assessment and intervention with young people. Whilst some models emphasise this element (e.g. Fonagy 2003) others make little explicit mention of it (e.g. Bailey 2002). Few models empathise the need for developmental evaluations to be culturally informed (Manassis 2014). However, because different cultures have different expectations of young people, subtle but distinct differences in development may need to be considered (see Bose and Sattar 2011). Assessment of the ways in which culture has contributed to the young person's attitudes towards conflict resolution, response to threats and perceptions of safety is also an important consideration when working with young people who have been violent (Harland 2011).

Developmental stage also has an impact upon the range of communication strategies that a child may choose to adopt (either as a conscious decision or through lack of capacity). For example, play, metaphor, tone of voice, facial expression, avoidance, responses to others, style of dress and movement are all ways in which children and young people communicate at different stages of their development (Lefevre 2010). The skill for the clinician lies in interpreting and deciphering this myriad of communication strategies. Likewise, the individual's developmental stage will also be significant in determining the appropriate intervention strategy. In part, this will relate to how the treatment is delivered (it must be comprehensible to the young person), but the individual's developmental age will also determine the focus of the violence intervention strategy.

Young people respond differently to risk and protective factors throughout their development (Manassis 2014). For example, Viljoen, Elkovitch and Ullman (2008) note that, in younger children, family and individual-level concerns are most significant in predicting recidivism. For older adolescents, community and peer concerns are more prominent. Moffitt's (1993) taxonomy of youth offending is also helpful in understanding how development impacts upon offending risk. It can also help with the selection of treatment strategies (Ogden and Hagen 2014). Individuals who demonstrate concerning behaviour from a young age tend to have a number of neurological, cognitive and behavioural risk concerns (such as poor impulse control, impaired problem-solving skills). These concerns are evident in a range of settings and can contribute to life-course persistent offending. In contrast, these deficits tend not to be seen in young people whose offending behaviour only emerges during adolescence. For such individuals, social and community risk factors appear more pertinent (Moffitt 2006).

Clinical concerns

This section relates to behavioural, cognitive or psychological aspects of a young person's functioning (such as mental health or intellectual disability (ID)). It is essential that clinicians consider the ways in which these may be revealed throughout the assessment and intervention process. Concerns do not need to be directly related to the offence behaviour in order to be clinically relevant.

Many young people who have engaged in violent behaviour have come from difficult and challenging backgrounds (Geldard and Geldard 2009). If they had no opportunity to develop a secure and safe relationship with a primary caregiver, they may have developed unhelpful relationships patterns. As such, they may feel fearful or anxious of rejection, or be dismissive or overly attached to others. For other individuals, their early experiences, such as being abused or witnessing domestic violence, community or war-related violence, may result in post-traumatic effects. They may persistently re-experience the event, and have recurrent memories, flashbacks or nightmares. External or internal cues to the traumatic experience (such as noises, smells or internal states) may trigger distressing memories. As a result, in an attempt to manage their anxiety they may avoid discussing, or encountering, stimuli which remind them of the trauma. When this includes failing to discuss their own violent actions, or the potential reactions of their victims, this can be mistaken for lack of empathy or disengagement. Therefore, it is useful to have a series of working hypotheses about ways in which clinical concerns may impact on assessment and intervention, and the associated elements within these constructs (such as the therapeutic relationship).

Quality of therapeutic relationship

A good therapeutic relationship is associated with a successful assessment and intervention outcome (Martin, Garske and Davis 2000). Duncan and colleagues show that the best therapeutic results are obtained when there is a high degree of trust between the clinician and client, and that both have a sense of hopefulness and optimism for the future. Problematic behaviour does not go unchallenged; clear consistent feedback is provided. But it is the behaviour that is disapproved of – not the client. The clinician should show empathy and genuinely try to understand the client. The client should be engaged in the assessment process, and feel listened to and accepted by the clinician. Both the clinician and client are active partners within the therapeutic process (Duncan et al. 2010).

However, there are a number of challenges to achieving such a relationship. These may relate to system variables (time pressures, imposed deadlines), clinician attributes (inexperience, lack of training, orientation), client variables or interactions between these. For example, the nature of adolescence, and the background characteristics and the behaviour of many young people who are violent, means that developing good therapeutic relationships can be particularly challenging. Negative experience of prior relationships can result in a distrust of others, and this reaction may be particularly common in young people who have experience of multiple transitions (in terms of location, caregivers and attachment figures). The nature of some of the violent acts the young person has committed may create difficulties for the practitioner in terms of the feeling elicited or the distress created. Consideration of how these and other elements within FAIV (such as developmental or clinical concerns) could impact upon the therapeutic relationship allows for potential strategies, to avoid or manage strain within assessment and intervention, to be developed. It also allows for the role of clinical supervision, professional development staff support and training to be explicitly considered and facilitated (Rose 2014)

Stability

Stability has been identified as a key concern when working with young people (Bailey 2002). Young people physically, emotionally and cognitively change, even when other factors in their lives remain constant. However, there are a myriad of factors within a young person's life which reduce consistency. For example, attempts by the school system to manage concerns means that relationships with teachers, peers and even the school may change. Relationships within the home may form and break. Parental relationships improve or deteriorate. Within secure forensic settings, peer groups, staff and procedures may vary, either as part of a planned change or as a reflection of unexpected circumstances. Such volatility needs to be considered within work with young people (Viljoen, Elkovitch and Ullman 2008).

Risk factors for violence: A social-ecological perspective

The causes of juvenile violence are multifaceted, complex and non-linear in nature (Borum and Verhaagen 2006); the literature is replete with lists of these concerns. An unintended side effect of this is that attention has tended to focus on the presence or absence of factors – not the mutually interactive nature of these concerns. In addition, these lists tend to refer to only one form of violence (e.g. general violence, sexual violence or dating violence). In part, this reflects definitional issues, but it also reflects the lack of integration between specialists working in different areas of concern. Finally, whilst many texts refer to the different levels at which the risk factors operate, few juvenile violence risk assessment texts present risk factors within an ecological framework (Bronfenbrenner 1979).

The social-ecological model is a key element of the FAIV. This model proposes that risk factors operate at different levels (Dahlberg and Krug 2002). *Social*-level variables reflect risks within the wider sociocultural environment (e.g. cultural and legal aspects), which contribute towards violence being seen as acceptable. *Community*-level variables encourage violent behaviour in settings in which social relationships are embedded (e.g. neighbourhood, school). *Relationship*-level risk variables characterise interpersonal relationship factors associated with increased risk of violence perpetration or victimisation. The final level, *individual*, encompasses biological, cognitive, psychological and personal history risk factors associated with violence. All of these risk domains are interconnected and nested within each other. Therefore, individual factors reflect and are affected by relationship concerns, which relate to community concerns and so on.

The social-ecological model is frequently discussed within literature relating to the prevention of youth violence. However, this focus has not generally extended to risk assessment texts (although please see Viljoen et al. 2014 for further discussion). There a number of reasons to place a social-ecological model at the centre of violence assessment and intervention:

- It provides a structure to conduct a comprehensive and holistic assessment. Looking at structural factors and pressures ensures that the young person's behaviour is not considered in isolation from their surroundings (Rich 2011).
- It encourages the clinician to look for a range of triggers and potential sources of risk factors, enabling the consideration of wider intervention plans and prevention strategies.
- It helps emphasise the interconnectedness of the risk concerns. This can highlight primary foci for intervention. For example, a history of trauma can result in neurological effects which can contribute to impulsiveness, substance misuse (SM) (as a form of self-soothing) and difficulties with applying intervention strategies that involve accessing the frontal cortex.

Figure 7.2 illustrates a social-ecological model of risk concerns associated with a range of violent acts by young people. It is not intended to be prescriptive or exhaustive. Not all risk concerns will relevant to each individual in each setting. Clinicians may need to consider additional variables (such as those explicitly relevant to culture, offence type or setting), especially as new research becomes

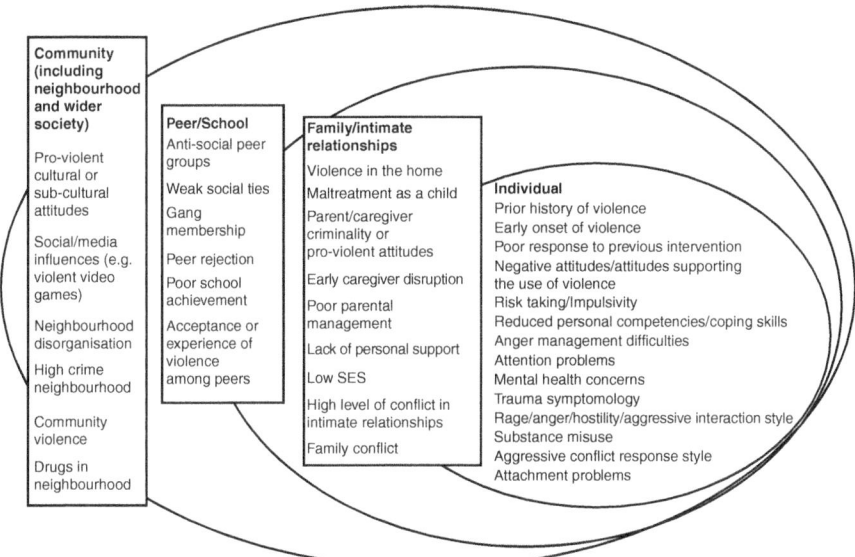

Figure 7.2 Social-ecological model of youth violence
Sources: Babic 2004; Bourm, Bartel and Forth 2006; Rich 2011; Leem et al. 2013; Office of the Surgeon General et al. 2001; van De Mere and Dawes 2007.

available. However, the list does reflect concerns highlighted by the literature (including the Structured Assessment of Violence Risk in Youth (SAVRY; Borum, Bartel and Forth 2006)) in relation to violence in a range of settings (community, home and institutions), victims (authority figures, peers, dating partners, strangers) and within different jurisdictions (e.g. the United States, Europe, UK). In line with other conceptualisations of youth violence (e.g. Williams et al. 2007), societal and community factors have been combined, and relationships outside of the family have been identified as presenting distinct risk concerns from those within the family.

Assessment, formulation and intervention

Within the FAIV, assessment, formulation and intervention are conceptually and practically linked. Whilst clinicians may be called upon to conduct just one element, each informs and is informed by the other aspects. The FAIV does not specify how to conduct assessments or formulations, or what interventions to apply. Rather, it highlights aspects and core principles significant to working with young people with a history of violence.

Assessment of violence risk

Within the FAIV, risk assessment is more than a list of concerns derived from the social-ecological model or a qualitative judgement of risk (high, medium, low). It is a complex, intellectually demanding and challenging task; a process that requires answers to the following type of questions:

- What is the function of the violent behaviour?
- What are the factors that have a causal link to the violent behaviour?
- How are the risk factors linked to each other?
- Under what circumstances is the violent behaviour likely to be repeated? When is risk likely to be reduced?
- How will affecting the risk factors change risk of violence?
- What risk factors are amenable to change at this current time? How might this situation change?
- How long will the assessment be valid for? Under what circumstances will it need to be reviewed?

Providing answers to these questions is challenging within any client group. However, with young people there are a number of additional contextual, ethical and scientific issues that need consideration.

Violence risk concerns. The identification of risk factors is only part of the process of risk assessment. The absence or presence of any particular risk factor is not as significant as its meaning or relevance. The social-ecological model helps the assessor see how risk factors are linked and how changes at one level affect other risk variables. For example, a new school placement or community location may serve to ameliorate relationship or family risk concerns. However, moving from one community to another may result in clients feeling aggrieved, lonely, hostile and fearful (increasing individual risk concerns). Situational factors are highly relevant to a young person's willingness to engage in risk behaviour, how they feel it will be perceived by others and their ability to control their actions (Baker and Kelly 2011). Therefore, the final assessment and treatment plan should actuate under what situations potential for risk is most likely to increase and under what circumstances risk will be reduced.

Who is at risk? Different risk concerns may relate to different potential victims. Factors that contribute to violence towards peers or strangers may be different to those related to violence towards parents, siblings or dating partners. Hence, when conducting a risk assessment all potential victim types should be incorporated into a management plan (Bailey 2002). In particular, violence against parents and siblings should be explicitly considered. Such violence has generally been less focused upon by both the scientific and empirical literature (Routt and Anderson 2011). Whilst precise prevalence figures for parental and sibling violence are difficult to come by, there is a growing body of work that suggests that such violence is frequent and clinically significant.

It is also infrequently recognised by agencies operating within the youth justice system (YJS) (Tew and Nixon 2010; Holt 2013).

Which risk assessment technique? Over the last 30 years, the science of risk assessment has expanded considerably. As a result, the clinician is presented with an array of risk assessment tools and opinions about which is the 'best' approach. The Risk Management Authority (RMA) of Scotland has an excellent Risk Assessment Tools Evaluation Directory (RATED-3), which provides a detailed breakdown of different assessment tools. The focus on the applicability to UK, as well as international populations, is particularly helpful.

However, even with this information available, the clinician will need to decide which assessment approach is best for each individual case. In coming to this decision, the scientific properties of the assessment technique (reliability and validity), and legal requirements, need to be evaluated and balanced against practicality. A number and range of assessment approaches can be deemed defensible when they reflect the different needs of a particular case, and are based upon an appropriate skill and knowledge base (Kemshall and Wilkinson 2011; Skeem and Monahan 2011; Chapter 5, this volume).

Informants. When working with young people, informants can provide access to data not otherwise available. For example, there may be relevant information the young person does not know or which, because of their developmental stage, they have been unable to correctly interpret (Cunningham and Baker 2004). Additionally, the young person may be unwilling to provide the information, may minimise their concerns or may exaggerate in an attempt to 'act tough' or to seek treatment (Rogers and Vitacco 2002).

However, careful consideration needs to be given as to who will be the best informant and what information is required of them (Herbert and Harper-Dorton 2002). For example, parents may be concerned about criticism of their parenting style. Mothers asked about their children's violent behaviour towards them have reported they feel that their parenting skills are being questioned (Tew and Nixon 2010). The use of historical documents and records can also be problematic. They may reflect a biased source of data (especially if they are based on subjective assessments) or reflect issues or concerns no longer current. They may reflect value-laden judgements and have the effect of stigmatising or labelling the young person (Hackett 2003). As a result, multiple sources of data should be accessed. Contradictions and differences in opinion should be noted, but treated with respect. It is also important to allow the young person to feel their voice is being heard – and that the opinions of others do not override their perspective.

Assessment-interfering behaviours. This refers to behaviours (from either the young person or the clinician) that derail the assessment process. For example, an emphasis by the clinician on the presence of risk concerns within the young person's life may result in an overly narrow focus. It can also result in the young person's voice and perceptions being marginalised (Baker and Kelly 2011). The young person themselves may have expectations of the process which serve to complicate the issue. The clinician will be judged not only on how they behave within the assessment process, but also on how other professionals have responded to the young person.

Other behaviours may relate to clinical concerns (as discussed earlier) interacting with the issues discussed within a violence risk assessment. For example, indicators such as apparent disinterest, lack of engagement or hostility, *may* serve to mask the extent of the psychological distress the young person is experiencing (Ardino 2011). Alternatively, subject matter discussion may result in the young person experiencing intrusive memories, thoughts or images (related to being a victim of violence, a perpetrator or both, Evans and Mezey 2007). Finally, trauma reactions during violent offences may mean that the young person genuinely does not have any memory of the event, and hence they are unable to provide a full account of their behaviour.

Formulation

Formulation lies at the heart of much psychological practice within forensic and mental health settings, and is a core competency of practitioner psychologists. It helps the clinician to organise complex and sometimes contradictory assessment information into a coherent explanation. It is a key element of the FAIV. A good formulation contains three main interlocking elements: an outline of the presenting concerns; hypothesised relationships between these concerns (which draw from psychological knowledge and theory); and links to the individual's difficulties. The formulation should act as an explicit link between assessment and intervention, and translate assessment information into a blueprint for intervention.

Theoretical orientation. Formulation should be based upon empirically supported theory relating to the presenting concern (Schwitzer and Rubin 2011). Ultimately, the specific theoretical perspective selected will reflect the clinician's training and personal theoretical orientation, as well as the specific nature of the case. However, because many pure approaches to conceptualisation were developed for use with adults, they often fail to incorporate the developmental issues or consider the range of variables that are significant in young people. Manassis (2014) suggests that, when formulating in relation to a young person, there is a need to integrate various disciplines and orientations – to adopt an eclectic approach. She proposes that only through adopting a range of perspectives (e.g. biological, psychological, cognitive, social) can the needs of individuals at different stages of development be incorporated. Many practitioner psychologists have background training in case formulation, and hence are well placed to assist practitioners to integrate multiple theoretical perspectives into complex formulations. Finally, the clinician needs to consider if any particular theoretical perspective focuses solely on the causes, aetiology and perpetuating factors that relate to client concerns. A significant difficulty with basing formulation on the problem, and not the entire individual, is that the client's strengths or areas of resilience are negated.

Individual or problem focus. Traditionally, in forensic settings, case formulation has focused on the presenting problem, negative behaviour or vulnerabilities (Kuyken, Padesky and Dudley 2008). However, recent models have called for the strengths of an individual to be incorporated. These may include specific behaviours or skills, interests or hobbies, beliefs, personal values, physical or mental abilities, character and emotional assets (Padesky, Kuyken and Dudley 2011; Manassis 2014). Through considering strengths (or protective factors) as well as risks, a more holistic and nuanced picture of the young person emerges (Viljoen et al. 2014). Factors that can reduce the likelihood of an adverse outcome are specifically focused upon. In turn, this allows for a greater range of interventions to be considered. The explicit consideration of strengths also allows for enhancement of the therapeutic relationship. Instead of the assessment focusing on what problems or concerns the client presents, the assessment can incorporate a more positive approach. It allows the client the opportunity to discuss aspects of their behaviour that are, or can be, prosocially reinforced. Focusing on strengths allows the clinician to feed back positive information to the client. This process is particularly beneficial for young people whose self-esteem is low or who are experiencing low mood; they may have not fully appreciated their strengths and positive aspects of their functioning. Even where this is not the case, the explicit inclusion of strength and resilience factors allows for the assessment to be more holistic in nature.

Formulation technique. Some theoretical approaches (such as cognitive behavioural therapy or cognitive analytical therapy) have clear structures and frameworks to support the formulation process. One model widely used is the four P's framework (predisposing, precipitating, perpetuating and protective; BPS 2011). This asks the clinician to articulate factors that contribute to, trigger and maintain the problematic behaviour, as well as those which may mitigate it. This approach has the advantage of being simple to use and understand. Whilst the four P's model can be applied to young people, it has not been explicitly designed for this purpose. An alternative is the approach outlined by Manassis (2014). This model has many similarities with the four P model; however, the differences may be helpful to the practitioner working with children and adolescents. It asks the clinician to consider both risk and protective factors within four main domains (biological, psychological, social and spiritual/cultural). As such, the social-ecological model can be explicitly considered and articulated. The development focus is evident in the differentiation across time periods (remote past, recent past, current). As with the four P's model, protective factors are considered, but this approach encourages clinicians to actively consider how protective factors operate within the different domains. This helps to identify potential areas of strength which may otherwise be overlooked, and avoids emphasising risk factors over protective factors (Manassis 2014).

Collaboration. It is important that formulation is a collaborative process. However, there are particular challenges in achieving this when working with children and adolescents, and particularly those who have engaged in violent behaviour. For example, young people find it hard to disagree with, or amend, formulations that are presented to them (BPS 2011). Where the clinician takes an 'expert' position and formulates about, rather than with, the young person, they can feel disengaged, disempowered, overwhelmed or upset (BPS 2011). To avoid this, the clinician should attempt to work alongside the young person and engage them in the process. Using the young person's own words, metaphors, mental images and constructs is helpful (Padesky, Kuyken and Dudley 2011), and enables the clinician to explicitly and implicitly consider cultural and spiritual considerations (Manassis 2014). These processes enable the young person to be an active participant in the process. It allows for the formulation to include the personal meaning of events and counteracts the tendency to produce a 'list of factors'. Furthermore, because it will be more easily comprehended by the young person, it facilitates the presentation of the formulation.

Communicating the formulation and recommendations. Sharing the formulation with others (including the client, family members and those that work with them) is an important aspect of any intervention plan (BPS 2011). It can help the young person themselves, their parents/carers and other staff understand the violent behaviours, the triggers and the impact the violence has on others. However, deciding what to share, and when, is particularly important with young people (Manassis 2014). When the formulation is first developed the young person may not yet have the psychological or cognitive skills required to understand the entire model. Hence, there may be times when a simpler version of the same conceptualisation will be required. As the young person develops, however, their ability to comprehend the issues will increase. Therefore, it is important to develop a model which could ultimately be shared with them. Likewise, it is useful to plan under what circumstances, when and in what manner this information will be shared. Factors that affect this decision include the stage of the therapeutic process, the client's level of insight and motivation, and the nature of the presenting concern (Padesky, Kuyken and Dudley 2010). Furthermore, the clinician may be called in to formulate with a team to help them with challenges they are experiencing when working with a young person. It may not be appropriate to share the results of this formulation with the young person directly. For example, the formulation may include staff team reactions or emotional responses to the client's behaviour. Under these circumstances, it is best to think of the formulation as part of a clinical supervision process, and treat the products in the same way as other supervision notes (BPS 2011).

Adaptations and changes. Formulation is best considered as a series of working hypothesis that can be adapted to incorporate new information (Manassis 2014). In some cases, this information might include elements not revealed to the practitioner until they were trusted (Winters, Hanson and Stoyanova 2007). Other information may relate to new or emerging issues; many of the issues in relation to stability in assessment will apply to formulation. For example, a young person's circumstances, motivation and priorities may change. Sometimes this will result in a refocusing of the model (elements which were present but not central before take on a new prominence). In other cases, it may be that new concerns emerge (e.g. a change of school location), which need to be included within the conceptualisation. Finally, developmental theories suggest that change in young people's lives reflects entirely normative processes. For example, family life models suggest that, as children age, families go through a number of transitions. These present challenges to both parents and children, and have the potential to increase stress within the family and the individual members (Golijani-Moghaddam 2014). Thus, it is good practice to regularly review the formulation to make sure it is still useful and relevant. Where changes are made this should be recorded, so that the formulation and reflection process is clear and transparent to all.

Intervention

FAIV proposes that client variables, assessment and formulation all contribute to the selection of an intervention strategy and prioritisation of interventions. However, the flow of this information should be bidirectional; the young person's reactions to treatment should also inform the other elements of the FAIV. Reactions and responses to interventions provide information which itself informs the clinician about the appropriateness of the assessment and formulation – this, in turn, can suggest alternative intervention strategies. Intervention should be informed by the formulation and the relevant evidence base or theory. In some cases, the supporting literature base may relate to the development of strengths (such as an improvement in socialisation skills, or prosocial recreational activities). In other instances, the relevant literature base may specifically relate to targeting violence concerns.

Over the years, a substantial evidence base has emerged in relation to interventions for young people who are violent (Guerra et al. 2008; Borduin, Dopp and Taylor 2013; Koehler et al. 2013). The blueprints programmes provide current details of evidence-based interventions (see http://www.blueprintsprograms.com). Whilst the precise focus and mechanism of delivery varies, effective interventions reflect the following features (Reid and Eddy 2002; Matjasko et al. 2012; Borduin, Dopp and Taylor 2013):

- They address known risk factors (both individual and systemic).
- They are rehabilitative (not punitive) in orientation.
- They include behavioural approaches within the environment in which the young person is based.
- They are well structured and defined.
- They support practitioners.
- They are developmentally informed to ensure that they meet the needs of young people (e.g. cognitive behaviour therapy (CBT) interventions have better results with older children; Reynolds et al. 2012).

The availability of particular interventions may vary according to location, jurisdiction, policy and resources. However, there are other important considerations (identified by the literature and incorporated into FAIV) which are central to intervention selection.

Systemic or individually-focused approaches. Matjasko and colleagues (2102) found that programmes that include the family had larger effect sizes (which suggests greater success) in reducing violence perpetrated by young people than programmes that did not. Likewise, the programmes that Borduin, Dopp and Taylor (2013) identified as most effective: multi-systemic therapy (MST; Borduin and Henggeler 1990); multidimensional treatment foster care (MTFC; Chamberlain 1990) and functional family therapy (FFT; Alexander and Parsons 1973) are systemic in nature. They do not focus on the individual in isolation, ignoring their environment. However, Kazdin (2011) notes that, in his clinical practice (working with severely aggressive and antisocial children), parents were not always available to engage in treatment; either because of their own clinical concerns such as mental health, or because of a lack of motivation. Strategies to address these parental concerns will differ across jurisdictions and settings. In some contexts, it may be possible to co-ordinate support for family members in line with that offered to the young person. In some cases, the difficulties the family face may be overwhelming for the young person and treatment may be best provided on an individual basis. As Rich (2011) notes, when working with a family, the focus must necessarily shift to towards family functioning and not that of the individual client. Therefore, in some cases the clinician may feel that the best intervention outcome will be served by an individually focused treatment that considers system-wide variables.

Risk management or risk reduction. When considering intervention goals, it is useful to be clear about the distinction between risk reduction and risk management. Risk reduction refers to interventions that serve to inherently reduce the level of concern a young person presents. For example, following intervention, the young person may have improved problem-solving skills or emotional management. As a result, they are less likely to react in a violent manner when they encounter high-risk situations. Ultimately, all interventions should work towards this goal. However, for reasons of capacity, motivation or insight, situational factors may have to be managed to prevent the young person encountering risk factors (risk management). The balance of risk management and risk reduction strategies needs careful consideration. Whilst the young person is learning new skills, or developing strengths, it will be helpful to mitigate them encountering risk situations. However, the ultimate goal is for the young person to learn to manage, or avoid, these triggers themselves. The notion of therapeutic (or positive) risk taking is a useful notion to consider under these circumstances. Where an individual is allowed to make decisions, which involves an element of calculated risk, they can learn from their experiences (both positive and negative). Where such an approach is applied within systems that recognise the value of therapeutic risk taking (Doyle and Dolan 2008) the benefits can be significant.

Treatment-interfering behaviours. Behaviours on the part of the clinician or client, which serve to interfere with treatment processes, have much in common with assessment-interfering behaviours. Some issues may reflect clinical concerns outlined at the beginning of the model. For example, experience of depression, anxiety and trauma, impact upon attentional skills and memory process (Pechtel and Pizzagalli 2011). These, in turn, may impact upon the individual's ability to engage in treatment. In other instances, treatment-interfering behaviours may relate to the young person's interpersonal style (such as being excessively demanding) or their motivational state (e.g. lack of engagement). Sometimes, addressing such behaviours may be a treatment target in itself. In other cases, the intervention provider may inadvertently trigger disruptive behaviour from the participant (e.g. through insensitivity, or failing to consider responsivity or cultural issues, Brodsky and Stanley 2013). In other instances, the treatment-interfering behaviours may reflect changes in the young person themselves. For example, a response to a change in their environment or anxiety about undertaking new behaviours. Treatment-interfering behaviours can be difficult to manage. However, the integrated nature of the FAIV will assist the practitioner to meet these challenges. For example, identification of *client variables*, will allow the clinician to predict, understand and plan for any issues that may arise. Establishment of a good *therapeutic relationship* will allow for an open discussion of these difficulties. *Supervision* and attention to clinician well-being (the foundation element of FAIV) will help the practitioner cope with the challenges that they meet.

Common factors in the therapeutic process. The phrase 'common factors' in therapy refers to a cluster of therapist–client variables which have a significant influence on therapy outcome (Lambert 2005). Literature from a range of psychological interventions shows that a good therapeutic relationship, empathy, positive expectancy and hope contribute to the success of interventions (Rich 2011). However, the central importance of this construct is sometimes overlooked in practice. Within youth offending services (YOSs), some treatments have been shown to have worse outcomes than no treatment at all (Matjasko et al. 2012). As a result, in some settings, there has been a drift towards focusing on 'what' needs to be delivered, at the cost of focusing on the interpersonal variables of treatment (Rich 2011). It is important to deliver *evidence-informed* treatment to young people in a way that is appealing to them (Geldard 2009) and responsive to their individual learning styles, personal needs and culture (Andrews and Bonta 2007). Contributing towards this process is an acceptance of diversity and difference; a recognition that there will be differences in how treatment is adopted and utilised by young people. Failure to place this at the heart of treatment selection and delivery will reduce the impact of any intervention (Geldard 2009).

Practitioner skills and well-being

In the plethora of advice about what to do with young people who have offended, how to assess them and what treatment strategies are best, it is easy to overlook the activities that the clinician needs to engage in to keep themselves healthy and appropriately grounded (see, for example, Rich 2011; Manassis 2014). It is this area that forms the foundation of the FAIV.

Monitoring, evaluating and adapting

Lack of stability, pace and rate of change when working with young people has been a key feature of much of what has been discussed in this chapter. Working with young people is often far from a smooth path. Developing perspective about this is helpful in assisting the practitioner to maintain a positive focus. The following strategies may be helpful to achieve this.

It is normal to experience setbacks. This should not reflect negatively on the young person or the clinician. It is the response to such 'detours in treatment' that is significant. It is useful to be prepared for 'one step forward and one step back'. However, it might be more useful to think of adolescents taking side roads. They may lose time in treatment (in that they do not take the most direct route), but they do not lose ground. Instead, they undertake their own route, learning as much from the routes that they did not find helpful, as the ones they did. Adolescence is a time of change, of trying to make your own way, of establishing independence from authority figures – this process will be reflected within intervention and within the relationship between the young person and the clinician. Not only is this normal, it is also healthy (Rich 2011).

Remember that there is more than one solution to any particular problem (Manassis 2014). When working with a young person, you are developing a set of working hypotheses. As such, it is appropriate to make changes and develop assessment and intervention strategies in line with new information. The ability to amend and change hypotheses as appropriate (i.e. after careful consideration and reflection) is a sign of clinical confidence. It should not be seen as an indication of a lack of clinical ability to get the answer 'right' in the first place.

Be realistic in what you expect. Whilst a key component of the therapeutic relationship is optimism, it is important to be realistic in what you are expecting of yourself and the young person. Sometimes apparently small changes can be clinically significant.

Remember, systemic variables will have a significant impact on the young person. The social-ecological is a key element of the FAIV. It is easy to lose sight of the impact of this once the assessment has been completed and the intervention plan agreed. Young people's reactions will reflect what is going on in their life. When they are experiencing a feeling of chaos they may well transfer that feeling to others. Knowledge of psychodynamic constructs of projection, transference and counter-transference will help the clinician recognise and understand these dynamics (even when they do not work within a psychodynamic paradigm) (Rich 2011).

Be creative in your interventions. Any intervention approach should be determined by the individual's formulation and other relevant evidence-based practice concerns. However, within these restraints it is useful to think about how learning objectives could be achieved in different and creative ways. For example, what could be achieved by using the strengths an individual has, or by focusing on the key points that are significant to them (Geldard 2009). The Good Lives Model (GLM) (Ward 2002) offers a useful new perspective on how to engage individuals within a strength-based focus. This approach allows for a range of intervention activities, in relation to the needs identified as relevant.

Clinical supervision

Working with young people who have committed violent acts, who have multiple problems and difficulties, who have experienced trauma and who demonstrate challenging behaviour is hard. Working with those who experienced trauma and have displayed violence can, at times, be traumatic itself. Regardless of level of experience, clinicians should not expect to undertake this work without access to support and clinical supervision. For example, if a young person feels unworthy of help they may accuse the clinician of disliking them, of patronising them or of being a 'fake'. Such challenges are difficult for clinicians to respond to unless they are aware of the underlying processes triggering the young person's behaviour. Supervision is a safe place to discuss such issues and to explore the relational dynamic between the young person and the clinician.

Supervision is essential, but the level of supervision and the format will depend upon the nature and type of work and the setting. In some cases, it may be appropriate that this is provided by more experienced clinicians. In other instances, it might usefully be provided by peers. Whilst the format may vary, the focus should remain the same, an opportunity to discuss and reflect upon cases and to receive direction or support as necessary (Rich 2011). This should be in a psychologically safe environment, where the clinician feels able to discuss situations that have not worked out as hoped.

Conclusion

There is a plethora of information relating to assessment and intervention with young people who have committed violent behaviour. Given the contrasting perspectives, the different foci and the strongly worded arguments within the literature, it is challenging for the clinician to identify, let alone manage, essential elements of this work. This chapter has presented a framework (FAIV) to assist practitioners achieve this goal when working with children and adolescents referred for violent behaviour. The FAIV does not advocate a single approach or solution to every case, but allows for incorporation of a variety of theoretical approaches. It recognises that each client–clinician interaction will have unique features, impossible to legislate for, and that settings, client and clinician variables will vary. When working with children and adolescents who have behaved violently there can be a tendency for the violent behaviour to become the sole focus of assessment and intervention work. The FAIV attempts to address this by suggesting that this focus is necessary but not sufficient – a holistic picture of the client, and the well-being of the clinician, are also essential elements of working with children and adolescents who have engaged in violent behaviour.

Notes

1. Where behaviour is of concern to others but the individual does not have the insight or ability to make choices about his/her actions, the clinician may prefer to refer to such actions as aggressive. Aggression can also refer to behaviours which are less harmful than those defined as violent (i.e. which cause discomfort but not fear or distress).
2. The interested reader is directed to Viljoen et al. (2014) for a discussion of assessment of multiple risk concerns.

References

Alexander, J. and Parsons, B. (1973) 'Short-term behavioral intervention with delinquent families: Impact on family process and recidivism', *Journal of Abnormal Psychology*, 81: 219–225.

Andrews, D.A. and Bonta, J. (2007) 'The risk-need-responsivity model of assessment and human service in prevention and corrections: Crime-prevention jurisprudence', *Canadian Journal of Criminology and Criminal Justice*, 49: 439–464.

Ardino, V. (2011) 'Post-Traumatic Stress in Antisocial Youth: A Multifaceted Reality', in V. Ardino (ed.), *Post-Traumatic Syndromes in Childhood and Adolescence: A Handbook of Research and Practice*. Chichester: Wiley-Blackwell, 211–230.

Bailey, S. (2002) 'Violent children: A framework for assessment', *Advances in Psychiatric Treatment*, 8: 97–106.

Baker, K. and Kelly, G. (2011) 'Risk Assessment and Young People', in H. Kemshall and B. Wilkinson (eds.), *Good Practice in Assessing Risk: Current Knowledge, Issues and Approaches*. London: Jessica Kingsley Publishers, 66–83.

Borduin, C.M. and Henggeler, S.W. (1990) 'A Multisystemic Approach to the Treatment of Serious Delinquent Behavior', in R.J. McMahon and R. DeV. Peters (eds.), *Behavior Disorders of Adolescence: Research, Intervention, and Policy in Clinical and School Settings*. New York: Plenum, 62–80.

Borduin, C.M., Dopp, A.R., and Taylor, E.K. (2013) 'Evidence-Based Interventions for Serious and Violent Juvenile Offenders', in L.A. Craig, L. Dixon and T.A. Gannon (eds.), *What Works in Offender Rehabilitation: An Evidence-Based Approach to Assessment and Treatment*. Oxford: John Wiley & Sons, Oxford, 192–210.

Borum, R. and Verhaagen, D.A. (2006) *Assessing and Managing Violence Risk in Juveniles*. New York: Guilford Press.

Borum, R., Bartel, P., and Forth, A. (2006) *Manual for the Structured Assessment of Violence Risk in Youth (SAVRY)*. Lutz, FL: PAR.

Bose, R. and Sattar, S. (2011) 'Culture and Child Development', in D. Skuse, H. Bruce, L. Dowdney, and D. Mrazek (eds.), *Child Psychology and Psychiatry: Frameworks for Practice*, 2nd edn. Chichester: Wiley-Blackwell, 13–17.

BPS (2011) *Good Practice Guidelines on the Use of Psychological Formulation*. British Psychological Society: Division of Clinical Psychology.

Brodsky, B.S. and Stanley, B. (2013) *The Dialectical Behavior Therapy Primer: How DBT Can Inform Clinical Practice*. Malden, MA: Wiley.

Bronfenbrenner, U. (1979) *The Ecology of Human Development*. Cambridge, MA: Harvard University Press.

Chamberlain, P. (1990) 'Comparative evaluation of specialized foster care for seriously delinquent youths: A first step', *Community Alternatives: International Journal of Family Care*, 2: 21–36.

Cunningham, A and Baker, L. (2004) *What About Me! Seeking to Understand a Child's View of Violence in the Family*. London: Centre for Children and Families in the Justice System.

Dahlberg, L.L. and Krug, E.G. (2002) 'Violence: A Global Public Health Problem', in E. Krug, L.L. Dahlberg, J.A. Mercy, A.B. Zwi, and R. Lozano (eds.), *World Report on Violence and Health*. Geneva: World Health Organization, 1–56.

David-Ferdon, C. and Simon T.R. (2014) *Preventing Youth Violence: Opportunities for Action*. Atlanta, GA: National Center for Injury Prevention and Control, Center for Disease Control and Prevention.

Dell, M.L. (2011) 'When Diagnosis is a Double-Edged Sword', *Virtual Mentor*, 13 (12): 856–860. Available at: http://virtualmentor.ama-assn.org/2011/12/ccas2-1112.html. Accessed on 01 May 2015.

Doyle, M. and Dolan, M. (2008) 'Understanding and Managing Risk', in K. Soothill, P. Rogers, and M. Dolan (eds.), *Handbook of Forensic Mental Health*. Collumpton: Willan, 244–266.

Duncan, B.L., Miller, S.D., Wampold, B.E., and Hubble, M.A. (2010) *The Heart and Soul of Change: Delivering What Works in Therapy*. Washington, DC: American Psychological Association.

Evans, C. and Mezey, G. (2007) 'The Nature of Memories of Violent Crime among Young Offenders', in S.Å. Christianson (ed.), *Offenders' Memories of Violent Crimes*. Chichester: John Wiley & Sons Ltd. 99–114.

Fonagy, P. (2003) 'Towards a developmental understanding of violence', *British Journal of Psychiatry*, 183: 190–192.

Geldard, K. (ed.) (2009) *Practical Interventions for Young People at Risk*. London: Sage.

Geldard, K. and Geldard, D. (2009) *Counselling Adolescents: The Proactive Approach for Young People*. London: Sage.

Golijani-Moghaddam, N. (2014) 'Applying family life cycle concepts in psychological practice with children and young people', *Applied Psychological Research Journal*, 1: 26–33.

Guerra, N.G., Williams, K.R., Tolan, P.H., and Modecki, K.L. (2008) 'Theoretical and Research Advances in Understanding the Causes of Juvenile Offending', in R.D. Hoge, N.G. Guerra, and P. Boxer (eds.), *Treating the Juvenile Offender*. New York: Guilford Press, 33–53.

Hackett, S. (2003) 'Evidence-Based Assessment: A Critical Evaluation', in M.C. Calder and S. Hackett (eds.), *Assessment in Child Care: Using and Developing Frameworks for Practice*. Lyme Regis: Russell House Publishing, 74–85.

Harland, K. (2011) 'Violent youth culture in Northern Ireland: Young men, violence, and the challenges of peacebuilding', *Youth & Society*, 43: 414–432.

Hart, H. and Rubia, K. (2012) 'Neuroimaging of child abuse: A critical review', *Frontiers in Human Neuroscience*, 6: 52.

Hazel, N. (2008) *Cross-National Comparison of Youth Justice*. London: Youth Justice Board.

Herbert, M. and Harper-Dorton, K.V. (2002) *Working with Children, Adolescents, and their Families*. Chicago, IL: Lyceum Books, Incorporated.

Hockenberry, S. and Puzzanchera, C. (2014) *Juvenile Court Statistics 2011*. Pittsburgh, PA: National Center for Juvenile Justice.

Holt, A. (2013) *Adolescent-to-Parent Abuse: Current Understandings in Research, Policy and Practice*. Bristol: Policy Press.

Howells, K., Daffern, M., and Day, A. (2008) 'Aggression and Violence', in K. Soothill, P. Rodgers, and M. Dolan (eds.), *Handbook of Forensic Mental Health*. Cullompton: Willan, 351–374.

Kazdin, A.E. (2011) 'Evidence-based treatment research: Advances, limitations, and next steps', *American Psychologist*, 66: 685.

Kemshall, H. and Wilkinson, B. (eds.) (2011) *Good Practice in Assessing Risk: Current Knowledge, Issues and Approaches*. London: Jessica Kingsley Publishers.

Koehler, J.A., Lösel, F., Akoensi, T.D., and Humphreys, D.K. (2013) 'A systematic review and meta-analysis on the effects of young offender treatment programs in Europe', *Journal of Experimental Criminology*, 9: 19–43.

Kuyken, W., Padesky, C.A., and Dudley, R. (2008) *Collaborative Case Conceptualization: Working Effectively with Clients in Cognitive-Behavioral Therapy*. New York: Guilford Press.

Lambert, M.J. (2005) 'Early response in psychotherapy: Further evidence for the importance of common factors rather than "placebo effects"', *Journal of Clinical Psychology*, 61: 855–869.

Leen, E., Sorbring, E., Mawer, M., Holdsworth, E., Helsing, B., and Bowen, E. (2013) 'Prevalence, dynamic risk factors and the efficacy of primary interventions for adolescent dating violence: An international review', *Aggression and Violent Behavior*, 18(1): 159–174.

Lefevre, M. (2010) *Communicating with Children and Young People: Making a Difference*. Bristol: Policy Press.

Manassis, K. (2014) *Case Formulation with Children and Adolescents*. New York: Guilford Publications.

Martin, D.J., Garske, J.P., and Davis, M.K. (2000) 'Relation of the therapeutic alliance with outcome and other variables: A meta-analytic review', *Journal of Consulting and Clinical Psychology*, 68: 438–450.

Matjasko, J.L., Vivolo-Kantor, A.M., Massetti, G.M., Holland, K.M., Holt, M.K., and Dela Cruz, J. (2012) 'A systematic meta-review of evaluations of youth violence prevention programs: Common and divergent findings from 25 years of meta-analyses and systematic reviews', *Aggression and Violent Behavior*, 17(6): 540–552.

Ministry of Justice (2014) *Youth Justice Statistics 2012/13 England and Wales: Youth Justice Board/Ministry of Justice Statistics Bulletin*. London: Ministry of Justice.

Moffitt, T.E. (1993) 'Adolescence-limited and life-course-persistent antisocial behavior: A developmental taxonomy', *Psychological Review*, 100: 674–701.

Moffitt, T.E. (2006) 'A Review of Research on the Taxonomy of Life-Course Persistent versus Adolescence-Limited Antisocial Behavior', in F.T. Cullen, J.P. Wright, and K.R. Blevins (eds.), *Taking Stock: The Status of Criminological Theory*. New Brunswick, NJ: Transaction Publishers, 277–311.

Muncie, J. (2008) 'The "punitive" turn in juvenile justice: Cultures of control and rights compliance in Western Europe and the USA', *Youth Justice*, 8: 107–121.

Nader, K. (2011) 'Evaluation and Diagnosis of PTSD in Children and Adolescents', in V. Ardino (ed.), *Post-Traumatic Syndromes in Childhood and Adolescence: A Handbook of Research and Practice*. Chichester: Wiley-Blackwell, 13–42.

Ogden, T. and Hagen, K.A. (2014) *Adolescent Mental Health: Prevention and Intervention*. Hove: Routledge.

Padesky, C.A., Kuyken, W., and Dudley, R. (2011) *Collaborative Case Conceptualization Rating Scale and Coding Manual. Version 5*. Available at: http://padesky.com/pdf_padesky/CCCRS_Coding_Manual_v5_web.pdf. Accessed 15 January 2015.

Pechtel, P. and Pizzagalli, D.A. (2011) 'Effects of early life stress on cognitive and affective function: An integrated review of human literature', *Psychopharmacology*, 214: 55–70.

Reid, J.B. and Eddy, J.M. (2002) 'Interventions for Antisocial Behavior: Overview', in J.B. Reid, G.R. Patterson, and J. Snyder (eds.), *Antisocial Behavior in Children and Adolescents*. Washington, DC: American Psychological Association, 195–201.

Reynolds, S., Wilson, C., Austin, J., and Hooper, L. (2012) 'Effects of psychotherapy for anxiety in children and adolescents: A meta-analytic review', *Clinical Psychology Review*, 32: 251–262.

Rich, P. (2011) *Understanding, Assessing and Rehabilitating Juvenile Sexual Offenders*. John New Jersey: Wiley & Sons.

Rogers, R. and Vitacco, M.J. (2002) 'Forensic Assessment of Malingering and Related Response Styles', in B. Van Dorsen (ed.), *Forensic Psychology: From Classroom to Courtroom*. New York: Springer, 83–104.

Rose, J. (2014). *Working with young people in secure accommodation: from chaos to culture (2nd ed)*. London: Routledge.

Routt, G. and Anderson, L. (2011) 'Adolescent violence towards parents', *Journal of Aggression, Maltreatment & Trauma*, 20: 1–19.

Schwitzer, A.M. and Rubin, L.C. (2011) *Diagnosis and Treatment Planning Skills: A Popular Culture Casebook Approach*. Los Angeles: Sage.

Seto, M.C. and Lalumiere, M.L. (2010) 'What is so special about male adolescent sexual offending? A review and test of explanations through meta-analysis', *Psychological Bulletin*, 136: 526–575.

Skeem, J.L. and Monahan, J. (2011) 'Current directions in violence risk assessment', *Current Directions in Psychological Science*, 20: 38–42.

Stader, D.L. (2011) 'Dating violence', *The Clearing House: A Journal of Educational Strategies, Issues and Ideas*, 84(4): 139–143.

Tew, J. and Nixon, J. (2010) 'Parent abuse: Opening up a discussion of a complex instance of family power relations', *Social Policy and Society*, 9: 579–589.

Tharinger, D.J., Gentry, L.B., and Finn, S.E. (2013) 'Therapeutic Assessment with Adolescents and their Parents: A Comprehensive Model', in D.H. Saklofske, V.L. Schwean, and C.R. Reynolds (eds.), *The Oxford Handbook of Child Psychological Assessment*. Oxford: Oxford University Press, 385–419.

Van der Kolk, B.A. (1989) 'The compulsion to repeat the trauma', *Psychiatric Clinics of North America*, 12: 389–411.

Van der Kolk, B.A. (2005) 'Developmental trauma disorder', *Psychiatric Annals*, 35: 401–408.

Viljoen, J.L., Elkovitch, N., and Ullman, D. (2008) 'Assessing Risk for Violence in Adolescents', in B. Jackson (ed.), *Learning Forensic Assessment*. New York: Routledge/Taylor & Francis, 385–416.

Viljoen, J.L., Nicholls, T.L., Cruise, K.R., Desmarais, S.L., and Webster, C.D. (with contributions from Beneteau-Douglas, J.) (2014) *Short-Term Assessment of Risk and Treatability: Adolescent Version (START:AV), User Guide*. Burnaby, BC: The Mental Health Law and Policy Institute, Simon Fraser University.

Ward, T. (2002) 'The management of risk and the design of good lives', *Australian Psychologist*, 37: 172–179.

Williams, K., Rivera, L., Neighbours, R., and Reznik, V. (2007). Youth violence prevention comes of age: Research, training, and future directions. Annual Review of Public Health, 28(195), 211.

Winters, N.C., Hanson, G., and Stoyanova, V. (2007) 'The case formulation in child and adolescent psychiatry', *Child and Adolescent Psychiatric Clinics of North America*, 16: 111–132.

8
Sexually Harmful Behaviour

Trudy Potter and Sarah Reeves

Introduction

The sexual activity of children can be hard to contemplate, let alone the notion that young people might engage in sexual acts that cause harm to others. Sexually harmful behaviour often takes place in secret, and may remain undetected and unreported. Positions of denial and minimisation of such behaviour in the public consciousness are hence understandable. However, when sexually harmful behaviour is discovered, it results in high levels of parental and professional anxiety, often associated with shame relating to the stigma attached to such behaviour, and fear about the future trajectory of the young person's life. These high levels of anxiety may permeate the other systems in which the young person lives. Professionals, however, need to react in ways that are measured and meaningful, responding to assessed levels of need, which then informs safety planning, subsequent intervention programmes and future life plans.

Workers in this area have struggled to find adequate models to make sense of such behaviour, alongside finding means to not only reduce reoffending, but also to support these young people to lead healthy, competent, social lives. Positive examples of successfully working with this client group are now emerging; juxtaposed with this is the awareness that work in this area continues to provoke strong feelings in the public mind, and presents a multitude of clinical, practical and systemic dilemmas.

This chapter will define what constitutes sexual offending in young people as well as what is considered sexually harmful behaviour. It will then go on to consider prevalence, including the complexities involved, such as underreporting. This is followed by an exploration of partnership working and its inherent dilemmas. The chapter then considers current research on the characteristics of this group of young people, and then discusses both international and national assessments and interventions. A composite case vignette, covering formulation and intervention, is presented. The chapter ends with a dialogue surrounding the complexities and dilemmas of working with this client group.

Terminology, definitions and prevalence

The National Children's Home (1992) introduced the issue of young people as perpetrators of abuse into the public domain, and opened possibilities, not only for professionals to share their anxieties, but also for discourses amongst professionals regarding how best to understand these young people and provide appropriate intervention. These professional debates were the impetus for policymakers to start to address significant unmet needs.

The definition of sexual abuse given in the document *Working Together* (HM Government 2013: 86) is abuse that:

> [I]nvolves forcing or enticing a child or young person to take part in sexual activities, not necessarily involving a high level of violence, whether or not the child is aware of what is happening. The activities may involve physical contact, including assault by penetration, (for example, rape or oral sex) or non-penetrative acts such as masturbation, kissing, rubbing and touching outside of clothing. They may also include non-contact activities such as involving children looking at, or in the production of, sexual images, watching sexual activities, encouraging children to behave in sexually inappropriate ways, or grooming a child in preparation for abuse.
>
> (including via the Internet)

However, there appears to be little consensus with respect to the appropriate terminology to describe young people who sexually abuse. UK policies include 'young people who display sexually harmful behaviour' (HM Government 2013) and 'young people who sexually abuse' (YJB 2008). Rich (2011) uses 'juvenile sexual offender', 'sexually abusive youth' and 'sexually troubled youth' interchangeably. It is not technically appropriate to use the term 'juvenile sexual offender' until the young person has been found guilty in a court of law (Ryan, Hunter and Murrie 2012). In this chapter we choose to use the term 'young people who display sexually harmful behaviour', as we believe that this separates the young person from their behaviour and promotes a whole-person focus. This term also recognises that harm has been done, without necessarily implying the intent to abuse.

Research in this area indicates that between a quarter and one-third of all childhood sexual abuse coming to the attention of authorities is perpetrated by adolescents (Lovell 2002; Erooga and Masson 2006; Finkelhor, Ormrod and Chaffin 2009; Radford et al. 2011). A study by Radford and colleagues (2011) found that two-thirds of contact sexual abuse (which includes physical touching) experienced by children aged 0 to 17 was perpetrated by someone aged under 18. Ten per cent of all offenders found guilty of sexual offences are aged under 18, with just under 32 per cent of all those cautioned also being below the age of 18 (YJB 2009). Langstrom (2001) suggests that the figures for adolescents who sexually harm, particularly females, are vastly underestimated, and many acts of sexual harm will not have gone through the court process or even been detected (Erooga and Masson 2006).

Most studies of adolescents who sexually harm indicate that the rates of sexual reoffending (5–14 per cent) are substantially lower than the rates for general offending (8–58 per cent) (Caldwell 2007; Zimring 2009). These discrepancies are possibly due to differences in definitions and length of follow-up. Research indicates that those who do reoffend tend to have significant histories of abuse, trauma or family dysfunction (Rich 2011).

Characteristics and risk factors

It is now increasingly accepted that adolescents who engage in sexually harmful behaviour are a heterogeneous population (Hackett 2007; Leversee 2007), who span a range of characteristics, including types of offending behaviours, extent of sexual knowledge, cognitive functioning, mental health issues, degree of social isolation and background experiences (Vizard, Monck and Misch 1995). In addition, the risk factors that have commonly been recognised when considering adult sexual offenders (e.g. deviant sexual arousal, lack of victim empathy) cannot easily be extrapolated to an adolescent population for a number of reasons. Firstly, there is a lack of clarity on what constitutes normal sexual development during adolescence (see Bancroft 2006). Secondly, adolescence is noted as a developmental stage where there is a high frequency of risk-related sexual behaviours (Henderson et al. 2002). In addition, applying adult models of sexual offending to a juvenile population fails to recognise the developmental needs and tasks of adolescence; in particular, both moral reasoning and the ability to empathise are skills that continue to change and develop throughout adolescence and into adulthood, and are affected by both neurodevelopment and puberty (e.g. Pfeifer et al. 2013).

There have been many attempts to describe subgroups of young people who display sexually harmful behaviour. Most studies, as noted by Worling (2001), have compared adolescents who offend against children with those who target peers or adults. However, a distinction that relies solely on victim age to indicate sexual abuse preference is problematic when considering adolescents, who are likely to exhibit fluidity in terms of sexual development and sexual preference. Worling (2001) suggested a personality-based typology, and, further to research with 112 male adolescent sexual offenders using the California Psychological Inventory (Gough 1987), described four personality-based subgroups. He noted no significant differences between the four groups in terms of victim age, gender or relationship. The four groups were as follows: (1) the 'antisocial/impulsive' subgroup showed high levels of delinquency and impulsivity (almost half of Worling's sample); (2) the 'unusual/isolated' group were described by Worling as being emotionally disturbed and insecure, with social isolation featuring strongly; (3) the 'overcontrolled/reserved' group were seen as emotionally overcontrolled, and shy and suspicious in social interactions; and (4) the 'confident/aggressive' group were depicted as being socially confident, and prone to interpersonal aggression. Of note is the fact that those in the first two groups were more likely to be charged with a subsequent criminal offence (sexual or otherwise).

Worling's (2001) study delineates two subgroups characterised by issues related to social and interpersonal difficulties; such young people may believe they are disliked or unlovable, fear they will be either rejected or humiliated by others and will never be able to establish friendships, and lack the social skills required to develop healthy relationships with peers. Indeed, Miner and Munns (2005) reported that juvenile sexual offenders feel more isolated from their peers than non-sexual juvenile offenders, and concluded that the inability to experience satisfaction in social relationships may be implicit in some adolescents turning to younger children to meet sexual and social needs.

Richardson and colleagues (2004) also described a personality-based taxonomy, using the Millon Adolescent Clinical Inventory (MACI; Millon, Millon and Davis 1993), and delineated five personality types, four of these being similar to the four groups delineated by Worling (2001): (1) a 'dysthymic/negativistic' group, characterised by oppositional traits and dysthymic mood, which they compared to Worling's 'antisocial/impulsive' group; (2) a 'dysthymic/inhibited' group, defined by social withdrawal and insecurity amongst peers, resembled Worling's 'unusual/isolated' group; (3) a 'submissive' group, characterised by subjugation of needs and dependence on others, matched Worling's 'overcontrolled/reserved' group; and (4) an 'antisocial' group, characterised by attempts to control and dominate others, corresponded to Worling's 'confident/aggressive' group. Notably, Richardson and colleagues (2004) found that 25 per cent of the sample obtained no clinically relevant scores on any of the personality scales. As in Worling's study, personality type did not correlate with the nature of the sexual offence.

Richardson (2007), in reviewing the literature on personality characteristics of adolescent sexual offenders, concluded that there is no evidence to support a personality subtype or profile of personality characteristics that is unique to adolescent young offenders. However, he proposed that there are two discernible groups of offenders: an antisocial group, who share characteristics associated with antisocial personality disorder and psychopathy; and an asocial group, characterised by interpersonal inadequacies and neurotic traits.

The relevance of personality disorder traits to offending behaviour is increasingly recognised in the literature (Frick et al. 2003), although research relating to the link between such traits and sexually abusive behaviour in adolescents is limited and inconclusive. Vizard, Hickey and McCrory (2007), studying a sample of 280 young people referred to a community treatment service, found that those with 'emerging severe personality disorder' were more likely to have abused multiple types of victims, and were more likely to engage in predatory sexual behaviour. Similarly, Lawing, Frick and Cruise (2010) found a relationship between self-report measures of callous and unemotional traits and characteristics of sexual crime (number of sexual offences, increased levels of violence and more planning with regard to sexual offences). A further study by Morrell and Burton (2014) aimed to assess how a variety of measures of psychopathy were related to characteristics of sexual offending in a sample of 191 incarcerated juvenile sexual offenders. In contrast with the findings of Lawing, Frick and Cruise (2010), only one measure, the Narcissism and Impulsivity Scale of the Antisocial Process Screening Device (Frick and Hare 2001), was significantly correlated to one particular characteristic of sexual crime: the number of victims. The majority of psychopathy scales were, however, related to non-sexual crime. Furthermore, a study by Gretton and colleagues (2001), using a sample of incarcerated juvenile sexual offenders, found that the presence of psychopathic personality disorder traits was not associated with sexual recidivism, but only with increased risk for violent and non-violent recidivism. This suggests that the trajectory for juvenile sexual offenders with such traits is more likely to be one of general offending behaviours, rather than just sexual offending.

In considering risk factors for the development of harmful sexual behaviour, prior sexual victimisation has been a consistent finding across the literature with regard to both adult (see, for example, Jespersen, Lalumiere and Michael 2009) and juvenile offenders (Burton 2008). In a review by Hackett and colleagues (2013) of 700 children referred to services for harmful sexual behaviour in the UK, there was clear evidence that 31 per cent had been sexually victimised in their childhoods, and strong professional suspicions of sexual victimisation in a further 19 per cent. Similar rates of sexual victimisation have been identified in earlier UK studies. For example, Dolan and colleagues (1996) found that 25 per cent of their sample had either a documented or self-reported history of sexual abuse. US studies have reported rates of between 40 per cent and 65 per cent (Becker, Cunningham-Rathner and Kaplan 1986; Worling 1995).

A further study by Ogloff and colleagues (2012) carried out a 45-year follow-up of victims of child sexual abuse: 5 per cent of male victims were subsequently convicted of a sexual offence, compared to 0.6 per cent in a control group. Furthermore, males who were victimised at age 12 or over were at even greater risk of committing a sexual offence. Sexual victimisation is hence a clear risk factor for sexual offending, particularly in males victimised during adolescence.

Veneziano and colleagues (2000) found that adolescent sexual offenders were more likely to repeat the behaviours they had experienced as victims, and that the characteristics of victims were more likely to be reflective of their own victim experiences. In each individual case, the mechanism by which this occurs may be different, and both social learning and classical conditioning theories have been put forward as explanatory models. Van der Kolk (1989) described the compulsion to re-enact, first studied by Sigmund Freud in 1914, which is common to trauma experiences, and refers to the seemingly unconscious need to revert to and repeat earlier situations, behaviour patterns and acts, even if such behaviours are experienced as unpleasant. This is a complicated psychological phenomenon, but if memories of traumatic experiences remain unprocessed and somatically stored (Van der Kolk, Burbridge and Suzuki 1997; Shapiro 2001), then sexual arousal is one aspect of this memory of sexual victimisation. This sexual arousal may then be unconsciously triggered by events in the present that are reminiscent of previous abuse experiences.

The study by Hackett and colleagues (2013) also found high rates of other abuse or trauma (i.e. physical or emotional abuse, neglect, parental rejection, family breakdown and conflict and domestic violence). In only 34 per cent of cases was there no known history of abuse or trauma (sexual or otherwise). Hunter, Figueredo and Malamuth (2010), found an association between exposure to violence and 'psychopathic and antagonistic attitudes', which have been shown to predict sexual recidivism in both juvenile and adult offenders. In addition, in line with research into the developmental trajectories which characterise general juvenile offenders, Hickey and colleagues (2013) found that those with early onset behaviour (i.e. onset of sexually abusive behaviour before the age of 11) were more likely than those with later onset behaviour to have experienced the following: inadequate family sexual boundaries, multiple forms of abuse, poorer parenting and insecure attachment. Those in the early onset group were also more likely to have abused a range of victims; Hickey and colleagues consider how early sexualisation, possibly through conditioning to diverse sexual stimuli, might explain this finding. This group was also characterised by a greater tendency to exhibit traits of emerging severe personality disorder (as measured by the Psychopathy Checklist: Youth Version (Forth, Kosson and Hare 2003)) and by higher rates of early onset of general antisocial behaviours.

It is hence not surprising, given this documented exposure to trauma, that much attention has recently focused on the relationship of attachment disruptions and disorders to harmful sexual behaviour, a topic which, historically, has received much attention in the adult sexual offender arena (see Rich 2006). Given that harmful sexual behaviour always occurs between two (or more) people, intuitively, attachment theory appears a relevant approach. In addition, the social isolation, social inadequacy and social anxiety reported by these young people (Miner and Munns 2005) may be linked to the hypothesised role of attachment in the development of self-agency and self-confidence. However, there is a lack of robust evidence to support attachment deficits as a primary cause of harmful sexual behaviour (Rich 2006); instead Rich proposes an attachment-informed model of harmful sexual behaviour which recognises attachment deficits as developmental vulnerabilities which impact on the developmental pathway, and which, when combined with other risk factors, may catalyse sexual aggression.

One of the hypothesised sequelae of secure attachment relationships is the development of empathy and, in turn, morality. Empathy is considered as a multistage process (Marshall et al. 1995), beginning with the ability to recognise emotional states in others, and then the ability to see situations from another's perspective. This is followed by emotional replication or the vicarious reproduction of the observed emotion, and then a decision on how to respond. A study by Varker and Devilly (2007) explored general empathy, general victim empathy and own victim empathy in a group of 16 adolescent sexual offenders. Compared to age-matched non-offending controls, the adolescent sexual offenders did not display general empathy deficits in terms of empathic concern and emotional distress, although they did show difficulties in perspective taking. In addition, they showed significant empathy deficits for their own sexual abuse victims compared to a general sexual abuse victim, a finding which has been replicated in other studies and is likely to have a self-serving effect (i.e. allowing the offender to overcome any emotional inhibitions that might otherwise be experienced). This is, however, a small study and it should be remembered that empathy is limited in all adolescents, and, as Rich (2006: 215) points out: 'if we think of empathy in adolescents in adult terms [...] we may indeed conclude that we are seeing callousness and unemotionality, rather than a developmental task in process'.

Exposure to pornography, another route towards sexualisation of young people, has also been considered as a risk factor, particularly in the presence of other risk factors, although, whether and how different risk factors might interact is uncertain. The ease of access to pornography has increased dramatically over the past ten years through access to the Internet. Wolak, Mitchell and Finkelhor (2007) found that 42 per cent of a sample of 10–17-year-olds had been exposed to pornography over the Internet in the prior year; college students reported even higher rates of exposure during adolescence (Sabina, Wolak and Finkelhor 2008). Research into the effect of pornography on young people is scarce; however, frequent use of internet pornography has been linked with more frequent thoughts about and a stronger interest in sex (Peter and Valkenburg 2008), as well as a propensity to view women as sex objects (Peter and Valkenburg 2009). There is also evidence for the role of social learning theory in influencing young people's sexual ideation, such that young people who watched pornography expressed a desire to try out the sexual positions they had viewed (Cowell and Smith 2009). In addition, exposure to such materials has also been related to a perceived social pressure to have sex (Bleakley, Henessy and Fishbein 2011).

In terms of a link between pornography and sexual offending, Burton, Leibowitz and Howard (2010) found that juvenile sexual offenders reported higher exposure to pornography before the age of 10 than non-sexual offenders. It is difficult to argue that exposure to pornography does not have an impact on sexual attitudes and beliefs. Furthermore, pornography, through exposing young people to a variety of sexual practices, increases awareness of sexual possibilities and heightens curiosity. Indeed, when pornography becomes a route to sexual gratification, not only might sexual gratification become conditioned to certain triggers (and it is highly plausible that the adolescent brain has more cortical vulnerability than the adult brain in this respect (Owens et al. 2012)), but, also, the notion of 'dating' a partner and spending time getting to know them without necessarily engaging in sexual activity may seem less attractive than the easier and quicker route to sexual gratification via watching pornography.

Further to this mounting evidence of the impact of pornography on young people's sexual behaviour and attitudes, a recent report from the Children's Commissioner (Horvath et al. 2013: 67) recommends that the:

> Youth Justice Board should include questions on exposure and access to pornography within the revised ASSET assessment tool, to better inform understanding of possible associations with attitudes and behaviour and improve the targeting of interventions for young people displaying violent, or sexually harmful behaviours.

With regard to the prevalence of harmful sexual behaviour perpetrated by females, the behaviour is often underreported and rarely prosecuted. In addition, there is a paucity of research in this area which adds to risk-averse decision-making. However, what research there is demonstrates that many females who sexually harm have been victims of sexual abuse themselves (Miccio-Fonseca 2000; McCartan et al. 2011). Masson and colleagues (2012) compared a sample of young males and females aged 8 to 16 referred to specialist services in England during the 1990s for their harmful sexual behaviour. Compared with the young men, young women tended to be referred at a younger age and had less criminal convictions at the point of referral. Females were more likely to have higher rates of historical sexual victimisation. They tended to have a lower number of victims, and were less likely to abuse their peers. Strickland (2008) suggests that the trauma of their own victimisation is pertinent in understanding the treatment needs of females who sexually harm.

In summary, understanding sexually harmful behaviour displayed by adolescents is complex and there is no single causal factor. It appears that it is a complex combination and interaction of multiple factors, which vary widely for each young person, and which culminate in young people engaging in sexually harmful behaviour. These factors include: a desire for social connection but lack of means to achieve this; the psychological and neuropsychological sequelae of trauma; exposure to sexual behaviour and imagery; and confusing societal sexual norms and values. We concur with Hackett (2007) that we must be careful to not demonise these young people, who share much in common with their non-offending peers. Above all we must remember that they are young people in need, showing the same anxieties and problems as other young people, and that issues of sexual offending need developmental and contextual understanding.

Partnership working and legal processes

Work with young people who display sexually harmful behaviour is carried out in a context of complex and confusing policies and legislation. In the document *Working Together* (DH 1999) it was first acknowledged that there was a need for agencies across child welfare and criminal justice in the UK to collaborate in the development of an operational framework, so that cases of young people who display sexually harmful behaviour can be assessed and managed effectively. Evidence from Hackett, Masson and Phillips (2005) suggested that the extent to which this guidance had been implemented was variable, and HM Inspectorate of Probation (2004) commented on the apparent lack of communication between youth offending teams (YOTs) and social services departments. Hackett, Masson and Phillips (2005) and Whittle, Bailey and Kurtz (2006) recommended the development of partnership working and the need for co-ordination of services for these young people, particularly focusing on the development of regional strategies and the appointment of lead local agencies.

However, a joint inspection across criminal justice services (HM Inspectorate of Probation 2013) continued to find a lack of comprehensive and co-ordinated multi-agency work. For instance, some of the cases they reviewed documented evidence of previous sexualised behaviour, which had not been addressed, possibly because the sexually harmful behaviour had been denied. Furthermore, some workers were reluctant to share information with education providers. The report makes recommendations to all agencies involved, and stresses the need for information to be shared in a timely manner, to inform comprehensive decision-making and to ensure delivery of interventions at the earliest stage possible.

Hence, to ensure that children receive appropriate responses tailored to individual need, there must be strong multidisciplinary partnerships supporting the child and their family from the beginning of any investigation through to its conclusion and beyond. All agencies must have a clear sense of their individual responsibilities, and an understanding of the underpinning child-focused legislation.

The United Kingdom is a signatory (1992) to the provisions of the UN Convention on the Rights of the Child. A child in this context means 'every human being below the age of 18 years, unless under the law applicable to the child, majority is attained earlier' (Article 1 of the Convention). In relation to work with children, Articles 19 and 37 are of particular note. Article 19 refers to the state taking all necessary steps to prevent and protect children from abuse and neglect, including sexual abuse, whilst Article 37 requires action to ensure the rights of the child are considered and protected in relation to the criminal justice system (CJS). Most importantly, in terms of working in this field, is the stated intention that imprisonment of children should only be used as a last resort.

Furthermore, responses should also fall within the guidelines disseminated by the Local Safeguarding Children's Board (LSCB), which dictates that safeguarding should be at the forefront of working with young people generally. All professionals should hence ensure that all practitioners working with, and on behalf of, children and families, take responsibility for ensuring everything possible is done to prevent the unnecessary escalation of issues or problems by seeking early intervention. Central to child welfare legislation is the Children Act (1989), which has a guiding principle that the welfare of the child is paramount. Sections 17 and 47 of the Children's Act are widely used when working with children with sexually harmful behaviour, as this ensures that a 'duty of care' is placed firmly with the local authority to promote the welfare of children.

Assessment

Professionals working with adolescents with sexually harmful behaviour are often asked to supplement treatment planning with a comprehensive assessment that makes some determination regarding future risk of sexual reoffending. Hanson (2000) noted that formal risk predictions for young people with sexually harmful behaviour are required for a number of reasons, including: sentencing, conditional release and decisions regarding family reunification. In general, three approaches to assessing risk are used: unstructured clinical judgement (UCJ); actuarial assessment and structured clinical judgement (see Chapter 5, this volume).

Professionals should guard against making unstructured clinical predictions, which largely rely on anecdotal experiences, much of which will be taken from the young person in interview. These predictions are notoriously open to challenge, as the conclusions are dependent on the level of training and professional competence of the person using the approach, and they are subject to professional bias.

Actuarial risk assessments (ARAs) use a structured and objective-rating system, providing a summation of scores linked to an overall risk level, correlated to a probabilistic assertion of future risk. They have structured procedures with precise instructions regarding variables to be considered. The Sex Offender Risk Appraisal Guide (Quinsey et al. 1998), Risk Matrix 2000 (Thornton et al. 2003) and the Rapid Risk Assessment for Sexual Recidivism (Hanson 1997) are three of a number of actuarial assessments validated for use with adult males. At this time there are no validated actuarial tools for use with adolescents who display sexually harmful behaviour; it is acknowledged that we cannot transfer our approach to assessing adult sexual offenders to young people, as this does not take account of the developmental aspect of their offending.

Structured clinical judgement combines actuarial and clinical methods (sometimes referred to as research-guided clinical judgement). Supporters advocate that this allows clinicians to integrate messages from research, and to be flexible in judgement, whilst using their experience to guide the process. Criticism of this approach argues that clinician bias and inconsistent administration is limiting (Hoge 2002).

The following presents a brief discussion of four promising risk assessment tools: Juvenile Sex Offender Assessment Protocol (J-SOAP-II), Estimate of Risk of Adolescent Sexual Offence Recidivism (ERASOR), Multiplex Empirically Guided Inventory of Ecological Aggregates for Assessing Sexually Abusive Adolescents and Children (MEGA) and Assessment, Intervention and Moving-On (AIM).

J-SOAP-II (Prentky and Righthand 2003) is a risk assessment tool for adolescent males aged 12–18 who have been prosecuted for sexual offences, or who are classed as having behaviour deemed to be sexually coercive. As with most of the approaches designed for young people, the model includes static (i.e. historical) and dynamic (i.e. potentially changeable, e.g. attitudes and beliefs) risk factors. The static factors are composed of two scales: the sexual drive/preoccupation scale and the impulsive/antisocial behaviour scale. The dynamic factors are also comprised of two scales: the intervention scale and the community stability scale. Fanniff and Letourneau (2012), in their review of J-SOAP-II, suggest that further evidence of its predictive properties is warranted. There are also no cut-off scores currently available for categories of risk.

ERASOR (Worling and Curven 2001) is an empirically guided approach to estimating risk of adolescent reoffending, for young people aged 12–18 years. Most items reflect dynamic risk factors, which can be targeted in treatment. The assessment provides a short-term estimate of risk (12 months), and could be potentially useful in assessing treatment needs and progress, but further cross-validation studies are needed (AIM Project 2012).

MEGA (Miccio-Fonseca 2009) is a developmentally sensitive, evidence-based, gender-specific risk assessment tool for assessing the level of risk of sexually abusive behaviours of male and female youth ages 4 to 19, including young people with low intellectual functioning. MEGA focuses on several domains, including: neuropsychological functioning, family history and dynamics, antisocial behaviours, and coercive and sexually abusive behaviours. This measure is designed for use every six months to monitor changes in risk. It is not widely used in the UK, largely because of the expense of the training, but it is used in Europe.

The AIM2 (Aim Project 2012) assessment is a 75-question 'clinically adjusted actuarial model' that takes empirically supported factors, but also incorporates other factors that are clinically supported by practitioners. The 2012 adaptation provides a universal model for use with females, black and Asian young men, and young people with intellectual difficulties, suggesting that practitioners should make use of interpreters and translating material, explore cultural and religious practices specific to the young person, and take account of the role of identity and ethnicity of the worker. The tool combines static and dynamic factors in four key domains: offence-specific factors, including offending history and the nature of the offence; developmental factors; family factors; and environmental factors. In each domain, strengths and concerns are explored, leading to a holistic assessment of the young person's risk, strengths, needs, capacity to change and the degree of support parents/carers can provide. The AIM model of assessment is the most commonly used model in the UK, supported by the youth offending service (YOS), the Ministry of Justice and social care.

It should be noted that it is difficult to assess risk accurately in a juvenile population, when not only are the risk factors being assessed subject to change during the developmental process (Hempel et al. 2013), but also personality itself may be expressed differently across the lifespan (Kernberg, Weiner and Bardenstein 2000). No psychological test can predict exactly how an individual will behave, particularly in the longer term (Prescott 2007).

Interventions

There is no standard intervention for young people who display sexually harmful behaviour, although the past 20 years has seen a growing recognition that interventions should be based on a developmental and contextual understanding of young people (Ryan 1999; Hackett 2007), rather than based on models of adult sexual offending. There is also increasing consensus that interventions should not just be offence specific, but should be holistic, focusing on the range of needs of the young person, with the aim of enabling the young person to become a confident healthy adult with a meaningful role in society. Furthermore, there is a growing recognition of the benefits of family involvement in this work with young people, the family playing a useful role in supporting, supervising and also challenging the young person, and hence playing a vital role in achieving sustainable outcomes (Ryan 1999; Johnson, Scott and Telford 2007).

Interventions should always be driven by individually tailored formulations. These formulations will necessarily be multifactorial, drawing on multiple areas of psychological theory to create hypotheses about the sexually harmful behaviour, its development, its triggers and its maintenance, as well as considering the protective factors and strengths within the system.

The following considers some promising models, and begins with a brief exploration of interventions outlined in the AIM manual. It then goes on to discuss the Good Lives Model (GLM), followed by an account of multi-systemic therapy – problem sexual behaviour (MST-PSB). The section ends with a description of restorative justice approaches, which may sit comfortably alongside any of the other intervention packages.

AIM

Following on from the AIM assessments detailed, the AIM interventions are holistic in nature and focused on demystifying the stigma in working with this population. The interventions are designed to address the concerns identified for the young person, the family and the wider community, including other professionals, for example, schools, youth groups and sporting clubs. Strong safeguarding plans are considered to be the starting point, and this begins at the point of first contact, particularly with young people who are engaged in the CJS. At point of referral, early intervention strategies should work to help reduce the risk of further allegations, support the young person, the family and any identified victim. This work can then be built upon in the intervention plan.

Interventions are practical, supportive and designed to be interactive for the young person, with lesson plans, homework tasks and review targets. The plan below is an example of an AIM 2 intervention:

1a. Induction: Old life – new life.

- An organising concept for the development of positive personal goals in therapeutic work.
- Identifying support strategies.
- Introduction of honesty line.

1b. Planning for change:

- Formulation of specific work goals and agreed areas of focus.
- Establishing order and priority of work.
- Construction of initial plan.

Topics include:

- Facing problems.
- Family.
- Relationships.
- Sexuality.
- Abusive behaviour.
- Other areas of difficulty.

2a. Healthy sexuality.
2b. Safe sexuality.
2c. What is abuse?
 3. Abusive behaviour:

- Fair and abusive continuum, explores specifically why the young person's behaviour was abusive.

 4. Steps to sexual abuse:

- Finkelhor's Four Preconditions Model; thoughts, feelings, behaviours.

 5. Exploring sexual interests:

- Application of Finkelhor's theory to personal experience/behaviour.

 6. The consequences of sexual abuse:

- Promotes an understanding of the potential practical and emotional consequences of further sexually abusive behaviour.
- Explores impact on family and victims.
- Cost-benefit analysis.

 7. Managing risk:

- Identifies personal risk factors.
- Develops strategies for management, support networks for management of risk of reabusing/reoffending.

 8. Communicating with others:

- Explores communication and relationships.

 9. Relationships with others:

- Communication, boundaries. Using the previous sessions to explore the impact of self upon relationships with others.
- Power within relationships – imbalance, control, safe relationships, harmful relationships.

10. Managing anger:

    - Cognitive behavioural therapy in application to anger.

11. Being assertive:

    - Exploring the difference between assertion and anger, looking at power imbalances.

The Good Lives Model (GLM)

The GLM of intervention (Ward and Marshall 2004) purports that intervention is most effective when young people learn to manage their risk of reoffending within the wider context of learning to live a better life. Collie and colleagues (2007) argue that the GLM incorporates risk management principles into a holistic and strengths-based approach.

The GLM views humans as goal-directed beings, whose actions seek to meet basic human needs, or 'primary human goods' (Ward 2002). Primary human goods are states of mind or being that are inherently beneficial or satisfying to humans, and are sought for their own sake rather than as a means to some other end. These primary goods, reclassified for young people as primary needs, include (Griffin and Price 2009; Wylie and Griffin 2013) being healthy, establishing a positive identity, gaining a sense of mastery and engaging in meaningful relationships.

In order to secure these primary goods or needs, individuals engage in a variety of activities, experiences and relationships, referred to as secondary goods. In order to attain the full range of primary needs in socially acceptable and personally satisfying ways, individuals require both the internal capacity (skills, knowledge, beliefs and values) and the appropriate external conditions (social support and opportunities). Individuals develop their own 'good life plan' that reflects their own strategies to achieve their desired goods.

The GLM suggests that individuals engaging in sexually harmful behaviour have difficulties in certain dimensions of their good life plan. For instance, they may lack the skills (e.g. through lack of social skills) or lack the opportunity (e.g. through being isolated) to meet their primary needs. They may also use socially unacceptable means to meet their needs (e.g. seek intimacy through abuse of children); sexually harmful behaviour is hence seen as an attempt to meet a primary human need, albeit in a destructive way. The aim of treatment is not to remove risk factors per se, but to equip individuals with the necessary psychological skills (internal factors) and social conditions to achieve their primary needs in socially acceptable ways. The model hence advocates that young people need to take chances and to have experiences, in line with their peer group.

The model can be used as a framework to identify what areas need to be targeted for change, and may rely on a range of models and interventions to achieve the objectives of treatment. However, further research is needed to demonstrate its efficacy (Wylie and Griffin 2013).

Multi-systemic therapy – problem sexual behaviour (MST-PSB)
MST is a treatment option that aims to assess and intervene with all of the relevant factors, within individual, family and community, that influence and drive sexually harmful behaviours (Borduin et al. 2003). It also aims to offer a holistic approach to treatment, considering the overall needs of the young person, with the aim of enabling the young person to establish a healthy identity, including achieving educationally and socially. The prime agent of change is viewed as the family, and hence caregivers are heavily involved in the intervention. Considerable emphasis is placed on building the parenting and communication skills of caregivers, such that they can address difficult issues with their child in a supportive manner, both during and subsequent to the intervention. Hence, in essence, it is a therapeutic approach that views the relationship between parents and child as crucial to achieving positive outcomes; and thus inevitably, but not explicitly, focuses on the attachment relationship between parents and child.

Two efficacy studies (Borduin et al. 1990; Borduin, Schaeffer and Heiblum 2009) and one effectiveness study (Letourneau et al. 2009) in the United States have demonstrated that recidivism is significantly reduced for young people who receive MST-PSB, compared with either individual therapy or treatment as usual (TAU) (group and/or individual therapy based on cognitive-behavioural premises). Interestingly, it seems that the positive impact of MST-PSB on the behaviour of young people is, in part, mediated by changes in caregiver discipline (Henggeler et al. 2009).

The MST intervention begins with establishing a risk reduction and safety plan, which includes the rules that the young person needs to abide by to reduce future risk. The responsibility for monitoring the plan, and delivering meaningful rewards and consequences to the young person, is placed with caregivers. This recognises that even though young people may hold good intentions to not commit further harmful sexual behaviour, their motivation will fluctuate. Risk reduction and safety planning must consider the needs of past and potential victims, as well as all family members, and must take into account the 'modus operandi' of the young offender. This can, in part, be ascertained from victim accounts and investigative reports, but can also be aided by the process of clarification (see the following paragraph). It is worth noting that, in our experience, most young people who engage in harmful sexual behaviour have not planned the event in any detail, at least considering their initial offence, and the offence is often viewed as impulsive. That being said, however, there must be a period, possibly very brief, during which young people overcome their inhibitions and give themselves permission to engage in such behaviour.

Assessing the multiple drivers to harmful sexual behaviour is achieved in a number of different ways: exploring the young person's sexual history, preferences and fantasies, including experience of abuse and access to pornography; exploring the family's sexual attitudes and behaviours (e.g. family rules about boundaries and privacy); and exploring in depth the offence profile, including what the young person was thinking and feeling prior to, during and after the offence (also known as clarification). Ideally, the majority of these 'clarification' conversations with the young person are led by the caregivers. As such, considerable time is spent preparing the caregivers, both in terms of improving their communication skills through modelling and role play, but also in exploring and working through their emotional reactions to what has happened. Common emotional response can include disgust, anger, shame and guilt. The intention is that caregivers will be able to hear whatever their child will disclose to them in a supportive and ultimately therapeutic manner. A containing relationship between caregiver and child is viewed as paramount to the success of the therapy.

Clarification itself has a number of purposes, which include having the young person acknowledge and take responsibility for the harmful sexual behaviour, as well as establishing the drivers to the behaviour, which will then contribute towards safety planning and risk reduction. Practitioners report that it is an incredibly emotive experience for everybody taking part; novice practitioners are usually very aware of their own trepidation in opening up this process, which is also shared by caregivers: our society in general is marked by strong reservations about discussing what is commonly seen as private (i.e. the whole range of sexual cognitions and impulses). However, in our experience, practitioners report that the process seems very cathartic, as if something, albeit intangible, is shifted by the very process itself; and possibly this is the letting go of some of the shame and guilt felt by young people when they expose the worst parts of themselves, but still realise that their family can be supportive and loving towards them.

Having established the drivers to the harmful sexual behaviour, evidence-informed approaches are used to target these drivers. Thus, distorted cognitions are challenged using the strategies of cognitive behaviour therapy (CBT) (see Westbrook, Kennerley and Kirk 2007 for an introduction); social isolation stemming from lack of social skills is managed by modelling, coaching and role play (Forman 1993). Techniques from structural and strategic family therapy (see, for example, Minuchin and Fishman 1981; Haley 1987) are also used as necessary to target subsystem boundaries, for instance, to promote both parental authority over the child as well appropriate levels of emotional connectedness. Weekly supervision on each case is essential to ensure both adherence to the model and also ethical therapeutic positioning, which is neither driven by the desire to punish nor by the urge to overprotect.

Restorative justice approaches

Restorative justice is both a way of thinking about crime and a process for responding to crime (Zehr 2002). The following is one of the many working definitions that have been developed. Restorative justice 'is a process to involve, to the extent possible, those who have a stake in a specific offence and to collectively identify and address harms, needs and obligations, in order to heal and put things as right as possible' (Zehr 2002: 37). Restorative processes bring those harmed by crime or conflict and those responsible for the harm into communication, enabling everyone affected by a particular incident to play a part in repairing the harm and finding a positive way forward. In criminal justice, restorative processes give victims the chance to tell offenders the real impact of their crime, and get answers to their questions and an apology. Restorative justice holds offenders to account for what they have done, helps them to understand the real impact of their behaviour, to take responsibility and to make amends.

Historically, restorative justice was developed from the family group conferencing (FGM) model used by Maori population of New Zealand (Zehr 2002). Adopted by professionals, and disseminated to Australia and the United Kingdom, the model has been generally used for those offences with a relatively minor sentence. The Youth Justice Board (YJB) for England and Wales has shown a strong commitment to restorative justice, including supporting the revision of the Victims' Code of Practice following the consultation by the Ministry of Justice entitled *Getting it Right for Victims and Witnesses* (Ministry of Justice 2012). This has set strategic targets at national and local level to ensure that practitioners adhere to the Restorative Justice Council (2011) principles – the ethical framework for restorative practice.

In the UK, the Criminal Justice Joint Inspection (2012) report, *Facing Up to Offending: The Use of Restorative Justice in the Criminal Justice System*, made specific reference to restorative justice and sexually harmful behaviour for the first time, recommending that each sexual offending case should be considered on a case-by-case basis. In many cases of sexual offending, restorative justice would be inappropriate because of concerns about the potential harmful impact upon the victim. Braithwaite (2002) also cautions about the need for appropriate standards in order to limit any reproduction of power relationships within restorative programmes, particularly within family group meetings. Other authors have highlighted the dangers of prescribing an apology from the perpetrator, since this would corrupt the nature and meaning of the apology (Jenkins 2006), and of inadvertently placing an expectation on the victim to forgive (James 2007).

This work clearly requires a high level of restorative skills in practitioners (Home Office 2004, 2011). In addition, this intervention should be guided by a multifaceted psychological formulation of the sexually harmful behaviour, not least to understand which factors might best be targeted and ameliorated as a prerequisite to the restorative justice process (e.g. power dynamics between victim and perpetrator, distorted cognitions and, particularly in cases of sexually harmful behaviour amongst siblings, the ability of the family to respond supportively to both children), but also to clarify the intended outcomes for the perpetrator (such as a better understanding of the impact on the victim and wider family system) and victim (e.g. feeling heard).

In the Australian context (Doig and Wallace 1999), the majority of cases involve victims who are already known to the perpetrator and whose paths are likely to cross in the future. In the UK, despite the growth in popularity of restorative justice, its use in cases of sexual and domestic violence remains controversial and views on its appropriateness polarises professionals (Daly 2008). However, Henniker and Mercer (2007), whilst highlighting both the potential benefits and downfalls of restorative justice to the victim, the perpetrator and the families, remain optimistic that the approach can balance the needs and rights of all concerned. Similarly, McNevin (2010) refers to the potential for intersubjective appreciations amongst family members, leading to increased openings for relationships to heal. However, there is a dearth of outcome research and the literature is mostly focused on individual case studies (Henniker and Mercer 2007; McNevin 2010). Further longitudinal research into the impact of restorative justice approaches on outcomes for young people who have sexually harmed, for the victims and for their families is clearly warranted.

Case study

The following presents a composite case study, detailing a case from first notification, through conviction and then on to subsequent intervention using MST-PSB. Inter-agency working is key throughout.

David is 15 years old and was arrested following an allegation of oral rape of his 6-year-old cousin, Amy. He lives at home with both parents, Reg and Sally, and a younger brother, Adam, who is 8. David has had no previous contact with the police. Academically, he functions at an average level. He has been provisionally offered an apprenticeship with a local electrical company, whose owners are friends of the family, when he turns 16. Both school and parents describe him as a bit of a loner; he has few hobbies, and spends much of his time at home either cooking or on the Internet. He is seen to be generally quite compliant with rules both at school and at home, but he has been involved in some fights at school, which he would justify by saying he was defending himself. He describes Louise, 13, who is Amy's older sister, as his best friend. He does not get on well with his brother, Adam, who has overheard many heated family conversations about the offence. Reg has a history of mild to moderate depression, which has fluctuated throughout his adult life; he has in the past received counselling and taken antidepressants. He works as a coach driver. Sally is a teaching assistant at the primary school attended by both her daughter and the victim. Sally was sexually abused as a child, although has not disclosed who the perpetrator is. The victim is Reg's brother's daughter. Reg and his brother, John, previously had a strong relationship, and the wives, Sally and Ann, had always been very good friends and grew up together.

David was initially referred to the Countywide Sexual Behaviour Service by the local police rape investigation team following his arrest. Due to the level of distress exhibited by the young man and concerns about the aggressive response towards him by his mother, the police officer in charge felt that it would be appropriate to initiate a dual response immediately, to both support the family, and to provide information regarding the ongoing investigation. The manager of the team was able to go out within two days to discuss how the investigation would proceed and to respond to questions from the family. This provided the parents and the young person with an understanding of the relevant legislation, and allowed the development of an appropriate safety plan. A safety plan was written up with support from the arresting officer, social care and the young person's school pastoral support officer; this safety plan was reviewed with the family and all relevant agencies on a monthly basis, to ensure safeguarding of David, the victim and their respective families. A Sexual Behaviour Service team member was also able to be present at all child protection meetings, and provided a conduit between the local authority, school and police, for instance, informing David about his bail conditions.

During the time the young person was on bail, the service was able to explore the family's attitude towards working post-court, to establish their levels of commitment and engagement, and to provide a working template of the services that could be offered to their son.

Following the entry of a guilty plea and prior to sentencing, David underwent an AIM-2 assessment, which would contribute to the pre-sentence report. It was not appropriate to carry out such a comprehensive assessment of the alleged behaviour until the police investigation had come to an end and David had submitted his plea, as the outcome of police investigations could have been compromised if the young person had been encouraged to discuss the offence, planning, motive or other mitigating factors prior to court disposal.

The AIM-2 assessment identified a 'medium' level of strengths within the system: both David and his family were positive about receiving help, and David himself had some clear goals for his own future. However, the family was historically very isolated, and were subject to community hostility as knowledge about David's offence leaked into the public arena. The AIM-2 assessment also recognised a high level of concerns: the highest concerns related in part to David's poor social skills (a dynamic risk factor), as evident from school and family reports, and in part to the hostility openly displayed by Sally towards David, subsequent to the offence (a further dynamic risk factor). There were also concerns in relation to David's apparent preoccupation with pornography, and his tendency to use pornography to cope with anger and frustration. Furthermore, the family frequently verbalised their anger towards the victim's family (stemming from entrenched patterns of mistrust and blaming of others) and David and his parents appeared to show little empathy for the victim. The high concerns/medium strengths indicated that David required intensive treatment, and had medium/high needs for supervision.

Parallel to this assessment process, a joint visit was arranged with the family by the YOT and the MST-PSB service manager. MST-PSB appeared the treatment of choice for a number of reasons: firstly, the parents were highly motivated to engage in the treatment process, and to be responsible for supervision and monitoring of David; secondly, the AIM-2 assessment had identified a number of dynamic risk factors in the family domain, which would clearly not be addressed if David were to receive individual work; and, lastly, David's social isolation was embedded within a family script of mistrust of others, which would be unlikely to shift without targeting the whole family system. The YOT produced a pre-sentence report, which included the findings of the AIM-2 assessment, as well as a recommendation to the judge that David and his family receive MST-PSB (alongside other possible courses of action) as a programme requirement of a Youth Rehabilitation Order (YRO – a generic community sentence for young offenders, which can include a number of requirements). This recommendation was followed by the judge.

Initial work with the family focused on establishing a robust safety plan to manage risk in home, school and community environments. Based on information obtained regarding the index offence, and on the outcome of the AIM-2 assessment, the practitioner worked with family and school to establish a set of rules, to be closely monitored by the adults, and with clear rewards and consequences. These rules initially were cautious, particularly because of high concerns in school about the risk David might pose to other pupils. However, it should be borne in mind that safety planning is a process, and that rules change over time, becoming more or less restrictive as new information comes to light. The rules were as follows:

1) David was not allowed unsupervised access with any female under the age of 13, and should remove himself from the situation should this arise.
2) David should not be allowed out unmonitored in the community, and parents were to know his whereabouts at all times.
3) David should not engage in play-fighting with Adam.

4) All family members should respect the privacy of others, lock bathroom doors and shut bedroom doors when getting dressed.

Although there was no evidence that David posed a risk to Adam, Sally and Reg agreed with the practitioner that rules 3 and 4 would, as well as protecting Adam, also protect David from any potential allegations made by Adam in the light of their difficult relationship.

The next step was to prepare the family for the process of clarification. Although all were persuaded of the many potential benefits of doing this, a major barrier to beginning this work was the fact that Sally's relationship with David had deteriorated significantly since his offence, and, as such, it was felt that carrying out clarification in such a hostile milieu would not be useful, and would likely deter David from opening up. Focusing on this relationship appeared to be one of the priorities. Individual sessions with Sally gave her the opportunity to acknowledge that she was disgusted with David for what he had done, and knew that he was experiencing her interactions to him as punishing. Further exploration revealed a number of drivers to Sally's emotional withdrawal and hostility towards David, including her belief that David deserved punishment and had not been sufficiently punished for what he had done, with an associated cognition that he had shown no remorse. Concomitantly, memories of her own abuse had resurfaced, along with anger that the perpetrator had never been brought to justice. In addition, her anger towards David was heightened by the extensive repercussions for the whole family following David's offence, which included the wedge that had been driven between her family and the victim's family as each tried to protect their own child, as well as Adam feeling ostracised by Amy and her family, which was evident as they attended the same school.

Whilst these repercussions for the family were not open to any timely resolution (although it would be hoped to address these issues later in the work), it was possible to intervene with some of the other drivers to Sally's anger, such as challenging Sally's ideas that David was not showing any remorse, and had not been punished. This was possible since the clinician knew that David had occasionally become distressed and been overwhelmed with shame about what he had done, although, as is often the case with young people, these moments appeared short-lived; he was also trying to make amends with his mother by attempting to be very helpful, attempts which Sally chose to dismiss. In relation to Sally's abuse, she was clear that she would not speak to the therapist about this and would not welcome any onward referral to adult mental health; however, she herself came to the conclusion that David was the target, to some extent, of the anger that she felt towards her own abuser. Sally agreed to work on this theme by writing unsent letters to her abuser. Having addressed these issues, the therapist was then able to gain Sally's alignment on responding to David in a more positive way, whilst also acknowledging Sally's position that she did not think she could forgive him. It should also be noted that Sally's relationship with David was a theme that was returned to throughout the course of MST-PSB involvement.

Sally and Reg agreed to work together in the process of clarification, and, aided by the therapist, identified a number of questions that they wanted to ask David to help clarify the sequence of his offence. They were particularly interested in whether David had planned the offence, or whether it was a more impulsive act. Having identified the questions, the parents experimented using them in role play, with the therapist role playing the part of David, hence teasing out any useful changes to the questions or the way in which they might be asked. This also allowed the parents to become, in part, desensitised to talking in a sexually explicit manner. David was understandably reluctant to engage in such a session, but Reg was gently able to explain to David why this conversation was so important, and to put in place an incentive (a takeaway meal in the evening). The preparation done with both Reg and Sally was pivotal in the clarification going well. The first session generated further questions, as often occurs, and hence further clarification sessions were also held.

Figure 8.1 details the 'fit' of David's offence; this takes into account the drivers identified during the process of clarification, such as the permission-giving thoughts (note that it appeared that this was more of a spontaneous act), as well as other drivers elucidated in conversations with David and his family, which focused on both family attitudes towards sexuality and on David's own sexual experience and knowledge. All of these drivers then became targets for intervention. Some of the drivers were already managed through the safety plan; others involved more extensive work. One of the priority drivers was deemed to be David's social isolation, which was also linked with a sense of hopelessness about never being able to have a girlfriend. A secondary fit on David's social isolation is illustrated in Figure 8.2, and suggests the impact of Sally and Reg's own world beliefs on David's developing schema about the world around him.

The following details the most prominent therapeutic interventions which target specific drivers on the PSB fit.

Social isolation

With respect to David's social isolation, Sally and Reg were clearly able to see how encouraging and empowering David to socialise more with his own peer group would be a protective factor for his future; however, it was harder for them to acknowledge how their own beliefs and approach to life might have had such a strong impact on David's own schema. The therapist was able to observe many interchanges between family members that clearly gave the message to David that others could not be trusted; over time, as these interchanges occurred in session, the therapist was able to help both Sally and Reg reflect on

190 *Sexually Harmful Behaviour*

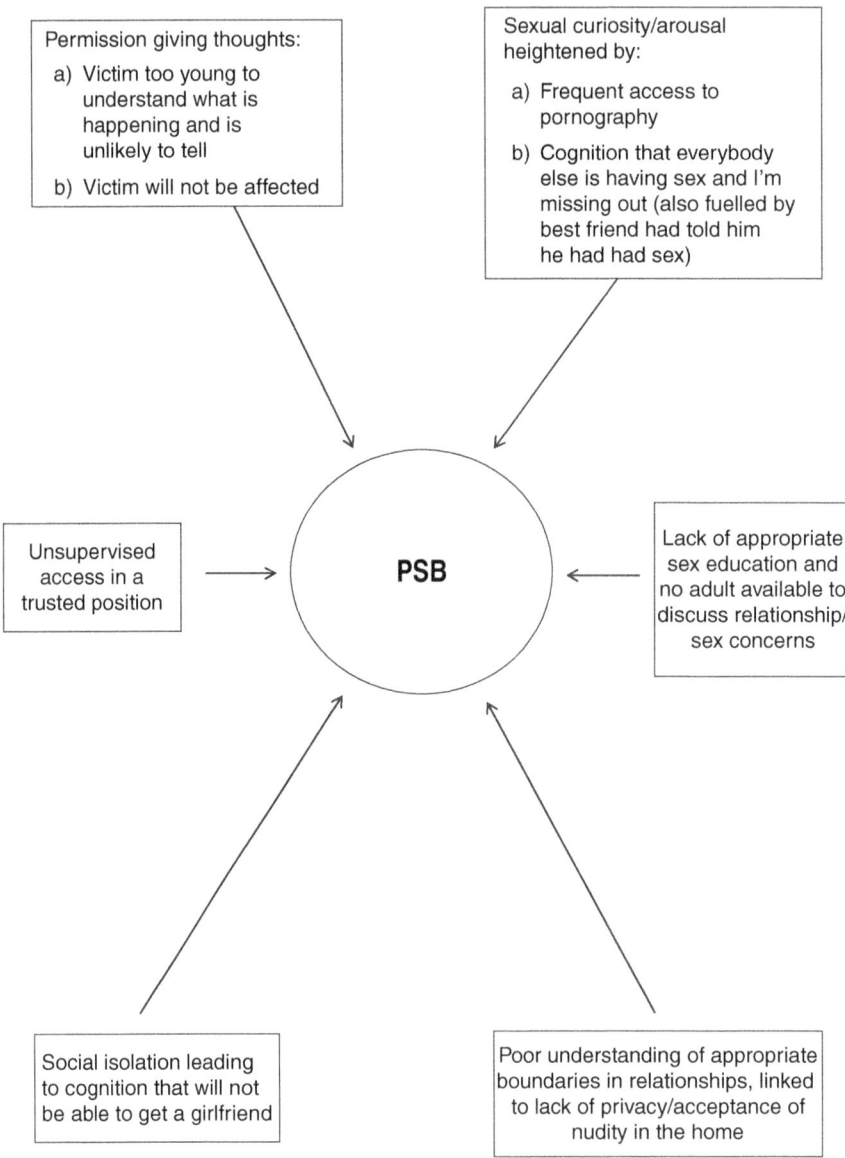

Figure 8.1 'Fit' for problem sexual behaviour

the impact of such messages, and, using enactment, help the family find other ways of communicating to David, hence challenging all of their beliefs about the trustworthiness of others.

This work was hampered by the breakdown in relationships between David's family and that of the victim. It seemed that Ann, the victim's mother, had

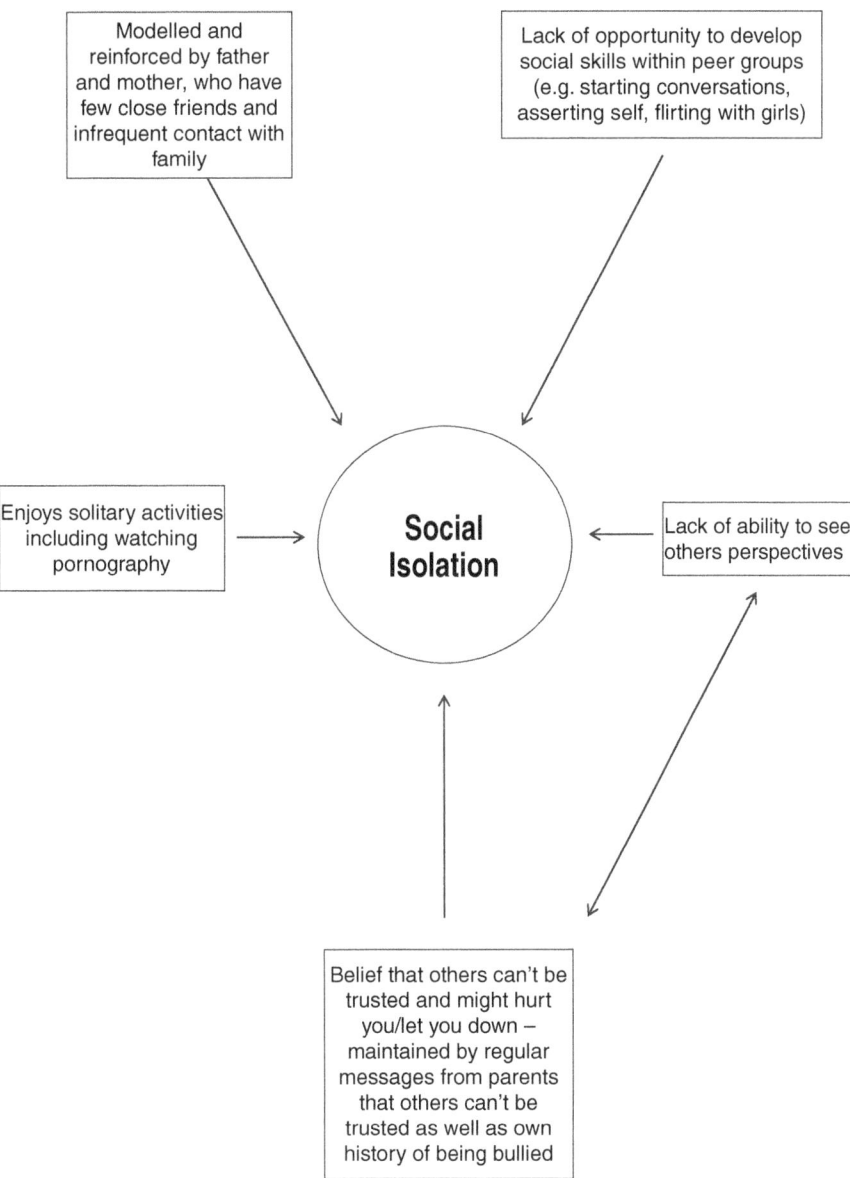

Figure 8.2 'Fit' for social isolation

confided to a friend about the offence, and this information had become known in the wider community. This not only fuelled ideas for David and his family of the world being an unsafe place, but the anger and blame directed towards the victim's family was shielding David from taking responsibility for the offence: any time the therapist referred to the victim, the family would begin to moan about her family. The therapist worked hard to help Sally, Reg and David see things from Ann's point of view, and to allow Sally and Reg to realise that their tirades about Ann were preventing David from developing his empathy towards the victim.

The work regarding increasing awareness and challenging unhelpful patterns of communication was supplemented with attempts to increase social activities for David, and the therapist worked alongside YOT to find meaningful activities for David where he could socialise with peers of his own age in a supervised environment. David initially joined a martial arts club.

Observations of David in these environments also highlighted some of his difficulties in social skills, such as his ability to start and maintain conversations with others, and his tendency to invade the personal space of others. It was clear that David was keen to make new friends, but also fearful of being rejected. The therapist involved the family in modelling and role playing social skills, combined with feedback to David of his successes, and also set goals for him to practise such skills in the live environment. Sally and Reg were also coached to help David problem-solve, and consider the perspectives of others when he experienced any problems in his attempts to build meaningful relationships with them.

Sex and relationship education

The clarification sessions and ongoing family work had already promoted Reg as somebody that David could go to talk to with any concerns that he might have about sex and relationships. The therapist helped Reg think about what messages he might want to give to David about healthy sexual and intimate relationships, and then facilitated a series of meetings between Reg and David to explore these areas. Topics ranged from exploring and understanding the concept of consent within relationships, to ways of starting up conversations with girls. Reg was also able to share some of his own teenage experiences with girls, thus normalising some of David's own worries. These conversations also focused on the impact of pornography on David and his beliefs about relationships. In the course of these conversations, David was able to acknowledge to Reg that he now felt guilty about having any sexual thoughts or fantasies, particularly during masturbation, and Reg was able to reassure David about the normalcy of such cognitions

Challenging unhelpful thoughts

Some of David's permission-giving thoughts had already been challenged by the process of being caught and charged with an offence. However, his understanding about the potential impact on the victim and his ability to empathise with her was, as previously discussed, limited by the anger felt by the whole family towards the victim's family, and this needed to be managed first. As Reg grew more able to see his brother's perspective, he felt able to meet with his brother and share their sadness about what had occurred. This opened up space for David to share his own remorse with Sally and Reg, and for Reg to feed back to David how Amy was coping. This led to David wishing to make an apology to Amy, and it was agreed that he would initially write an unsent letter to Amy that could feasibly be given to her when her own family felt it was timely.

Challenges in this work

There is no doubt that working with young people who display harmful sexual behaviour, and supporting their families, is clinically stretching. For instance, the deconstruction of themes such as denial, minimisation and victim blame, which are often demonstrated by both the young person and their families, presents one pertinent challenge for workers. Workers may find themselves feeling shocked and at times disgusted by some of the offences committed, and deeply troubled by and contemptuous of a young person's apparent lack of remorse and failure to take responsibility for harm caused to others. Workers may hence be surprised by the strength of some of their urges to denigrate or humiliate the young person in an attempt to have him or her 'see sense'. This is an example of a parallel process, whereby the perpetrator blaming the victim can be mirrored by the therapist and family blaming the perpetrator.

Ultimately, humiliation of a young person who may already be fearing rejection by others and feeling socially inadequate – some of the very factors which may have contributed towards their harmful sexual behaviour in the first place – will only exacerbate their sense of not belonging, and of feeling unloved and unacceptable. Hence, one of the founding principles of any intervention is to constructively work through the shame of the young person without further shaming them in this process. This entails understanding that denial and victim blame may be driven by self-protective factors, such as protection from shameful emotions and negative identity conclusions. Regular supervision to support workers, to enable them to reflect on the impact of the work on themselves, and to constructively critique the work is thus vital to ensure that they are striving to practise from an ethical position (see Jenkins 2009). The therapeutic process should not be, whether wittingly or not, a mode of punishing the young person.

At the opposite end of the spectrum to the urge to punish, lies the drive to rescue and protect young people from the awfulness of their actions. This may be evidenced, for instance, by therapists often unknowingly failing to challenge victim blame, or by colluding with mindsets held by families that the perpetrator has learnt his lesson, will hence not offend again and thus needs no intervention. Alongside this, therapists may recoil from naming what has taken place, for instance, referring to 'the incident' rather than labelling what has happened as 'abuse', hence trivialising and minimising such behaviour. Part of the therapeutic journey involves enabling families to acknowledge what their child might have done, which might previously have been too horrific for them to contemplate, in order that they will be sufficiently motivated to support and safeguard their child. Again, clinical supervision needs to adequately address the therapeutic pitfalls, including the issue of disguised compliance that may serve to neutralise the professional's authority (Reder, Duncan and Gray 1993: 106–107).

Work with young sexual offenders can also impact upon practitioners in complex ways, particularly because it forces us to consider issues of sex, violence and children. This can be distressing but can also bring aspects of workers' own sexuality sharply into focus. Workers may be shocked and surprised by their own sexual responses as clients discuss their abusive behaviour. Moulden and Firestone (2007, 2010) also recognise the potential for vicarious traumatisation of clinicians. Such issues clearly have implications for the therapeutic alliance and for therapist burnout. It is therefore essential that all workers have access to supervision that is reflective, supportive and grounded in an understanding of transference and counter-transference (Vizard and Usiskin 2006; Moulden and Firestone 2007). In addition, research into work with adults who sexually harm suggests that clients do best when they perceive their therapist to be sympathetic, warm and confident (Ward, Mann and Gannon 2006).

Therapists should also think of themselves as 'accountable' to those who have been abused, holding in mind the impact of abuse, and the needs of victims, in order to inform practice with perpetrators. This can be achieved more generally through ongoing reading and research, but there also needs to be case-specific understanding of victimology, through access to victim statements where available.

The issue, however, of the importance of treatment or rehabilitation versus punishment and incarceration for young people who display harmful sexual behaviour, remains contentious. Clearly, there are long-term repercussions for young people who are found guilty of sexual offences, with regard to employment possibilities and to future relationships. The decision to incarcerate should be based on assessed levels of supervision, the young person's willingness to comply with available community intervention programmes, and an acknowledgement by the court that alternative community-based programmes have greater efficacy than traditional custodial sentences that typically do not include family interventions. In any case, the custodial provision nationally for juvenile sexual offenders has been reduced (YJB 2013).

Furthermore, there is a precarious balance between promoting and fulfilling the developmental needs of the young person whilst also protecting the community as a whole, including victims and potential victims. This necessarily involves close liaison with and joint decision-making between various agencies, including education, social care and YOTs, and is fraught with tensions in professional relationships as each party seeks to ensure that their safeguarding duties are fulfilled. For example, creative solutions need to be found to ensure integration of a young person who has displayed sexually harmful behaviour into a school environment. Whilst this may be deemed essential to promote social and educational success (and hence reduce long-term risk of offending), schools have a duty to safeguard all of their pupils, and are likely to require intensive support with managing their responses to the young person and safely managing risk.

The stigma associated with sexual offending, and increased likelihood of the perpetrator themselves being victimised should information about the harmful sexual behaviour come to light, means that careful consideration needs to be given to the question of *who* needs to know *what* about the circumstances of the harmful sexual behaviour. The overriding premise is safeguarding, to protect past victims and any potential future victims. The issues of confidentiality will always be contentious; there is further contention about which professional holds the responsibility for deciding who else needs to be told. Such decisions may have major ramifications for the young person, which could lead to exclusion from education or employment. Our position is that such decisions should be shared and made in a multidisciplinary environment, with professionals trained to understand the complexities of the law and its application to safeguarding, and with recourse to an objective assessment and formulation of risk. Of course, there will always be situations where convictions for sexual offences must be reported by law, for instance, job applications requiring a Disclosure, Barring and Vetting form, or planned education moves.

Conclusion

The past two decades have been witness to shifts in our formulations and understandings of sexually harmful behaviour by young people, with a concomitant development of empirically guided risk assessment instruments, and a drive to evaluate the efficacy of specialised treatment programmes. The embedding of evidence-based practice in the field has become increasingly apparent.

There now appears to be a consensus amongst academics, practitioners and policymakers that treatment models of adult sexual offending cannot be indiscriminately applied to young people who engage in sexually harmful behaviour; instead, conceptualisation of such behaviour by young people needs to be mindful of the developmental and social-ecological context in which such behaviour takes place. It is also recognised that these young people are a heterogeneous group, with varied levels of risks, but also with the needs, difficulties, hopes and anxieties that are generally present during adolescence. As such, treatment should be multifaceted and address the range of needs presented, rather than focus solely on sexually harmful behaviour. Emerging models (e.g. MST-PSB, GLM) all appear to be driven by multifactorial formulations that draw on multiple theoretical perspectives and focus on overall quality of life, rather than committing to interventions that solely emphasise risk management. These models must strike a balance between managing risk and enabling the young person to live as normal a life as possible, this tightrope being highly conspicuous, for example, when reintegrating a young person who has sexually harmed a peer into the school environment, or when deciding that a young person who has sexually harmed a sibling can remain or move back into the family home.

Despite such progress, it has yet to be determined which treatment modalities yield the most promising outcomes, or what interventions are most efficacious with differing presentations. Further research is merited into the efficacy of the emerging models, and, in the case of MST-PSB, how a model developed in the United States can be successfully implemented in the UK. We should also bear in mind the issue of desistance, as most young people who engage in sexually harmful behaviour do not continue perpetrating into adulthood, and may desist without any formal intervention (e.g. Worling and Langstrom 2006). However, as yet there are no models for predicting who these young people might be, and hence the emphasis should be on a holistic response, targeting all of the developmental and ecological needs of the young person and their families.

Inter-agency collaboration is rightly seen as an underlying philosophy, to ensure that we respond appropriately to young people and their families. This reduces duplication of services and allows for transparency and consistency. All families should have the opportunity to access a needs-led assessment and appropriate interventions, with a lead agency holding case responsibility and co-ordinating responses.

Budgetary constraints remain a concern. For instance, MST-PSB is an expensive commodity compared with peer-group interventions; it is not expensive when compared with the cost of residential care or custody. However, which agency should meet the costs for an intensive service is unclear. Traditionally, costs for young people who go into residential units are met by either the local authority or by the NHS via clinical commissioning groups; costs for custody are met nationally in the UK. Hence, whilst MST-PSB might be an effective alternative to custody for some young people, there is no local benefit for funding such a service. Whilst the debates about funding continue, families are often left on the perimeter of services, feeling uncontained and unsupported.

There remains a paucity of treatment centres within the custodial environment; similarly, with regard to residential care, local authorities tend to rely on private providers, due in part to the apparent lack of intensive foster care placements, but also due to the closure of local authority residential units. There is a clear need for private providers to demonstrate evidence-based practice, underpinned by comprehensive psychologically informed formulations.

Interventions must also consider that a number of perpetrators are also victims of abuse; the needs of the young person as a victim should be paramount, and addressed as a priority. Again, consideration needs to be given to the funding of services that work with such young people, who may be excluded from traditional child and adolescent mental health services (CAMHS).

Our knowledge base of how to assess and work effectively with young people who engage in sexually harmful behaviour, and their families, is hence expanding; whilst the field remains in its infancy, it nevertheless provides us with increasing hope of being able to achieve positive outcomes for these young people, who have historically been misunderstood and mislabelled, and who have fallen outside the remit of traditional services for young people. We recognise, however, that there is a paucity of research into the application of these treatment models to specific populations, such as those with cognitive difficulties, and young females who sexually harm; and further adaptation of treatment paradigms, alongside rigorous outcome research, is clearly warranted.

References

AIM Project (2012) Available at: http://www.aimproject.org.uk. Accessed on 1 May 2015.

Bancroft, J. (2006) 'Normal Sexual Development', in H. Barbaree and W. Marshall (eds.), *The Juvenile Sex Offender*. 2nd edn. New York: Guildford Press, 19–57.

Becker, J.V., Cunningham-Rathner, J., and Kaplan, M.S. (1986) 'Adolescent sexual offenders: Demographics, criminal and sexual histories', *Journal of Interpersonal Violence*, 1: 431–445.

Bleakley, A., Henessy, M., and Fishbein, M. (2011) 'A model of adolescents' seeking of sexual content in their media choices', *Journal of Sex Research*, 48: 309–315.

Borduin, C.M., Schaeffer, C.M., and Heiblum, N. (2009) 'A randomized clinical of multisystemic therapy with juvenile sexual offenders: Effects on youth social ecology and criminal activity', *Journal of Consulting and Clinical Psychology*, 77(1): 26–37.

Borduin, C.M., Henggeler, S.W., Blaske, D.M., and Stein, R. (1990) 'Multisystemic treatment of adolescent sexual offenders', *International Journal of Offender Therapy and Comparative Criminology*, 34: 105–113.

Borduin, C.M., Letourneau, E.J., Henggeler, S.W., and Swenson, C.C. (2003) 'Treatment manual for multisystemic therapy with sexual offenders and their families'. Unpublished manuscript. University of Missouri, Columbia.

Braithwaite, J. (2002) 'Setting standards for restorative justice', *British Journal of Criminology*, 42(3): 563–577.

Burton, D. (2008) 'An exploratory evaluation of personality and childhood sexual victimization to the development of sexually abusive behaviour', *Sexual Abuse: A Journal of Research and Treatment*, 20(1): 102–115.

Burton, D.L., Leibowitz, G.S., and Howard, A. (2010) 'Comparison by crime type of juvenile delinquents on pornography exposure: The absence of relationships between exposure to pornography and sexual offense characteristics', *Journal of Forensic Nursing*, 6: 121–129.

Caldwell, M.F. (2007) 'Sexual offense adjudication and sexual recidivism among juvenile offenders', *Sexual Abuse: A Journal of Research and Treatment*, 19: 107–113.
Collie, R., Ward, T., Ayland, L., and West, B. (2007) 'The Good Lives Model of Rehabilitation: Reducing Risks and Promoting Strengths with Adolescent Sexual Offenders', in M.C. Calder (ed.), *Working with Children and Young People Who Sexually Abuse: Taking the Field Forward*. Lyme Regis: Russell House, 53–64.
Cowell, A. and Smith, E. (2009) *Streetwise Pornography Research*. Newcastle upon Tyne: Streetwise Young People's Project.
Criminal Justice Joint Inspection (2012) *Facing up to Offending: Use of Restorative Justice in the Criminal Justice System*. No place of publication.
Daly, K. (2008) 'The Limits of Restorative Justice', in D. Sullivan and L. Tifft (eds.), *Handbook of Restorative Justice: A Global Perspective*. Abingdon: Routledge, 134–146.
DH (Department of Health) (1999) *Working Together to Safeguard Children: A Guide to Interagency Working to Safeguard and Promote the Welfare of Children*. London: Department of Health.
Doig, M. and Wallace, B. (1999) 'Family Conference Team'. Paper presented to Restoration for Victims of Crime Conference, Australian Institute of Criminology, September 1999.
Dolan, M., Holloway, J., Bailey, S., and Kroll, L (1996) 'The psychosocial characteristics of juvenile sexual offenders referred to an adolescent forensic service in the UK', *Medical Science Law*, 36(4): 342–352.
Erooga, M. and Masson, H. (2006) 'Children and Young People with Sexually Harmful or Abusive Behaviours: Underpinning Knowledge, Principles, Approaches and Service Provision', in M. Erooga and H. Masson (eds.), *Children and Young People Who Sexually Abuse Others: Current Developments and Practice Responses*. 2nd edn. Abingdon: Routledge, 3–17.
Fanniff, A.M. and Letourneau, E.J. (2012) 'Another piece of the puzzle: Psychometric properties of the J-SOAP-II', *Sexual Abuse: A Journal of Research and Treatment*, 24: 378–408.
Finkelhor, D., Ormrod, R., and Chaffin, M. (2009) *Juveniles Who Commit Sex Offenses against Minors*. Washington, DC: Office of Juvenile Justice and Delinquency.
Forman, S.G. (1993) *Coping Skills Interventions for Children and Adolescents*. San Francisco, CA: Jossey-Bass.
Forth, A.E., Kosson, D., and Hare, R.D. (2003) *The Hare Psychopathy Checklist: Youth Version*. Toronto: Multi-Health Systems.
Frick, P.J. and Hare, R.D. (2001) *Antisocial Process Screening Device*. Toronto: Multi-Health Systems.
Frick, P.J., Cornell, A.H., Bodin, S.D., Dane, H.A., Barry, C.T., and Loney, B.R. (2003) 'Callous-unemotional traits and developmental pathways to severe conduct problems', *Developmental Psychology*, 39(2): 246–260.
Gough, H.G. (1987) *California Psychological Inventory*. Palo Alto, CA: Consulting Psychologists Press.
Gretton, H.M., McBride, M., Hare, R.D., O'Shaughnessy, R., and Kumka, G. (2001) 'Psychopathy and recidivism in adolescent sex offenders', *Criminal Justice and Behaviour*, 28(4): 427–499.
Griffin, H.L. and Price, S. (2009) 'Good Lives approach evaluation tools'. Unpublished G-map, Manchester.
Hackett, S. (2007) 'Just How Different Are They? Diversity and the Treatment of Young People with Harmful Sexual Behaviours', in M.C. Calder (ed.), *Working with Children and Young People Who Sexually Abuse: Taking the Field Forward*. Lyme Regis: Russell House, 9–22.

Hackett, S., Masson, H., and Phillips, J. (2005) *Services for Young People Who Sexually Abuse: A Report on Mapping and Exploring Services for Young People Who Have Sexually Abused Others*. London: Youth Justice Board.

Hackett, S., Masson, M., Balfe, M., and Phillips, J. (2013) 'Individual, family and abuse characteristics of 700 British child and adolescent sexual abusers', *Child Abuse Review*, 22(4): 232–245.

Haley, J. (1987) *Problem-Solving Therapy*. 2nd edn. San Francisco, CA: Jossey-Bass.

Hanson, R.K. (1997) *The Development of a Brief Actuarial Risk Scale for Sexual Offense Recidivism*. Ottawa: Department of the Solicitor General of Canada.

Hanson, R.K. (2000) *Risk Assessment*. Beaverton, OR: Association for the Treatment of Sexual Abusers.

Hempel, I., Buck, N., Cima, M., and van Marle, H. (2013) 'Review of risk assessment instruments for juvenile sex offenders: What is next?' *International Journal of Offender Therapy and Comparative Criminology*, 57(2): 208–288.

Henderson, M., Wight, D., Raab, G., Abraham, C., Buston, K, Har, G., and Scott, S. (2002) 'Heterosexual risk behaviour among young teenagers in Scotland', *Journal of Adolescence*, 25: 483–494.

Henggeler, S.W., Letourneaus, E.J., Chapman, J.E., Bourduin, C.M., Scheew, P.A., and McCart, M.R. (2009) 'Mediators of change for multisystemic therapy with juvenile sexual offenders', *Journal of Consulting and Clinical Psychology*, 77(3): 451–462.

Henniker, J. and Mercer, V. (2007) 'Restorative Justice: Can It Work with Young People Who Sexually Abuse', in M.C. Calder (ed.), *Working with Children and Young People Who Sexually Abuse: Taking the Field Forward*. Lyme Regis: Russell House, 230–244.

Hickey, N., Vizard, E., McCrory, E., and French, L. (2013) *Links between Juvenile Sexually Abusive Behaviour and Emerging Severe Personality Disorder Traits in Childhood*. London: Department of Health.

HM Government (2013) *Working Together to Safeguard Children*. London: Department for Education.

HM Inspectorate of Probation (2013) *Examining Multi-Agency Responses to Children and Young People Who Sexually Offend*. London: HM Inspectorate of Probation.

Hoge, R.D. (2002) 'Standardised instruments for assessing risk and need in youthful offenders', *Criminal Justice and Behaviour*, 29(4): 380–396.

Home Office (2004) *Best Practice Guidance for Restorative Practitioners*. London: Home Office.

Home Office (2011) *New Best Practice Guidance for Restorative Practice*. London: Home Office.

Horvath, M.A.H., Alys, L., Massey, K., Pina, A., Scally, M., and Adler, J.R. (2013) *Basically Porn is Everywhere: A Rapid Evidence Assessment on the Effects that Access and Exposure to Pornography Has on Children and Young People*. London: Office of the Children's Commissioner.

Hunter, J.A., Figueredo, A.J., and Malamuth, N.M. (2010) 'Developmental pathways into social and sexual deviance', *Journal of Family Violence*, 25(2): 141–148.

James, K. (2007) 'The Interactional Process of Forgiveness and Responsibility: A Critical Assessment of the Family Therapy Literature', in C. Flaskas, I. McCarthy, and J. Sheehan (eds.), *Hope and Despair in Narrative and Family Therapy: Adversity, Forgiveness and Reconciliation*. London: Routledge, 127–138.

Jenkins, A. (2006) 'Shame, realisation and restitution: The ethics of restorative practice', *Australian and New Zealand Journal of Family Therapy*, 27(3): 153–162.

Jenkins, A. (2009) *Becoming Ethical: A Parallel Journey with Men Who Have Abused*. Lyme Regis: Russell House.

Jespersen, A.F., Lalumiere, M.L., and Michael, C.S. (2009) 'Sexual abuse history among adult sex offenders and non-sex offenders: A meta-analysis', *Child Abuse and Neglect*, 33(3): 179–192.

Johnson, T., Scott, J., and Telford, P. (2007) 'Working with the Families of Children and Young People Who Sexually Harm: It Shouldn't Be an Optional Extra', in M.C. Calder (ed.), *Working with Children and Young People Who Sexually Abuse: Taking the Field Forward*. Lyme Regis: Russell House, 103–109.

Kernberg, P.F., Weiner, A.S., and Bardenstein, K.K. (2000) *Personality Disorders in Children and Adolescents*. New York: Basic Books.

Langstrom, N. (2001) *Young Sex Offenders: A Research Overview*. Stockholm: National Board of Health and Welfare.

Lawing, K., Frick, P.J., and Cruise, K.R. (2010) 'Differences in offending patterns between adolescent sex offenders high or low in callous-unemotional traits', *Psychological Assessment*, 22: 298–305.

Letourneau, E.J., Henggeler, S.W., Bouduin, C.M., Schewe, P., McCart, M., Chapman, J., and Saldana, L (2009) 'Multisystemic therapy for juvenile sexual offenders: 1-year results from a randomized effectiveness trial', *Journal of Family Psychology*, 23: 321–336.

Leversee, T. (2007) 'Using Typologies to Individualise the Assessment, Treatment and Supervision of Sexually Abusive Youth', in M.C. Calder (ed.), *Working with Children and Young People Who Sexually Abuse: Taking the Field Forward*. Lyme Regis: Russell House, 38–52.

Lovell, E. (2002) *Children and Young People Who Display Sexually Harmful Behaviour*. London: NSPCC.

McCartan, F.M., Law, H., Murphy, M., and Bailey, S. (2011) 'Child and adolescent females who present with sexually abusive behaviours: A 10-year UK prevalence study', *Journal of Sexual Aggression*, 17(1): 4–14.

McNevin, E. (2010) 'Applied restorative justice as a complement to systemic family therapy: Theory and practice implications for families experiencing intra-familial adolescent sibling incest', *Australian and New Zealand Journal of Family Therapy*, 31(1): 60–72.

Marshall, W.L., Hudson, S.M., Jones, R., and Fernandez, Y.M. (1995) 'Empathy in sex offenders', *Clinical Psychology Review*, 15: 99–113.

Masson, H., Hackett, S., Phillips, J., and Balfe, M. (2012) 'Developmental markers of risk or vulnerability? Young females who sexually abuse – characteristics, background, behaviours and outcomes', *Child and Family Social Work*, 20(1): 19–29.

Miccio-Fonseca, L.C. (2000) 'Adult and adolescent female sex offenders: Experiences compared to other females and male sex offenders', *Journal of Psychology and Human Sexuality*, 11(3): 75–88.

Miccio-Fonseca, L.C. (2009) 'MEGA: A new paradigm in protocol assessing sexually abusive children and adolescents', *Journal of Child and Adolescent Trauma*, 2: 121–141.

Millon, T., Millon, C., and Davis, R. (1993) *Millon Adolescent Clinical Inventory Manual*. Minneapolis, MN: National Computer Systems.

Miner, M.H. and Munns, R. (2005) 'Isolation and normlessness: Attitudinal comparisons of adolescent sex offenders, juvenile offenders, and nondelinquents', *International Journal of Offender Therapy and Comparative Criminology*, 49(5): 491–504.

Ministry of Justice (2012) *Getting It Right for Victims and Witnesses*. London: Ministry of Justice.

Minuchin, S. and Fishman, C. (1981) *Family Therapy Techniques*. Cambridge, MA: Harvard University Press.

Morrell, L.M. and Burton, D.L. (2014) 'An exploration of psychopathy in self-report measures among juvenile sex offenders', *International Journal of Offender Therapy and Comparative Criminology*, 58(5): 550–566.

Moulden, H.M. and Firestone, P. (2007) 'Vicarious traumatization: The impact on therapists who work with sexual offenders', *Trauma, Violence, Abuse*, 8(1): 67–83.

Moulden, H.M. and Firestone, P. (2010) 'Therapist awareness and responsibility in working with sexual offenders', *Sex Abuse*, 22(4): 374–386.

National Children's Home (1992) *Report of the Committee of Enquiry into Children and Young People Who Sexually Abuse Other Children*. London: National Children's Home.

Ogloff, J.R.P., Cutajar, M.C., Mann, E., and Mullen, P. (2012) 'Child sexual abuse and subsequent offending and victimisation: A 45-year follow-up study', *Trends and Issues No 440*, Australian Institute of Criminology. Available at http://aic.gov.au/media_library/publications/tandi_pdf/tandi440.pdf. Accessed on 1 May 2015.

Owens, E.W., Behun, R.J., Manning, J.C., and Reid, R.C. (2012) 'The impact of internet pornography on adolescents: A review of the research', *Sexual Addiction and Compulsivity*, 19: 99–122.

Peter, J. and Valkenburg, P.M. (2008) 'Adolescents' exposure to sexually explicit internet material and sexual preoccupancy: A three wave panel study', *Media Psychology*, 11: 207–234.

Peter, J. and Valkenburg, P.M. (2009) 'Adolescents' exposure to sexually explicit internet material and notions of women as sex objects: Assessing causality and underlying processes', *Journal of Communication*, 59: 407–433.

Pfeifer, J.H., Kahn, L.E., Merchant, J.S., Peake, S.J., Veroude, K., Masten, C.L., Lieberman, M.D., Mazziotta, J.C., and Dapreto, M. (2013) 'Longitudinal change in the neural bases of adolescent social self-evaluations: Effects of age and pubertal development', *Journal of Neuroscience*, 33(17): 7415–7419.

Prentky, R. and Righthand, S. (2003) *Juvenile Sex Offender Assessment Protocol-II (J-SOAP-II) Manual* (NCJ 202316).

Prescott, D. (2007) 'Adolescent Risk Assessment: Practice, Policy, Language and Ourselves', in M.C. Calder (ed.), *Working with Children and Young People Who Sexually Abuse: Taking the Field Forward*. Lyme Regis: Russell House, 134–147.

Probation (2004) Joint Inspection of youth offending teams: The first phase. Annual report, London: Home Office.

Quinsey, V.L., Harris, G.T., Rice, M.E., and Cormier, C.A. (1998) *Violent Offenders: Managing and Appraising Risk*. Washington, DC: American Psychological Association.

Radford, L., Corral, S., Bradley, C., Fisher, H., Bassett, C., Howat, N., and Collishaw, S. (2011) *Child Abuse and Neglect in the UK Today*. London: NSPCC.

Reder, P., Duncan, S., and Gray, M. (1993) *Beyond Blame: Child Abuse Tragedies Revisited*. London: Routledge.

Restorative Justice Council (2011) *Best Practice Guidance for Restorative Practice*. London: Restorative Justice Council.

Rich, P. (2006) *Attachment and Sexual Offending*. Chichester: John Wiley.

Rich, P. (2011) *Understanding, Assessing and Rehabilitating Juvenile Sexual Offenders*. New Jersey: Wiley.

Richardson, G. (2007) 'Emerging Personality Disorders in Sexually Harmful Young People', in M.C. Calder (ed.), *Working with Children and Young People Who Sexually Abuse: Taking the Field Forward*. Lyme Regis: Russell House, 65–95.

Richardson, G., Kelly, T.P., Graham, F., and Bhate, S.R. (2004) 'A personality-based taxonomy of sexually abusive adolescents derived from the Millon Adolescent Clinical Inventory (MACI)', *British Journal of Clinical Psychology*, 43: 285–298.

Ryan, E.P., Hunter, J.A., and Murrie, D.C. (2012) *Juvenile Sex Offenders: A Guide to Evaluation and Treatment for Mental Health Professionals*. Oxford: Oxford University Press.

Ryan, G. (1999) 'Treatment of sexually abusive youth: The evolving consensus', *Journal of Interpersonal Violence*, 14(4): 422–436.

Sabina, C., Wolak, J., and Finkelhor, D. (2008) 'The nature and dynamics of internet pornography exposure for youth', *CyberPsychology and Behaviour*, 11(6): 691–693.

Shapiro, F. (2001) 'Trauma and Adaptive Information-Processing: EMDR's Dynamic and Behavioral Interface', in M.F. Solomon, R.J. Neborsky, L. McCullough, M. Alpert, F. Shapiro, and D. Malan (eds.), *Short-Term Therapy for Long-Term Change*. New York: W.W. Norton & Co, 112–129.

Strickland, S. (2008) 'Female sexual offenders: Exploring issues of personality. Trauma and cognitive distortions', *Journal of Interpersonal Violence*, 23(4): 474–489.

Thornton, D., Mann, R., Webster, S., Blud, L., Travers, R., Friendship, C., and Erikson, M. (2003) 'Distinguishing and Combining Risks for Sexual and Violent Recidivism', in R.A. Prentky, E.S. Janus, and M.C. Seto (eds.), *Annals of the New York Academy of Sciences*: *Vol. 989*. New York: New York Academy of Sciences, 225–235.

Van der Kolk, B. (1989) 'The compulsion to repeat the trauma: Re-enactment, revictimisation and masochism', *Psychiatric Clinics of North America*, 12(2): 389–411.

Van der Kolk, B.A., Burbridge, J.A., and Suzuki, J. (1997) 'The psychobiology of traumatic memory: Clinical implications of neuro imaging studies', *Annals of the New York Academy of Sciences*, 821: 99–113.

Varker, T. and Devilly, G.J. (2007) 'Types of empathy and adolescent sexual offenders', *Journal of Sexual Aggression*, 13(2): 139–149.

Veneziano, C., Veneziano, L., and LeGrande, S (2000) 'The relationship between adolescent sex offender behaviour and victim characteristics with prior victimization', *Journal of Interpersonal Violence*, 15: 363–374.

Vizard, E. and Usiskin, J. (2006) 'Individual Psychotherapy for Young Sexual Abusers of Other Children', in M. Erooga and H. Masson (eds.), *Children and Young People Who Sexually Abuse Others: Current Developments and Practice Responses*. Abingdon: Routledge, 131–144.

Vizard, E., Hickey, N., and McCrory, E. (2007) 'Developmental trajectories associated with juvenile sexually abusive behaviour and emerging severe personality disorder in childhood: A 3-year study', *British Journal of Psychiatry*, 190(49): 27–32.

Vizard, E., Monck, P., and Misch, P. (1995) 'Child and adolescent sex abuse perpetrators: A review of the research literature', *Journal of Child Psychology and Psychiatry*, 36(5): 731–756.

Ward, T. (2002) 'Good lives and the rehabilitation of offenders: Promises and problems', *Aggression and Violent Behaviour*, 7: 513–528.

Ward, T. and Marshall, W.L. (2004) 'Good lives, etiology and rehabilitation of sexual offenders: A bridging theory', *Journal of Sexual Aggression*, 10: 153–169.

Ward, T., Mann, R.E., and Gannon, T.A. (2006) 'The Good Lives Model of offender rehabilitation: Clinical implications', *Aggression and Violent Behaviour*, 12: 87–107.

Westbrook, D., Kennerley, H., and Kirk, J. (2007) *An Introduction to Cognitive Behaviour Therapy: Skills and Applications*. London: Sage.

Whittle, N., Bailey, S., and Kurtz, Z. (2006) *The Needs and Effective Treatment of Young People Who Sexually Abuse: Current Evidence*. Joint Department of Health and National Institute for Mental Health in England (NIMHE), Victims of Violence and Abuse Prevention Programme (VVAPP). London: Department of Health.

Wolak, J., Mitchell, K., and Finkelhor, D. (2007) 'Unwanted and wanted exposure to online pornography in a national sample of youth internet users', *Pediatrics*, 119(6): 247–257.
Worling, J.R. (1995) 'Sexual abuse histories of adolescent male sex offenders: Differences on the basis of the age and gender of their victims', *Journal of Abnormal Psychology*, 104(4): 610–613.
Worling, J.R. (2001) 'Personality-based typology of adolescent male sexual offenders: Differences in recidivism rates, victim selection characteristics and personal victimization histories', *Sexual Abuse: A Journal of Research and Treatment*, 13(3): 149–166.
Worling, J.R. and Curven, T. (2001) *The ERASOR: Estimate of Risk of Adolescent Offence Recidivism (Version 2.0)*. Toronto: Sexual Abuse Family Education and Treatment (SAFE-T) Program.
Worling, J.R. and Langstrom, N. (2006) 'Risk of Sexual Recidivism in Adolescents Who Offend Sexually: Correlates and Assessment', in H.E. Barbaree and W.L. Marshall (eds.), *The Juvenile Sex Offender*. 2nd edn. New York: Guilford Press, n.p.
Wylie, L.A. and Griffin, H.L. (2013) 'G-map's application of the Good Lives Model to adolescent males who sexually harm: A case study', *Journal of Sexual Aggression*, 19(3): 345–356.
YJB (Youth Justice Board) (2008) *Young People Who Sexually Abuse*. London: Youth Justice Board.
YJB (Youth Justice Board) (2009) *Youth Justice Annual Workload Data 2007/2008*. London: Youth Justice Board.
YJB (Youth Justice Board) (2013) Available at: http://www.justice.gov.uk/news/press-releases/yjb/yjb-reduces-number-of-commissioned-places-in-youth-custody. Accessed 01 May 2015.
Zehr, H. (2002) *Little Book of Restorative Justice*. Intercourse, PA: Good Books.
Zimring, F.E. (2009) *An American Travesty: Legal Responses to Adolescent Sexual Offending*. Chicago, IL: University of Chicago Press.

9
Fire-Setting in Adolescence
Abigail Willis

Introduction

The balance between the appeal and risk of fire has resulted in its use as a metaphor ('playing with fire', 'flying close to the flame', 'having one's fingers burnt'). Understanding the fire-setting of adolescents is a pertinent concern. Many young people engage in fire play (MacKay et al. 2009), and it is estimated that between 40 and 50 per cent of arson offences are carried out by young people (Office of the Deputy Prime Minister 2003; Arson Prevention Bureau 2006). Engagement with fire is associated with inherent risks and these are amplified in fires set by young people without adult awareness. Young people may be less likely to properly identify, report or escape from fire (Kafry 1980; Jones and Haney 1985; Jones et al. 1989). Indeed, some young people will die accidentally from fires that they have set (MacKay, Ruttle and Ward 2012).

Appraisal of fire-setting behaviour in adolescents relies upon thorough assessment methods being used to develop a comprehensive formulation underpinned by knowledge of recidivistic indicators. Psychological intervention for fire-setting in young people requires a stepped approach that is responsive to the risks posed, with attentiveness to the multifactorial range of factors that may contribute. This chapter aims to provide an introduction to each of these areas, using client examples for illustration.

Defining terms

There is discrepancy in the use of definitions in the literature. Discrepancies in the terms can lead to confusion when interpreting findings across research studies. The following terms distinguish the focus of the studies described in this chapter, and are informative in considering individual research studies in the area.

Fire play concerns behaviours involving fire, but that lack intent for damage or disturbance. For many younger children it may involve lighting matches without parental permission (Kafry 1980). The term is frequently used in the literature referring to younger children. The term 'play' does not exclude the potential for significant damage or injury.

Fire-setting refers to intentional setting of fire that targets property or person, ignited without supervision or permission from authority. The term is common in the adolescent-based literature.

Fire deviant behaviour includes fire-setting and behaviours such as excessive interest in fire, threats involving fire, and explosives and behaviours aimed at activating the fire brigade.

Arson is the legal term applied to fire-setting that results in criminal conviction. Only 8 per cent of reported incidents result in prosecution or caution (Official Statistics from the Office of the Deputy Prime Minister 2003). The term is more commonly used in the adult literature.

Prevalence of fire play and setting among young people

The majority of young people engaged in fire play do not cause significant levels of damage or injury by their behaviour; their behaviour may not come to the attention of others. The behaviour in adolescence is often conducted outside of the home (Strachan 1981; Perrin-Wallqvist and Norlander 2003), and involves setting fire to grass, sticks, paper or rubbish, or experiments involving wastebaskets and gasoline (Kolko and Kazdin 1994; Perrin-Wallqvist and Norlander 2003). Del Bove and colleagues (2008) observed only 28.3 per cent of parents were aware of their child's fire-setting. Kolko and Kazdin (1994), with a younger sample, found nearly a third of parents of children aged 6 to 13 years had been unaware of their fire-setting. A lack of adult awareness of fire play and setting can lead to underestimation of the frequency of the behaviour. Further prevalence studies using self-report methods often fail to sufficiently discriminate fire-setting from fire-play behaviour. The prevalence figures reported in studies therefore vary depending on the item definition, sampling (nationality, age, specific groups) and methodology applied (self, parental report).

Examples of variations in study findings include those by Chen, Arria and Anthony (2003), who administered a version of Achenbach's Child Behavior Checklist to 4,595 North American young people aged 12–17 years. The Checklist focuses on the previous six months, and includes the item 'I have set fires'. The prevalence was found to be 6.3 per cent and the behaviour was more common in boys. In contrast, Del Bove and colleagues (2008), using a similar methodology with an Italian sample of young people, found a much higher prevalence rate, with 29 per cent endorsing the item. MacKay and colleagues (2009) found 27 per cent of 364 Canadians aged 11–19 years endorsed that they 'set something on fire that [they] weren't supposed to' in the last year. Perrin-Wallqvist and Norlander (2003) interviewed fifty 18-year-old males and forty-five 18–19-year-old females. Seventy per cent of young men and 44 per cent of young women had played with fire as children, mainly at primary school age but also between the ages of 12 and 15.

These prevalence studies indicate that, despite differences in methodology and definition, a significant proportion of adolescents engage in fire play. Many more young people are exposed to this behaviour, as it is frequently conducted with other young people present (Kafry, Block and Block 1981; Strachan 1981; Icove and Estepp 1987). Studies consistently highlight a very clear predominance of boys involved (82 per cent across childhood meta-analysis, Kolko 1985). Young men in a qualitative study described motivations for fire-setting as including curiosity and distraction (Perrin-Wallqvist and Norlander 2003). Pinsonneault (2002: 25) notes that 'the fact that setting a fire *is* inherently dangerous, *is* against the law, and yet *is* relatively easy to rationalize as victimless, is *exactly* what makes it developmentally appealing to an adolescent' (emphasis in original). The studies described indicate a peak in the behaviour during mid-adolescence and a decline prior to 18 years (Chen, Arria and Anthony 2003; Del Bove et al. 2008). Note that some authors do describe high frequency of fire play in earlier childhood (Kafry 1980; Jacobson 1985; Kolko 1985; Dadds and Fraser 2006), but this is not the focus of this chapter.

Del Bove and colleagues (2008) found 85 per cent of young people that had engaged in fire-setting at initial assessment had not re-engaged in that behaviour two years later. In younger samples, with mixed clinical and non-clinical groups, higher recidivism rates have been observed: 35 per cent over one year (Kolko and Kazdin 1992) and 59 per cent over two years (Kolko et al. 2001). Perrin-Wallqvist and Norlander's (2003) interviews saw young people describe desisting from fire-setting due to parental influence, greater knowledge, other interests or having become afraid of fire. The behaviour was regarded as 'abnormal' and 'not suitable' for 18 year olds.

One can conclude that, for many adolescents, fire-setting is not a frequently repeated or escalating behaviour; rather, the behaviour reflects aspects of their developing maturity and is anticipated to decline with approaching adulthood. The increased frequency may reflect more general elevated risk taking in the adolescent period, a trend likely to be underpinned by neurological, developmental and social factors (see Siegel 2014). For a minority, however, fire-setting will result in significant damage. Perrin-Wallqvist and Norlander's (2003) study found 14 per cent of young men had experienced uncontrolled fires, with some resulting in significant damage. The Diagnostic Statistical Manual V (APA 2013) criteria for conduct disorder includes fire-setting with intent to cause serious damage; prevalence rates in a community sample using this definition are much lower, from 0.1 per cent in females to 0.4 per cent in males (Gelhorn et al. 2009). Some young people will engage in repetitive fire-setting; Hanson and colleagues (1994) compared 25 young people with criminal fire-setting behaviour with delinquent controls, and observed that 95 per cent had a history of previous fire-setting compared with only 28 per cent of the controls. MacKay and colleagues (2009) found 13.5 per cent of young people had engaged in the behaviour more than three times in the past year. There is a group of young people that set fires, whose behaviour or co-morbid presentation will attract the attention of adolescent forensic services. The fire-setting behaviour of these young people may be different from that seen among their peers; the contextualising factors may increase concern or the visibility of their fire-setting, reduced intellectual function or impulsivity may impair concealment, caregiver concern may be provoked by unusual behaviour or multifaceted complex needs.

Psychosocial characteristics associated with fire-setting

Early psychoanalytic interpretations of fire-setting offered by Freud (1932) identified the penis as having two functions: the evacuation of urine (associated with water and the potential to extinguish fire) and the sexual act (associated with flame and fire). Man's relationship to fire was interpreted as the ability to overcome the id or instinctual passions. Psychoanalytic authors linked the behaviour with libidinal excitement (Kaufman, Heims and Reiser 1961) and highlighted its association with enuresis.

More recent studies comparing young people that set fires with those that do not have observed higher levels of psychopathology (Moore, Thompson-Pope and Whited 1996; Del Bove et al. 2008; Mackay et al. 2009), alcohol and substance misuse (SM) (Repo and Virkkunen 1997; MacKay et al. 2009), overt antisocial behaviours including delinquency and aggression (Kolko, Kazdin and Meyer 1985; Chen et al. 2003; Becker et al. 2004; Del Bove et al. 2008) and covert antisocial behaviours (e.g. shoplifting, stealing, lying and cheating – aggressive fire setters; Del Bove et al. 2008). Among peers, they experience increased levels of interpersonal difficulties, lower social skills, hostile rumination and peer rejection (Kolko, Kazdin and Meyer 1985; Chen et al. 2003; Del Bove et al. 2008). Indeed, young people that set fires have been conceptualised as a subsample of the conduct disordered population (Forehand et al. 1991). Fire-setting behaviour has also been observed to be significantly associated with hyperactivity (Kolko et al. 1985) and attention deficit disorder (Kuhnley, Hendren and Quinlan 1982; Kolko et al. 1985). Fire-specific variables with significant association, discriminatory or predictive value to adolescent fire-setting include history of fire involvement and excitement, interest and attentional bias to fire stimuli (see summary of studies by Mackay et al. 2012).

Young people that set fires have family histories characterised by instability, harsh or inconsistent discipline, parental psychopathology, parental alcohol misuse, parental violence, lower parental monitoring and disrupted family relationships (Moore et al. 1996; Bradford and Dimock 1986; Kolko and Kazdin 1986; Bailey, Smith and Dolan 2001; Becker et al. 2004; MacKay et al. 2009). Young people that set fires experienced more emotional neglect and physical abuse (Bradford and Dimock 1986; Showers and Pickrell 1987) and sexual abuse (Moore, Thompson-Pope and Whited 1996).

The associated variables represent the psychological and environmental context for fire-setting. There is an incremental link between the contextualising variables and severity of fire-setting. MacKay and colleagues (2009) observed an elevated profile among higher frequency fire setters on a wide range variables,[1] in comparison with those with no or lower frequency fire-setting (one to two instances in the past year). The number of risk indicators was positively associated with fire-setting. Previous maltreatment (physical abuse, physical neglect or sexual abuse) has been associated with increased frequency of fire-setting (estimated by caregiver) and versatility according to range of ignition and targets (Root et al. 2008). Sakheim and Osborn (1994) found young people who engaged in 'severe' intentional and purposeful fire-setting experienced higher concerns in a range of areas[2] compared with those engaged in 'non-severe' fire behaviour motivated by curiosity, experimentation, attention seeking or accident.

Identifying subgroups of young people setting fires and their different motivations

A number of authors have sought to identify subgroups within the fire-setting population. The categories usually discriminate groups according to motivation for fire-setting. For example, Fineman (1995) identified two subgroups: non-pathological, which includes accidental and curiosity-driven fire-setting, and a broader pathological group. The pathological group includes delinquent (including fire for profit and to cover another crime), severely disturbed (including sensory reinforcement controlled and self-harm), cognitively impaired, sociocultural (those that receive support for setting fires from within their communities and in civil unrest) fire-setting, and those setting fires to wild land or as a cry for help. Swaffer and Hollin (1995) interviewed young people resident in a secure accommodation service with criminal charges. All but one young man's reason for setting fire could be categorised under one of the following: revenge, crime concealment, peer group pressure, accidental and fascination.[3] The young man who could not be categorised by one domain reported fire-setting including both revenge and crime concealment. The Office for the Deputy Prime Minister (2002) describe the classifications used by the Arson Scoping Study for categorising arson offences as follows: youth disorder (children playing with fire and fire vandalism – an antisocial disruptive behaviour), malicious (fire used as a weapon, usually for revenge), emotional expression (fire used as a means of communication) and criminal (fire used to cover up evidence of another crime, and for financial gain).

A number of findings suggest the fire-setting by young women may be different to that by young men. Apart from lower involvement in the behaviour by girls (MacKay et al. 2009), qualitative descriptions include a less obvious decline in fire-setting prior to 18 years and include different motivations: seeking excitement, amusement and the 'bizarre'. 'Bizarre' included fire-setting motivated by expression, power and escape from reality (Perrin-Wallqvist and Norlander 2003). Fritzon, Canter and Wilton (2001) identified a theme of higher emotional and psychological disorder associated with female arsonists. Swaffer and Hollin (1995) also found the young women's motivation for fire-setting was different: an attempt to harm themselves.

It is probable that different subgroups are associated with specific contextualising factors. Motivational classifications such as 'severely disturbed' point towards emotional and coping factors, 'delinquent' suggests wider antisocial behaviours and pressures. Research studies tend to utilise broad samples of fire setters rather than subgroups within the population. It is probable that specific groups of fire setters share stronger association between variables than observed in the research literature.

In summary, clinicians assessing young people with fire-setting behaviour should be aware of the high prevalence and characteristic typology of adolescent fire-setting behaviour, and the psychosocial variables and subgroups associated with more problematic fire-setting behaviour.

Introducing composite case examples

To assist the reader in considering the different presentations and subgroups of young people presenting fire-setting, a composite case example are used. The case examples that make up the composite comprise elements from a number of real clinical examples and are therefore based on clinical work. However, given the case example presented is a composite, no one client can be identified. The cases used have been chosen to enable consideration of assessment, formulation and intervention, with attentiveness to the background research presented in earlier in this chapter.

Jake is aged 17 and lives with his mother. He has set fires on wasteland with peers, experimenting using paint, aerosols and petrol, and jumping over the fire. He is suspected to have set fire to a neighbour's shed; he was in dispute with the neighbour. He is currently supervised under a Youth Referral Order by the Youth Justice Service (YJS). He has not engaged with child and adolescent mental health service (CAMHS) since the age of 12, but has a previous diagnosis for conduct disorder and attention deficit hyperactivity disorder (ADHD).

The foster parents of Tom, aged 11 years, have found repeated burns to furnishings in his bedroom. He secretly collects matches and lighters. His drawings include repetitive elements of fire and the fire brigade. He experiences high levels of anxiety, difficulties in his peer relationships and has a diagnosis of autism spectrum disorder (ASD); the professionals working with Tom receive consultation from the CAMHS.

Aaron, aged 14 years, held a lit match to a hedge which caught fire. He and his friends attempted to extinguish the fire, but it resulted in damage. A complaint to the police was received from the home owner. Aaron has not previously received input from the CAMHS or YJS. He is currently attending school and a youth group.

Seth, aged 16 years, is currently in custody on a Youth Detention Order. He lit a fire in his stepfather's garage following a family dispute where he perceived his mother sided against him. The fire escalated due to petrol machinery. In custody, he appears anxious and reports being verbally bullied. He has threatened to set fire to his room and states he has knowledge of how to construct an explosive with the materials he has access to.

Assessment

The cases described may receive a variety of health services. Universally available health-care services, such as that of a general practitioner, might be sought in response to injury. Referral to a youth justice mental health worker might be activated through the YJS. Co-morbid mental health complaints may trigger involvement of the CAMHS in the community or custody environments. The health worker in each of these settings should include the seriousness of the fire-setting behaviour and whether further specialist assessment is required, either by them or a by a more specialist service.

Triage and assessment of fire-setting within a specialist mental health service requires information that is behaviour specific and descriptive of its context. A number of comparative sources of information are required (young person, their family/carer, justice organisations, including any accounts of fire-setting from fire agency investigations, education and mental health services). A young person's self-report of their fire setting behaviours may include minimisations or exaggerations, depending on the function their behaviour. Young people may not fully understand the impact and potential impact of their behaviour, or be aware of contextual factors that may be involved.

An initial triage for assessments should consider if the behaviour demonstrated constitutes fire play or fire-setting, that is, does the behaviour represent single-incident fire play without intent for damage, which is frequently seen in the adolescent population, or is the behaviour repetitive, or with intent to cause damage? What were the circumstances of the behaviour and the levels of risk associated? To what extent does the information indicate co-morbidities which indicate that fire-setting might be more probable to be repeated, risky or likely to become so? A thematic opinion should be utilised integrating different information sources and risk factors. A number of triage tools have been developed by different professional groups to assist in this process, although these have yet to be validated (e.g. Federal Emergency Management Agency Juvenile Fire Setter Handbook, see DiMillo 2002).

In the case examples described, only Aaron at triage would clearly not be referred for a forensic adolescent service assessment. For young people such as Aaron, who are identified as engaging in fire play or normative adolescent fire behaviour, the risks of this behaviour should not be ignored or dismissed. Rather, these young people presenting with a frequently observed behaviour without additional co-morbidity or risk indicators should be provided with an education-based intervention programme (more detail is provided under intervention) (Figure 9.1).

For young people presenting fire-setting behaviour or fire play with co-morbidities or additional risks indicative that the behaviour may escalate, a full assessment is required. This might be conducted by a forensic CAMHS. Risk-management contingencies will be required at least for the period of assessment (e.g. agreement for levels of supervision, reduced access to fire-setting materials). The assessor should work collaboratively with the young person, their family and wider services to implement this, and to begin to collate and formulate detailed information for assessment.

The assessor will address a wide range of variables. Below is a list of relevant areas but additional areas will be salient, dependent on specific presentations.

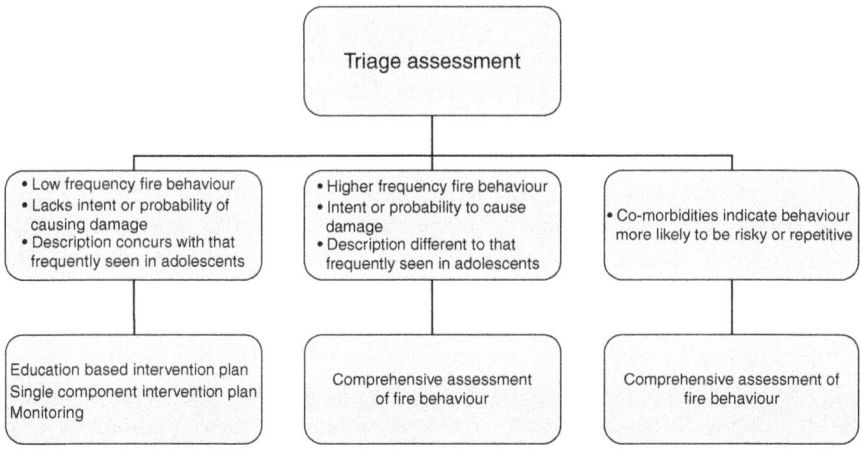

Figure 9.1 Triage assessment pathways

Fire-setting – All incidents known and disclosed, onset, frequency, timing, location of fire, method of ignition, individuals present, impact of behaviour (anticipated by them, and the actual impact and how discovered); potential impact of behaviour (e.g. risk to life and property); antecedents (including emotional and social); consequences (including emotional, responses by others); behaviour at scene of fire (e.g. watching fire, awaiting response of emergency fire service); and retrospective view on incident (acceptance of responsibility, remorse, learning, self-gratifying rehearsal or intrusive memories of the event).

Fire-related factors – fire interest, match play, fire play and experimentation with inflammatory items; involvement or interest with emergency fire services; presentation when discussing fire; undisclosed indicators of fire-setting (e.g. damaged furnishings, tampered electrical items); exposure to fire-setting and involvement of others; understanding of fire risks and how to address; and understanding of potential risks by carers, initial attempts to manage potential risks in immediate environment and willingness to engage in intervention.

Behavioural context – engagement in conduct-disordered, antisocial and reckless behaviours; impulsivity; rigidity in behaviour profile; substance and alcohol use; engagement in prosocial behaviours that may be protective; and engagement with authorities and support agencies (including justice, education and health).

Social context – peer relationships; experiences of marginalisation or bullying; exposure or involvement in antisocial peer groups; position in any antisocial or older peer groups or gangs (e.g. leader, conformist, subordinate); and emotional tone of interpersonal relationships (e.g. hostility).

Developmental context – ability to regulate emotions; ability to manage own recreational times; ability to self-impose boundaries and manage impulsive responses; ability to social problem-solve and apply social skills; ability to anticipate consequences of own behaviours; cognitive ability; mental health, neurodisability and developmental disorder; developing personality traits and temperament; and history of fire behaviour or injury by self or caregiver.

Family factors – family functioning, including relationships between adults, relationships between adults and young people, experience of abuse and disruption in family relationships, levels of supervision and support, approaches to managing behaviour, parental skills and barriers to appropriately support tasks of young adulthood, understanding and attitudes towards young person's fire-setting; and experiences of being 'looked after', residing in foster, residential or adoptive placement.

Community factors – levels of community disorganisation and crime, levels of supervision in community, recreations available and attended in local community.

A number of authors have sought to support the method of assessment through heuristic tools and checklists (see summary by MacKay et al. 2012). The Firesetting Risk Interview (Kolko and Kazdin 1989a) lists psychometrically supported items, which are administered as a questionnaire or interview to the parent. Results are interpreted by comparing sample scores for those with and without a fire-setting history, in addition to thematic analysis. A shorter version is available for children, and has good reliability and validity for use with young people aged 6 to 13 years (Kolko and Kazdin 1989b). Gallagher-Duffy and colleagues (2009) describe development of a Fire Stroop (stroop tests are commonly used computer based reaction time tasks to examine information processing biases) which enables assessment of information-processing bias for fire-related stimuli.

Formulation

Jackson, Glass and Hope (1987), in describing their work with adult arsonists, provide a developmental formulation that can be usefully adapted to young people. Figure 9.2 uses the template with the content adapted to consider issues more frequently presented by young people.[4] The antecedents 'Dissatisfaction with life and self' is replaced with 'Current lifestyle'. Many young people do not voice dissatisfaction with their life and some advocate that they value involvement in antisocial behaviour. The antecedent also attempts to highlight lifestyle aspects that are frequently reported by young people, or are of increased significance due to their youth, for example, use of alcohol and substances, involvement with antisocial peers, and disaffection or exclusion from local community activity and resources. 'History of social ineffectiveness' is replaced with 'Adolescent development factors' to enable focus on whether the adolescent is achieving developmental goals and to consider factors that might be specific to this particular developmental phase, such as neurological development, managing increasing responsibilities for free time and ability to self-impose behavioural boundaries. The figure omits consequences of restrictions severely limiting access to fire-setting and the opportunity to develop a more healthy approach to fire, which are more evident in high secure populations on which the model was developed.

Figure 9.3 provides an example of a formulation considering the issues presented by Jake, who was introduced in the case examples. Formulation of his fire-setting behaviour brings the proximal and distal contributing factors into clear focus to allow consideration of how these might influence risk appraisal and indicate intervention approaches.

An alternative model to that described for consideration is the Dynamic Behavioural Model by Fineman (1995).

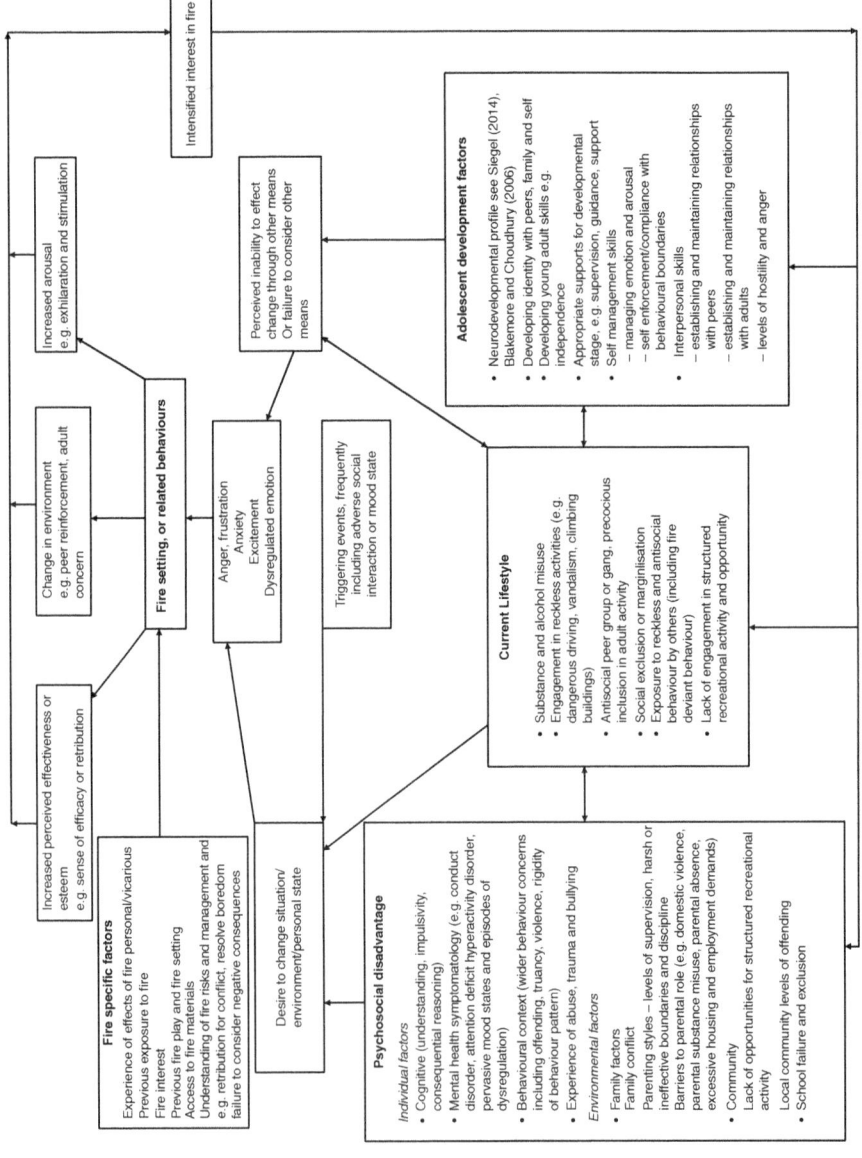

Figure 9.2 Developmental formulation

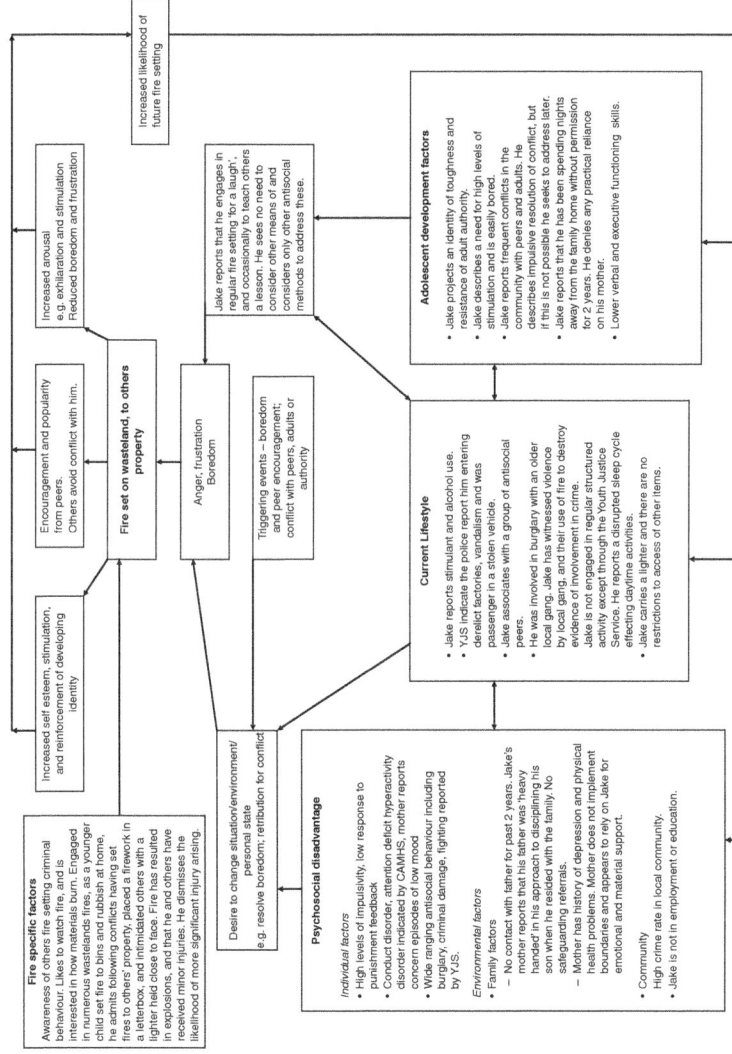

Figure 9.3 Formulating Jake

The formulation of fire-setting should achieve four key aims:

- Identify the presence (or absence) of evidence-based risk indicators (a description of these is included in the section 'Predicting risk and risk-management approaches').
- Hypothesise the factors predictive of further incidents of fire-setting (a description of proximal and distal factors likely to modulate the probability).
- Hypothesise those factors that are likely to be the focus of a successful intervention approach (both in short and medium term).
- Act as a template that can be modified to reflect new information and change over time.

In the developmental formulation adopted, each of these areas will be attended to and depicted in the diagram developed.

Predicting risk and risk-management approaches

Accurate prediction of recidivistic fire-setting behaviour is complex as there is a lack of a robustly validated structured professional judgement (SPJ) tool (Doley and Watt 2012; MacKay et al. 2012), and fire-setting is usually a low frequency behaviour. Sakheim and Osborn (1994) provide a worksheet covering 25 variables that they have consistently found to be associated with juvenile fire-setting risk, and 5 variables seen to indicate reduced risk; however, the support for this tool is limited.

Kolko and colleagues have conducted a number of studies on recidivism in younger children aged 6 to 13 years. Predictors include fire-specific factors (frequency, attraction, knowledge, curiosity, involvement, community complaints), child factors (hostility, externalising behaviours, covert antisocial behaviour) and family factors (lax discipline, family conflict, limited parental acceptance, family affiliation and organisation) (Kolko and Kazdin 1992, 1994; Kolko et al. 2001; Kolko, Herschell and Scharf 2006). However, given the limited evidence base, particularly for older adolescents, such predictors are unlikely to be applicable across all subgroups of young people. In clinical practice, adolescent risk indicators may include variables with empirically supported association with fire-setting, but that have not been demonstrated as predictive of future fire-setting.

Risk assessments of young people's fire-setting behaviour should be developed in accordance with national and professional guidance for best practice (e.g. DH 2007). A risk summary should include a summary of all risks identified currently or if escalation is likely (behavioural outline and potential consequences), the factors which are hypothesised to increase and reduce the likelihood of such risks (both short and medium term, internal and external factors). The conclusions of a risk assessment should be shared with the young person, their family and the services supporting the young person, to ensure awareness of concerns and to develop risk-management approaches. Risk assessment is a dynamic process. The risk assessment is only valid whilst conditions remain constant and not for a period longer than six months. The need to frequently review risk is even more pronounced in an adolescent population, given the rapid changes that are characteristic of this development stage.

Returning to Jake's case scenario, this indicates a number of risks: risk to self (through reckless accident); risk to others (through violence and fire); and risk to property (through fire). Fire-setting behaviour can be separated into functionally distinct behaviours, including setting fire for stimulation/arousal on wasteland and to discarded property, and setting fire for retribution/intimidation in response to conflict. Both can be increased by use of explosives and accelerants. Factors likely to increase the probability of stimulation/arousal fire-setting include substance and alcohol misuse, lack of structured activity/boredom, lack of supervision, encouragement by antisocial others. Factors likely to increase the probability of intimidation and retribution fire-setting include interpersonal conflict with Jake or his associates, opportunity for targeted behaviour, anger, substance and alcohol use.

Intervening with fire-setting behaviour

Reflecting the breadth of young people involved in the behaviour, and the different means by which the behaviour is brought to adult attention, the literature describes a variety of approaches that have been applied to intervention by both mental health professionals and fire service personnel. Fritzon, Cantor and Wilton (2001) highlight the fact that the subgroups deriving from the heterogeneity of those involved in fire-setting, and the behaviour evidenced, are likely to indicate the requirement of different intervention approaches for effective outcomes. The most frequently described approaches can be divided into the following categories.

Fire safety education

In 2002, more than three quarters of United Kingdom fire brigades ran some form of intervention or education programme (Office for the Deputy Prime Minister 2002). Fire safety education (FSE) provides instruction and practise in the dangers and effects of fire, personal safety strategies and prevention practices. Bumpass, Brix and Preston (1985) highlight the fact that fire services can be in the best position to offer an intervention promptly and with face validity for young people and their families. However, many programmes have lacked standardisation or evaluation (Office for the Deputy Prime Minister 2002). There are some positive indicators for the effectiveness of such programmes: for example, Kolko and colleagues (2006) observed in young fire setters (aged 5 to 13 years) that FSE impacted on fire knowledge and safety measures, and the frequency of reported match play and fires at a one-year follow-up. The approach can be provided as a single intervention or supplemented. Bumpass, Brix and Preston (1985) described how fire department staff successfully utilised a graph to depict the antecedents and consequences of fire-setting incidents. However, Adler and colleagues (1994), studying outcomes, were less optimistic about the impact of additional behavioural components by fire service personnel to interventions.

Behavioural and cognitive behavioural approaches

These approaches seek to functionally analyse fire-setting behaviour and to address the factors that control it and its opposing behaviours incidence. Early studies utilised behavioural models, including aversion therapy, overcorrection satiation procedures and contingency management, to facilitate appropriate behaviour incompatible with fire-setting. The studies supporting this tend to be based on single case studies, often with children younger than the focus of this chapter (e.g. Welsh 1971; Denholtz 1972; Kolko 1983; Wolff 1984; Daniel 1987; Hardesty and Gayton 2000). Similarly, there are early references to systemic approaches; for example, Morrison (1969) describes a family therapy approach to working with the system surrounding a 5-year-old with fire-setting behaviour.

More recent interventions tend to incorporate cognitive approaches. Kolko (2002) provides descriptions of a number of specific techniques that might be adopted, including graphing, affect identification, anger expressiveness and control, challenging distorted cognitions, problem solving and sensitisation to the negative consequences of fire. Kolko and colleagues (2006) observed that a cognitive behavioural intervention of generalised self-control and establishing environmental conditions that encourage behaviours other than fire-setting increased positive problem solving in children aged 5 to 13 years. Kolko (2001) found this approach resulted in fewer children setting a fire after treatment and less match play than those receiving a home visit by a fire fighter or FSE.

There is a lack of large-scale studies evaluating what works in addressing fire-setting in young people (Office of Deputy Prime Minister 2005) and no studies addressing the types of intervention that might be differentially suited to subgroups of fire setters. Choosing between the interventions outlined has frequently led to the following heuristic:

> FSE [Fire Safety Education] is more efficacious with children exhibiting heightened curiosity about fire or who are exposed to fire setting materials, and that CBT [Cognitive Behavioural Therapy] is more effective with

children presenting with heightened psychopathology or with dysfunctional parents or families.

(Kolko et al. 2006, p.228)

The authors, however, highlight the fact that the assumptions on which these statements are based have not been evaluated. Whilst it is recognised that intervention approaches need to be stepped in accordance with the level of risks presented, there is a lack of interventions for young people with more serious fire-setting behaviours (MacKay et al. 2012).

Integrated approaches

In clinical practice and with young people presenting significant risk, a combination of approaches is adopted and tailored to the specific behaviours and contextualising presentation. Interventions and risk-management approaches are underpinned by a multifactorial psychological formulation of the presenting difficulties. Examples of a few multicomponent intervention approaches are available in the literature. Hollin and Epps (1996) provide an example of a formulation-based cognitive behavioural approach. The Good Lives Model (GLM), proposed by Ward (2002), assumes those engaged in offending are seeking to achieve 'primary human goods', with offending behaviour the flawed attempts to gain these goods. The approach has been applied to a fictionalised case of a 17-year-old male arsonist. The application was to illustrate a step-by-step basis of how a multicomponent intervention plan can be designed and implemented to reduce risk of further offending and support new ways of living (Chu, Ward and Willis 2014).

The types of work applied in integrated approaches are likely to include adaptations and extensions to the types of work described in the literature. The areas of work include those completed directly with the young person, and those with the wider system (including caregivers and agencies). The system work is of importance in supporting individual intervention (particularly when accessibility and motivation of young people may be low) and in the management of risks. This support is likely to be essential in sustaining placements when fire-setting has targeted residential properties, or risked spreading to them.

For young people for whom fire-setting occurs within the context of a mental health diagnosis, attentiveness should be given to recommendations for interventions specific to the diagnosis. For example, Jake's fire-setting occurred within a previous diagnosis of conduct disorder and ADHD. The fire-setting intervention would best be positioned within an individualised multisystemic intervention for conduct disorder (NICE 2013).

Although idiosyncratic, interventions reliably include the areas detailed in Table 9.1. Sharing and developing the risk formulation enables a shared understanding of the fire-setting behaviour, a tool for communication with the young

Table 9.1 Areas of work for high-risk fire-setting, to be completed with individual and wider system

Intervention approach	Description
Sharing and developing the risk formulation	Development of an individual formulation of previous fire-setting behaviour, with consideration of how this might apply to future scenarios. The work should identify: situations, cognitions and emotions that precipitate fire-setting; the goal of fire-setting; behaviours involved in fire-setting scenarios; possible outcomes in short and medium term. This type of individual work requires attentiveness to ensure the accessibility of the approach. Some young people may wish to use images or writing to convey their labels for the contributing and triggering factors to fire-setting behaviour. The wider system also requires familiarity with the formulation, and opportunity to add observations.
Addressing proximal antecedent and consequence factors	The identified proximal triggers, including types of scenario, cognitions and emotions, can be used as targets of intervention. The target may be to reduce exposure to factors which increase the probability of fire-setting, or to change the response to exposure to these to reduce the probability that fire-setting will occur. Interventions can seek to modify the consequences of fire-setting. This might include addressing attitudes and emotions associated with having set fires or changing the response of the system to implement a new consequence, e.g. legal consequence.
Addressing distal factors	The distal contributing factors may have a less immediate or direct impact on the probability of fire-setting. However, attentiveness to these can increase the robustness of the overall intervention.
Developing protective attitudes and skills	Developing attitudes, behaviours and goals inconsistent with future fire-setting.

person and wider system, and a means of encouraging engagement in other areas of intervention. The later stages of the intervention comprise methods of risk monitoring and reduction, addressing the factors that are hypothesised to increase the likelihood of fire-setting in the short and medium term.

Returning to the case scenarios, Seth may benefit from an individual assessment to enable a comprehensive consideration of his mental health and functioning in custody, and to begin to develop the individual formulation of his fire-setting behaviour. It is likely that an intervention would include attentiveness to the triggering factors: interpersonal conflict, perceived marginalisation and bullying, anxiety and helplessness. He may benefit from work to consider how he responds to these triggers and skills to manage these externally and internally. Encouragement to reappraise the outcome of his use of fire to gain short-term empowerment to include medium-term consequences (i.e. authorities intervene, resulting in further disempowerment) may assist. The success of any individual work is likely to depend on wider systemic work to ensure, within custody, that any use of new skills is supported and bullying is addressed, and to consider the transition to a return to his home environment upon release.

Conclusions

Fire play and setting is seen among the adolescent population in relatively high frequency. The behaviour can be 'high cost', a cause of significant injury and property damage. There is a lack of robust tools to assist professionals predicting which young people will engage in higher risk or repetitive behaviours. Decisions about the probability of future risky fire-setting requires comprehensive assessment, psychologically informed formulation, and awareness of the available research literature on associated and recidivism factors. A range of interventions are proposed from which a stepped and targeted intervention approach can be utilised. However, much more research is required to support assessments in this area and the success of interventions when applied to different subgroups of young people engaged in fire-setting behaviour.

Notes

1. Binge drinking, frequent cannabis use, illicit drug use, delinquent behaviour, sensation seeking and psychological distress.
2. Strong feelings of anger at maternal rejection, neglect, abandonment or abuse; fantasies of revenge or retaliation; inadequate superego development; sexual conflicts or disturbance; identity confusion; sexual excitement or pleasurable arousal associated with fires; impulsivity; poor self-control; poor social judgement; rage at insults, disrespect or humiliation; fire preoccupation, attraction, curiosity or fantasy; past history of fire play; lower feelings of guilt, shame or remorse re: fire-setting incident; castration anxiety, fear of body damage; shows cruelty to children or animals; lack of empathy with others.
3. This category was combined with a denial of fire-setting history.
4. Many thanks to Dr Howard Jackson for his comments on a previous version of this chapter.

References

Adler, R., Nunn, R., Northham, E., Lebnan, V., and Ross, R. (1994) 'Secondary prevention of childhood firesetting', *Journal of the American Academy of Child and Adolescent Psychiatry*, 33: 1194–1202.

APA (American Psychiatric Association) (2013) *Diagnostic and Statistical Manual of Mental Disorders*, 5th edn. (DSM-IV). Washington, DC: American Psychiatric Association.

Arson Prevention Bureau (2006) 'Arson control forum annual report', *Arson Prevention Bureau*. Available at: http://webarchive.nationalarchives.gov.uk/20061209022624/ http://www.communities.gov.uk/index.asp?id=1504163. Accessed on 01 May 2015.

Bailey, S., Smith, C. and Dolan, M. (2001), 'The social background and nature of "children" who perpetrate violent crimes: A UK perspective', *Journal of Community Psychology*, 29: 305–317.

Becker, K.D., Stuewig, J., Herrera, V.M., and McCloskey, L.A. (2004) 'A study of firesetting and animal cruelty in children: Family influences and adolescent outcomes', *Journal of the American Academy of Child and Adolescent Psychiatry*, 43(7): 905–912.

Blakemore, S.J. and Choudhury, S. (2006) 'Development of the adolescent brain: implications for executive function and social cognition', *Journal of Child Psychology and Psychiatry*, 47: 296–312.

Bradford, J. and Dimock, J. (1986) 'A comparative study of adolescents and adults who wilfully set fires', *Psychiatric Journal of the University of Ottawa*, 11: 228–234.

Bumpass, E.R., Brix, R.J., and Preston, D. (1985) 'A community-based program for juvenile firesetters', *Hospital and Community Psychiatry*, 36: 529–533.

Chen, Y.H., Arria, A.M., and Anthony, J.C. (2003) 'Firesetting in adolescence and being aggressive, shy, and rejected by peers: New epidemiologic evidence from a national sample survey', *Journal of the American Academy of Psychiatry and Law*, 31: 44–52.

Chu, C.M., Ward, T., and Willis, G.M. (2014) 'Practising the Good Lives Model (GLM)', in I. Durnescu and F. McNeill (eds.), *Understanding Penal Practice*. Oxford: Routledge, 206–222.

Dadds, M.R. and Fraser, J.A. (2006) 'Fire interest, fire setting and psychopathology in Australian children: A normative study', *Australian and New Zealand Journal of Psychiatry*, 40: 581–586.

Daniel, C.J. (1987) 'A Stimulus Satiation Treatment Programme with a Young Male Firesetter', in B.J. McGurk, D.M. Thornton, and M. Williams (eds.), *Applying Psychology to Imprisonment: Theory and Practice*. n.p., 239–246.

Del Bove, G., Caprara, G.V., Pastorelli, C., and Paciello, M. (2008) 'Juvenile firesetting in Italy: Relationship to aggression, psychopathology, personality, self-efficacy and school functioning', *European Child and Adolescent Psychiatry*, 17: 235–244.

Denholtz, M.S. (1972) 'At Home: Aversion Treatment for Compulsive Fire Setting Behaviour: Case Report', in R.B. Rubin, H. Fensterheim, J.D. Henderson, and L.T Ullman (eds.), *Advances in Behavior Therapy*. New York: Academic Press, n.p.

DH (Department of Health) (2007) *Best Practice in Managing Risk: Principles and Evidence for Best Practice in the Assessment and Management of Risk to Self and Others in Mental Health Services*. London: Department of Health

DiMillo, J. (2002) 'Screening and Triage Tools', in D. Kolko (ed.), *Handbook on Firesetting in Children and Youth*. California: Academic Press, n.p.

Doley, R.M. and Watt, B.D. (2012) 'Assessment of Firesetters', in G.L. Dickens, P.A. Sugarman, and T.A. Gannon (eds.), *Firesetting and Mental Health*. London: RCPsych Publications, n.p.

Fineman, K.R. (1995) 'A model for the qualitative analysis of child and adult fire deviant behaviour', *American Journal of Forensic Psychology*, 13(1): 31–60.

Forehand, R., Wierson, M., Frame, C.L., Kemptom, T., and Armistead, L. (1991) 'Juvenile firesetting: A unique syndrome or an advanced level of antisocial behavior?', *Behaviour Research and Therapy*, 29(2): 125–128.

Freud, S. (1932) 'The acquisition of power over fire', *International Journal of Psychoanalysis*, 13: 705.

Fritzon, K., Canter, D., and Wilton, Z. (2001) 'The application of an action system model to destructive behaviour: The examples of arson and terrorism', *Behavioural Sciences and the Law*, 19: 657–690.

Gallagher-Duffy, J., MacKay, S., Duffy, J., Sullivan-Thomas, M., and Person-Badali, M. (2009) 'The pictorial Fire Stroop: A measure of processing bias for fire-related stimuli', *Journal of Abnormal Child Psychology*, 37: 1165–1176.

Gelhorn, H., Harman, C., Sakai, J., Mikulich-Gilbertson, S., Stallings, M., and Young, S. (2009) 'An item response theory analysis of DSM-IV conduct disorder', *Journal of Child and Adolescent Psychiatry*, 48: 42–50.

Hanson, M., MacKay-Soroka, S., Staley, S., and Poulton, L. (1994) 'Delinquent firesetters: A comparative study of delinquency and firesetting histories', *Canadian Journal of Psychiatry*, 39: 230–232.

Hardesty, V.A. and Gayton, W.F. (2000) 'The Problem of Children and Fire: An Historical Perspective', in D. Kolko (ed.), *Handbook on Firesetting in Children and Youth*. California: Academic Press, n.p.

Hollin, C.R. and Epps, K.J. (1996) 'Adolescent Firesetters', in C.R. Hollin and K. Howells (eds.), *Clinical Approaches to Working with Young Offenders*. Oxford: John Wiley and Sons, 197–207.

Icove, D.J. and Estepp, M.H. (1987) 'Motive-based offender profiles of arson and fire related crime', *FBI Law Enforcement Bulletin*, 56: 17–23.

Jackson, H.F., Glass, C., and Hope, S. (1987) 'A functional analysis of recidivistic arson', *British Journal of Clinical Psychology*, 26: 175–185.

Jacobson, R.R. (1985) 'Child firesetters: A clinical investigation', *Journal of Child Psychology and Psychiatry and Allied Disciplines*, 26(5): 759–768.

Jones, R.T. and Haney, J.I. (1985) 'Behavior therapy and fire emergencies: Conceptualization, assessment and intervention', in M. Hersen, R. Eisler, and P. Miller (eds.), *Progress in Behaviour Modification*, Volume 19, 128–135. Orlando, Fl: Academic Press.

Jones, R.T., Ollendick, T.H., McLaughlin, K.J., and Williams, C.E. (1989) 'Elaborative and behavioural rehearsal in the acquisition of fire emergency skills and the reduction of fear of fire', *Behavior Therapy*, 20: 93–101.

Kafry, D. (1980) 'Playing with Matches: Children and Fire', in D. Canter (ed.), *Fires and Human Behaviour*. Chichester: Wiley, n.p.

Kafry, D., Block, J.H., and Block, J. (1981) *Children's Survival Skills: A Basis for Functioning in Society: Final Report Prepared for the Maternal and Child Health and Crippled Services Research Program*. Rockville, MD: Bureau of Community Health Services. (This reference is no longer available but is cited by other authors)

Kaufman, I., Heims, L.W., and Reiser, D.I. (1961) 'A re-evaluation of the psychodynamics of firesetting', *American Journal of Orthopsychiatry*, 31(1): 123–136.

Kolko, D. (1983) 'Multicomponent parental treatment of firesetting in a six-year-old boy', *Journal of Behavior and Experimental Psychology*, 14: 349–354.

Kolko, D. (1985) 'Juvenile firesetting: A review and methodological critique', *Clinical Psychology Review*, 5: 345–376.

Kolko, D.J. (2001) 'Efficacy of cognitive-behavioural treatment and fire safety education for children who set fires: Initial and follow-up outcomes', *Journal of Child Psychology and Psychiatry*, 42: 359–369.

Kolko, D.J. (2002) 'Child, Parent, and Family Treatment: Cognitive-Behavioral Interventions', in D. Kolko (ed.), *Handbook on Firesetting in Children and Youth*. California: Academic Press, n.p.

Kolko, D.J. and Kazdin, A.E. (1986) 'A conceptualization of firesetting in children and adolescents', *Journal of Abnormal Child Psychology*, 14(1): 49–61.

Kolko, D.J. and Kazdin, A.E. (1989a). 'Assessment of dimensions of childhood firesetting among patients and nonpatients: The Firesetting Risk Interview', *Journal of Child Psychology and Psychiatry*, 29: 157–184.

Kolko, D.J. and Kazdin, A.E. (1989b) 'The children's firesetting interview with psychiatrically referred and nonreferred children', *Journal of Abnormal Child Psychology*, 17(6): 609–624.

Kolko, D.J. and Kazdin, A.E. (1992) 'The emergence and recurrence of child firesetting: A one-year prospective study', *Journal of Abnormal Child Psychology*, 20(1): 17–37.

Kolko, D.J. and Kazdin, A.E. (1994) 'Children's descriptions of their firesetting incidents: Characteristics and relationship to recidivism', *Journal of the American Academy of Child and Adolescent Psychiatry*, 33(1): 114–122.

Kolko, D.J., Herschell, A.D., and Scharf, D.M. (2006) 'Education and treatment for boys who set fires: Specificity, moderators and predictors of recidivism', *Journal of Emotional and Behavioural Disorders*, 14(4): 227–239.

Kolko, D.J., Kazdin, A., and Meyer, E.C. (1985) 'Aggression and psychopathology in childhood firesetters: Parent and child reports', *Journal of Consulting and Clinical Psychology*, 53: 377–385.

Kolko, D.J., Bridge, J.A., Day, B.T., and Kazdin, A.E. (2001) 'Two-year prediction of children's firesetting in clinically referred and nonreferred samples', *Journal of Child Psychology and Psychiatry*, 42(3): 371–380.

Kuhnley, E.J., Hendren, R.L., and Quinlan, D.M. (1982) 'Fire setting by children', *Journal of the American Academy of Child Psychiatry*, 21: 560–563.

MacKay, S., Ruttle, E.M., and Ward, A.K. (2012) 'The Developmental Aspects of Firesetting', in G.L. Dickens, P.A. Sugarman and T.A. Gannon (eds.), *Firesetting and Mental Health*. London: RCPsych Publications, n.p.

MacKay, S., Feldberg, A., Ward, A.K., and Marton, P. (2012) 'Research and practice in adolescent firesetting', *Criminal Justice and Behaviour*, 39(6): 842–864.

MacKay, S., Paglia-Boak, A., Henderson, J., Marton, P., and Adlaf, E. (2009) 'Epidemiology of firesetting in adolescents: Mental health and substance use correlates', *Journal of Child Psychology and Psychiatry*, 50: 1282–1290.

Moore, J.M., Thompson-Pope, S.K., and Whited, R.M. (1996) 'MMPI-A profiles of adolescent boys with a history of firesetting', *Journal of Personality Assessment*, 67(1): 116–126.

Morrison, G. (1969) 'Therapeutic intervention in a child psychiatric emergency service', *Journal of American Academy of Child Psychiatry*, 8: 542.

NICE (National Institute for Health and Care Excellence) (2013) 'Antisocial behaviour and conduct disorders in children and young people: recognition, intervention and management', *NICE Clinical Guideline 158*.

Office for the Deputy Prime Minister (2002) *The Burning Issue: Research and Strategies for Reducing Arson*. London: OPDM Free Literature.

Office of the Deputy Prime Minister (2003) *Arson Control Forum Annual Report*. London: OPDM.

Office of the Deputy Prime Minister (2005) *Evaluation of Interventions with Arsonists and Young Firesetters*. London: ODPM.

Perrin-Wallqvist, R. and Norlander, T. (2003) 'Firesetting and playing with fire during childhood and adolescence: Interview studies with 18-year-old male draftees and 18–19-year-old female pupils', *Legal and Criminal Psychology*, 8: 151–157.

Pinsonneault, I. (2002) 'Developmental Perspectives on Children and Fire', in D. Kolko (ed.), *Handbook on Firesetting in Children and Youth*. California: Academic Press, n.p.

Repo, E. and Virkkunen, M. (1997) 'Young arsonists: History of conduct disorder, psychiatric diagnoses and criminal recidivism', *Journal of Forensic Psychiatry*, 8(2): 311–320.

Root, C., MacKay, S., Henderson, J., Del Bove, G., and Warling, D. (2008) 'The link between maltreatment and juvenile firesetting: Correlates and underlying mechanisms', *Child Abuse and Neglect*, 32: 161–176.

Sakheim, G.A. and Osborn, E. (1994) *Firesetting Children: Risk Assessment and Treatment*. Washington, DC: Child Welfare League of America.

Showers, J. and Pickrell, E. (1987) 'Child firesetters: A study of three populations', *Hospital and Community Psychiatry*, 38: 495–501.

Siegel, D.J. (2014) *Brainstorm: The Power and Purpose of the Teenage Brain*. New York: Penguin Group.

Strachan, J.G. (1981) 'Conspicuous firesetting in children', *British Journal of Psychiatry*, 138: 26–29.

Swaffer, T. and Hollin, C.R. (1995) 'Adolescent firesetting: Why do they say they do it?', *Journal of Adolescence*, 18: 619–623.

Ward, T. (2002) 'Good lives and the rehabilitation of offenders: Promises and problems', *Aggression and Violent Behavior*, 7: 513–528.

Welsh, R.S. (1971) 'The Use of Stimulus Satiation in the Elimination of Juvenile Firesetting Behaviour', in A.M. Graziano (ed.), *Behavior Therapy with Children*. Chicago: Aldine Atherton. 283–289.

Wolff, R. (1984) 'Satiation in the treatment of inappropriate firesetting', *Journal of Behavioural Therapy and Experimental Psychiatry*, 15: 337–340.

10
Self-Harming Behaviour

Joel Harvey, Alison Sillence and Kirsty Smedley

Introduction

Working as a practitioner psychologist with young people who self-harm, in both secure and community forensic settings, can be a psychologically demanding but rewarding job. It is essential for psychologists to have an understanding of self-harming behaviour and how to carry out comprehensive assessments (including an analysis of risk), devise formulations, deliver – or oversee the delivery of – interventions, and develop safety plans. Psychologists need to understand not only the young person's individual and systemic strengths and difficulties, but, crucially, the context in which the self-harm takes place. Psychologists, as well as other forensic practitioners, must consider the function of the self-harm and think about how the function of self-harm may change over time and place. Indeed, young people who are in contact with forensic services may make transitions to and from different spaces. For example, they may move in and out of prison, or move wing within a prison, or move from a prison to a secure hospital setting. Other transitions may include being taken into care and moving to live in a children's home, or being asked to leave home by a caregiver and moving into hostel accommodation, or, indeed, sleeping rough on the streets. Young people who are in contact with forensic services often have a combination of enduring and complex social and psychological needs and multiple temporary 'transition' experiences, where they have to adapt to different places at different times. Different environments and carers will stimulate a range of attachment behaviours and evoke emotions in the young person, which they may struggle to manage. For example, a young person entering custody may have previously coped with their social anxiety by using alcohol – a strategy that is no longer available to them in a prison setting, resulting in the re-emergence of psychological distress. This can lead to the young person searching for new ways to cope with distressing thoughts and feelings, and often finding self-harm to be effective initially. It is the practitioner psychologist's role to understand the different social contexts in which young people exist, and how these contexts play a role in shaping self-harming behaviour.

Young people who have thoughts of self-harm, or who have self-harmed, become known to psychologists, and other forensic practitioners, at various times and from various sources. The issue of self-harm may become known through disclosure by a young person during the course of an assessment or psychological intervention. However, it has been noted that young people may be reluctant to disclose thoughts of self-harm to a mental health professional (Berman and Jobes 1999), and often the knowledge that a young person may have self-harmed comes from a different source. Indeed, it is often through the conduit of a positive relationship that the young person has built up with another professional that the psychologist learns about the current concerns in relation to self-harm. Or, it may be that a friend or caregiver has concerns and informs a member of the multidisciplinary team (MDT). This 'second-order disclosure' of course adds complexity to engaging with the young person, and there is a need for careful thinking, attention to detail and sensitivity, in order to ensure that the young person does not feel alienated or disempowered by the disclosure of another person, but can appreciate the possibility that others are genuinely concerned about their well-being. This is but one challenge that the psychologist must hold in mind.

This chapter sets out to examine the challenges and complexities of working with young people who may have thoughts of self-harm or may self-harm within the context of forensic community and secure settings. The chapter begins with defining self-harm and then moves on to consider the prevalence of self-harm. We will then consider the individual and systemic risk factors for self-harm, and think about where this information fits with clinical forensic practice. Following this, we will explore assessment in relation to self-harm before moving on to examining psychologically informed formulation and intervention. A composite vignette will be presented to elucidate core aspects of practice, and ethical considerations will be highlighted.

Defining self-harm

Harming the self can be a relatively normal feature of adolescence, and, arguably, adult life. Smoking, drinking alcohol, taking recreational drugs and engaging in risky activities like casual sex and driving too fast are often considered 'typical' teenage behaviour. Farberow (1980) defined behaviours like these as 'indirect' self-harm, where there is no clear self-destructive intention, but cumulative damage can be caused. In such cases it may be helpful to consider the young person as having a disregard for their own health and safety and perhaps placing themselves in risky situations in the knowledge that they may be hurt by their own actions or those of others. This kind of harm to self can be viewed as existing on a continuum with other behaviours that adults in society may consider to be quite normal. For example, drinking too much after a hard week at work, or working very long hours to cope with the break-up of a relationship. However, for some, risk taking can become more frequent and more harmful and can develop into more deliberate forms of self-harm. 'Direct' self-harm can range from immediate and intentional self-injury through to suicide. The most common forms of self-harm that lead to hospital admissions among young people in the community are self-poisoning, most commonly with paracetamol, and self-cutting (Hawton et al. 2010). Other forms include self-hitting, self-burning, self-biting, jumping from a height, head banging, inserting objects and scratching.

From the personal accounts of young people who self-harm, evidence suggests that self-harm can be a way of coping with overwhelming feelings in order to stay alive, or it can be meant as a way to end life (Walsh 2006). It can also be a way to feel again, in the face of numbness and dissociation, or a way to stop feeling. The different motivations behind self-harm have meant that there is no single recognised definition and there are a confusing set of terms: including parasuicide, attempted suicide, self-mutilation, non-suicidal self-injury (NSSI) and self-injury. Terms like 'attempted suicide' and 'parasuicide' seem to imply suicidal intent. Basing definitions around the presence or absence of suicidal intent is problematic because suicidal intention exists along a continuum (Harris, Hawton and Zahl 2005). It can be difficult to establish intention after the event, especially with young people, who may be reluctant to talk about their reasons, feel confused about why they did what they did, or be unable to remember. As a result, definitions for self-harm often describe the behaviour itself, rather than the motivation behind it.

The National Institute for Health and Care Excellence (NICE) has defined self-harm as: 'self-poisoning or self-injury irrespective of the apparent purpose of the act' (NICE 2004: 17). This guidance does not use the word 'deliberate' because acts of self-harm can happen out of the person's awareness and seemingly out of their control at times of dissociation. The purpose of this definition is to guide clinical care, and so a broader definition of self-harm might be more helpful. In contrast, researchers have used much more detailed definitions because these are more likely to be interpreted in the same way by different people and so have greater validity (Stanford and Jones 2011). The Child and Adolescent Self-Harm in Europe (CASE) Study was a seven-country collaborative investigation of deliberate self-harm in school children aged 16–18, with a sample size of over 30,000 (Madge et al. 2008). It used the following definition of self-harm:

A report of at least one of the following acts deliberately undertaken with non-fatal outcome: Initiated behaviour (e.g. self-cutting, jumping from a height), which they intended to cause self-harm; Ingested a substance in excess of the prescribed or generally recognised therapeutic dose; Ingested a recreational or illicit drug that was an act that the person regarded as self-harm; Ingested a non-ingestible substance or object.

(Madge et al. 2008: 669)

Both the NICE and CASE definitions encompass suicide attempts, as well as self-harm with other motivations. It must be borne in mind that definitions of self-harm differ and that these differences in definitions affect findings relating to prevalence rates, risk factors and reasons for self-harm. They also have implications for identifying people who have self-harmed. Defining and identifying self-harm is important: people who deliberately self-harm are at a much greater risk of suicide, particularly in the months following a self-harm episode (Cooper et al. 2005). Hawton and Harriss (2007) looked at mortality in a 20-year cohort of young people presenting to hospital having self-harmed. They found that 1.7 per cent went on to commit suicide.

Prevalence of self-harm

In a survey of over 6,000 school children aged 15–16 in England, 6.9 per cent said that they had self-harmed in the past year, and 13.2 per cent had self-harmed at some time in their life; similar rates have been found in Scotland (Hawton et al. 2002; Brock et al. 2006; Platt et al. 2006; O'Connor et al. 2009). A study of 30,000 European school children, using the same definition of self-harm, found an average prevalence of 5.8 per cent, with rates varying across countries (Madge et al. 2011). These large-scale studies relied on anonymous questionnaires. Young people were asked whether they had deliberately undertaken a number of different harmful behaviours (including: self-cutting, jumping from a height, overdosing, ingesting a non-ingestible object), with the intention of causing themselves harm. Around 45 per cent of young people in England who had self-harmed in the past year said they had wanted to die and more than half (54 per cent) had self-harmed multiple times. Self-cutting (64.4 per cent) and self-poisoning (30.7 per cent) were the most common methods. Only a relatively small number of adolescents who self-harmed went to hospital: 6.3 per cent of those who self-cut and 22.9 per cent of those who self-poisoned.

Self-harm is rare in children under 12 and then rates begin to increase sharply (Fox and Hawton 2004). A national survey of the mental health of children aged 5 to 15 in the UK found that 13–15 year olds were 1.5 times more likely to self-harm than 11–12 year olds (Meltzer et al. 2001). This survey found that the number of young people presenting to hospital having self-harmed increases between ages 10 and 17 for both males and females.

Young people seem to be at particular risk of self-harm. The largest numbers of females presenting to hospital with self-harm are in the 15–19 age group and the largest number of males in the 20–24 age group. Females in Europe were twice as likely to say they had self-harmed as males, and, in England, they were more than three times as likely (11.2 per cent vs 3.2 per cent) (Madge et al. 2011).

Research into self-harm in young people in forensic settings has found significantly higher rates than the general population, but the quality and quantity of research is limited. A recent review of suicide and self-harm in juvenile correctional facilities found 45 peer-reviewed studies, of which four were UK-based (Casiano et al. 2013). Between 2004 and 2012, 23 per cent of all recorded self-injury in prison was by 15–20 year olds (Ministry of Justice 2012b). Morgan and Hawton (2004) used the same definition of self-harm as Hawton and colleagues (2002) to measure self-harm in the community. They found that 15.6 per cent of adolescent males aged 16–18 entering a juvenile detention centre had a history of self-harm. This is double the lifetime prevalence found for males in the community (7 per cent). Suicidal ideation (13.2 per cent) was also higher than in the community sample (8.5 per cent). A major drawback to this study was the small sample size of 45. The study was terminated early by the prison governor, who was concerned that asking about self-harm would result in emotions and behaviours that the institution would be unable to cope with because of staff shortages. This highlights the difficulties in researching and treating self-harm in prison. A reluctance to ask questions about self-harm may risk failing to identify young people who self-harm or are at risk of doing so. Morgan and Hawton (2004) found that only half of the subjects who reported deliberate self-harm had this noted in their medical records. They point out that young people may deny or forget about suicidal behaviour when they are asked directly.

In 1997, the Office for National Statistics undertook a large study of psychiatric morbidity in prisoners, across a wide range of ages and categories (Meltzer et al. 1997). This study attempted to separate self-harm and attempted suicide. Deliberate self-harm was assessed using the question: 'Since you have been in prison, have you deliberately harmed yourself in any way but not with the intention of killing yourself?' (Meltzer et al. 1997: 8). The study found rates of self-harm ranging from 7 per cent for male on-remand prisoners to 11 per cent for female sentenced prisoners aged 16–20. Other studies have found that prisoners on remand are at greatest risk of suicide, particularly within the first seven days of entering prison (Shaw et al. 2004). The difference is probably because the question asks about self-harm 'since entering prison'. Remand prisoners have spent less time in prison and sentenced offenders will be including the time they spent in remand, making it difficult to compare the two. Results are also difficult to compare with those of community studies, which typically ask about one year and lifetime rates. The question also tries to rule out suicidal intent, investigating attempted suicide with a separate question. The highest rate of attempted suicide for prisoners was in the 16–20 age group: 28 per cent of male remand young offenders and 20 per cent of female remand young offenders had attempted suicide in the past year. Female sentenced respondents had a lifetime prevalence of a third for suicide attempts, twice that of male sentenced offenders.

Risk factors for self-harm

When considering 'risk factors' for self-harm among people it is important to recognise that young people are not 'mini-adults' and therefore we cannot simply apply risk factors from research with adults (see Chapter 1, this volume). Evidence suggests that stressful life events and broader social factors can be risks for self-harm in community and forensic populations of young people. Physical and sexual abuse, drug and alcohol use, time spent in local authority care and social disadvantage are risk factors for self-harm in both community and prison samples of young people, as is female gender (Hurry and Storey 1998; Meltzer et al. 2001; Koplin and Agathen 2002; Hawton et al. 2010; Madge et al. 2011; Casiano et al. 2013). These risk factors are at very high levels in young offender samples (Meltzer et al. 1997). A UK-wide survey of psychiatric morbidity among prisoners found that a quarter of adolescent prisoners had suffered abuse at home, 96 per cent had experienced a stressful life event, such as running away from home or being expelled from school, and 60 per cent had used an illegal drug in the month before coming to prison (Lader, Singleton and Meltzer 2003). Although fewer than 1 per cent of children in England are in care, 30 per cent of girls and 40 per cent of boys in custody were looked after children (LAC), even prior to their detention (Murray 2012). This suggests high rates of family disruption and trauma.

Experiencing the suicide or self-harm of others has been found to be a risk factor in community populations (Koplin and Agathen 2002; Hawton et al. 2010; Madge et al. 2011). Young people in prison are much more likely to know someone who has attempted suicide. Hales and colleagues (2003) found that 43 per cent of young men in a youth offender institution knew someone who had attempted suicide. Most of them had had this contact in prison, and the most important factor that increased the chance of knowing a suicide attempter was time spent in prison.

Exposure to violence has also been shown to be a risk factor for self-harm among young people in prison (Howard, Lennings and Copeland 2003). Again, this exposure is more likely to occur in prison, which has higher rates of assault than the community (Ministry of Justice 2012a). Thus, somewhat unsurprisingly, the prison environment itself is likely to be a risk factor for self-harm.

There are also a number of internal risk factors for self-harm. Research in forensic settings has found that severity of self-harm in young people is associated with mental health diagnoses including depression, anxiety and borderline personality disorder traits (Alessi et al. 1984; Plattner et al. 2007; Abram et al. 2008) and attention deficit hyperactivity disorder (ADHD). Psychological characteristics such as impulsivity and low self-esteem are also risk factors for self-harm (Plattner et al. 2007; Madge et al. 2011). Mental health difficulties, including affective disorders and personality disorders, as well as ADHD and impulsivity, are more common in young people in prison (Rohde, Seeley and Mace 1997; Fazel and Danesh 2002; Eme 2008). Moreover, self-harm has been associated with trauma-related distress (Weierich and Nock 2008; Ferentz 2014).

Self-harm is often used as a coping strategy to manage intense feelings and relieve tensions. A frequently reported motive for self-harm in young people in the community and young offenders is: 'to get relief from a terrible state of mind' (Knowles, Townsend and Anderson 2011: 487). Research suggests that 80–94 per cent of people who self-harm feel better afterwards (Bennum and Phil 1983; Coid 1993). Some studies have found that adolescents who self-harm use less effective coping strategies to manage difficult emotions than their peers (Evans, Hawton and Rodham 2005; Hall and Place 2010). Young people in prison who self-harm have been found to perform worse on a problem-solving task and commit more violations of prison rules than young offenders who do not self-harm (Casiano 2013). Chapman, Gratz and Brown (2006) point out that impulsivity, combined with difficulties generating other strategies, might increase the tendency to choose self-harm over more adaptive coping strategies that take longer to alleviate distress. Young people in a prison environment may have a greater tendency to self-harm as well as less access to alternative coping strategies, such as seeking social support, or distraction.

Young offenders serving their sentence in the community also have high rates of self-harm and high levels of risk factors. Knowles, Townsend and Anderson (2011) found a lifetime prevalence of 55 per cent for self-harm behaviour in this group. Chitsabesan and colleagues (2006) compared self-harm in community and prison samples of young offenders. This study found high levels of family disruption and mental health problems, which did not differ between groups; overall, 37 per cent had been in care and 74 per cent came from households where the family structure had broken down, whilst 31 per cent of young people were identified as having a mental health need. The community sample had greater needs in relation to substance abuse, possibly because of more restricted access in prison. Knowles, Townsend and Anderson also found high levels of substance use in young offenders in the community; over 80 per cent of young people had a history of drug use. However, in offender samples, they point out that levels of risk factors, like drug and alcohol abuse, family disruption and social disadvantage, are much higher than in community samples, so they are not as helpful in identifying individuals who may be at risk. In their relatively small study, none of these risk factors differentiated between young offenders in the community who self-harmed and those who did not.

Self-harm and social media

Knowles (in preparation) reviewed the literature on social networking and self-harming behaviour. She draws our attention to the fact that websites on self-harm have increased significantly in recent years and that these websites include:

> [Y]oung people sharing their experiences through personal websites, communication amongst those who self-harm in virtual communities (e.g. message forums) and major social networks (e.g. Facebook) and sharing videos and images through popular e platforms such as YouTube.
>
> (Knowles, in preparation)

On the one hand, it has been acknowledged that social media sites can have a potential positive impact for young people who engage in self-harming behaviour, but, on the other hand, it has been acknowledged that they can serve to reinforce self-harming behaviour (Lewis and Baker 2011). Given the suggestion that social media can influence young people in different ways, it is essential that we include it within an assessment of self-harm, in order to understand the potential role it might play.

Assessment and formulation

Psychological assessment is a dynamic and careful process that moves with the young person towards developing an understanding of their thoughts and feelings in relation to their behaviour (rather than providing a simplistic diagnostic explanation – e.g. you are depressed). The aim of an assessment is to develop a psychological formulation and to work towards developing interventions and a robust safety plan to ensure that the young person remains safe. A forensic formulation has been defined as 'a conceptual model representing an offender's various problems, the hypothesized underlying mechanisms, and their interrelationships' (Vess and Ward 2011: 179). A psychological formulation should:

> [S]ummarize the client's core concerns; show how the client's difficulties may relate to one another, by drawing on psychological theories and

principles; explain, on the basis of psychological theory, why the client has developed these difficulties, at this time and in these situations; give rise to a plan of intervention which is based on the psychological processes and principles already identified; are open to revision and re-formulation.

(Johnstone and Dallos 2006: 11)

A prerequisite to all assessments of self-harm is the need for the *service* in which the psychologist works to acknowledge that this is a complex and emotionally charged area, and that practitioners need support and guidance in understanding and responding to the needs of young people. The individual psychologist, or other forensic practitioner, in both community and secure settings, needs to be aware of the local protocols that are in place and have support from their host organisation so they do not feel isolated and are able to respond to the young person in a careful manner.

When carrying out assessments with young people, it is important to first think about the *manner* in which the assessment is carried out and how the young person is asked questions. Nixon and colleagues (2009) state that only a small proportion of young people will disclose self-injury. Bearing this in mind, we need to think about our interpersonal style in enabling young people to disclose. A delicate balance is required between carrying out a comprehensive assessment of risk, but, at the same time, not interacting in an intrusive and inquisitorial manner. It is therefore necessary for the psychologist to think about the pace of the assessment and the cognitive and emotional capacity of the young person with whom they are working. As in most clinical assessments, it is beneficial to use open questions, but it may also be necessary to intersperse these with some closed questions (which only elicit a 'yes' or 'no' answer); an assessment that is comprised solely of open questions may be overwhelming for a young person. Reflective listening and summarising back to check that the message conveyed by the young person has been correctly interpreted by the practitioner is vital, and demonstrates to the young person that an attempt is being made to genuinely understand their position. It is important to validate the feelings of a young person and not to carry out an assessment in a manner that feels rushed or leads to the young person feeling not listened to.

Also, the use of eye contact is an important consideration. Whilst making eye contact is a component of effective listening, it can also be intense, and for young people who have not had the opportunity to engage often in one-to-one conversations, sitting with someone making eye contact could potentially inhibit them. In fact, two of the authors, when working as part of a youth offending team (YOT), found that carrying out assessments in the car or walking along side by side in a park was often effective in terms of generating conversation and allowing a young person to express themselves. This also only involved making eye contact from time to time.

The place an assessment is carried out is also an important consideration. Community work allows more flexibility in this regard, and assessments can take place at the young person's home or public location, such as a café (following a risk assessment) or at the office base. It is important that the young person feels safe and that the service is accessible both physically and psychologically. Within secure settings, although the choices may be more limited, it is important to think about this too.

Areas of assessment

NICE (2011) put forward recommendations for assessing self-harming behaviour. The guidance states that an assessment should take into account the method and frequency of current and past self-harm, current and past suicidal intent, depressive symptoms and the relationship between these symptoms and self-harm, any psychiatric illness (diagnosis) and the relationship between these difficulties and self-harm, the personal and social context of the individual and any specific factors preceding the self-harm, specific risk and protective factors, the individual's coping strategies, significant relationships that might be supportive or pose as a therapy, and an assessment of immediate and longer-term risk. Similar to this guidance, Berman and Jobes (1999) argue that an assessment should be multifocal and should cover the following six areas: (1) imminent risk – evaluate imminent versus longer-term risk of self-harm; (2) lethality and intent – desired and expected outcome; (3) precipitants and predisposing factors; (4) psychopathology; (5) compliance; and (6) coping skills and resources.

It is important to establish intent and to gain an appreciation of the lethality of the method used. There is not a direct relationship between intent and lethality, and we therefore cannot use lethality alone as a guide for intent. Indeed, a young person may use a potentially highly lethal method but not have high intent, or they can use a method that has lower lethality but their intent to die was high. Both need to be assessed, but a direct relationship cannot be assumed. It is essential, however, that such questions are not asked in a rote-like fashion and that the young person does not feel interrogated. The psychologist must also begin to tentatively formulate the function of the behaviour.

When attempting to establish the function of self-harm, clinicians may worry that identifying how self-harm is helpful is akin to condoning self-harm. However, it is vital to demonstrate a compassionate and non-judgemental approach. Young people may have been told that self-harming behaviour is 'wrong' or 'bad' in some way, and this does not contribute to a shared understanding of the difficulty and may confirm or exacerbate the young person's already highly negative view of themselves, which may, in turn, lead to an increase in self-harm. Many young people who harm themselves have been coping in the best way they knew with emotions and experiences that they do not have the capacity to process. Recognition of their survival, by whatever means, is an important part of the engagement process.

As indicated, the assessment would also need to consider reasons for living, levels of hopelessness and depression. Asking the young person whether or not they have told someone how they are currently feeling is important and especially useful for safety planning. Indeed, knowing who knows and who does not know is crucial when thinking about *how* to share information and develop a robust safety plan. Another important area to examine is the young person's willingness to seek support from others. It may be the case that some forms of support are available, but that young people vary in their willingness to access such support. It is important to assess what seeking support represents to a young person and the extent to which they feel able to place their trust in others. These factors need to be taken into account in the case formulation.

When carrying out an assessment of current thoughts of self-harm and self-harming behaviour it is also important to know whether the young person has thought about self-harm or has self-harmed in the past. If they have self-harmed in the past, it is important to know how often they have self-harmed, if they can identify any further triggers, whether there have been times when they have felt in a similar psychological state but have not self-harmed, and any times when the self-harm is worse for them or times when it is better. It is essential that the young person is asked about this rather than solely relying on collateral information (e.g. from clinical notes). This new information, if it comes to light, can then be included within an integrated up-to-date chronology.

In general, whilst there does not appear to be any evidence to suggest that talking about self-harm increases the overall risk of self-harm, there might be times when the initial discussions of self-harm can itself be a trigger for self-harming behaviour. Although it is important to assess this behaviour, such an assessment must be carried out at a pace and level that does not overwhelm the young person. Indeed, the practitioner psychologist needs to think about dissociation and emotional dysregulation during sessions. The level of emotional tolerance must be gauged carefully, and it is the psychologist's responsibility to be aware of the young person's emotional and behavioural presentation during the session and to adjust in order for the young person to remain in a zone whereby they can tolerate emotional distress.

Use of assessment tools

There are some assessment tools available that may aid an assessment. However, these assessment measures should not be a substitute for a clinical interview. Clouther and Humphreys (2009) argue that using a standardised measure can aid case conceptualisation and that it might help the young person make sense of the function of their self-harm. Indeed:

[A]dolescents may not have a clear understanding of the functions of their NSSI if asked generally during a clinical interview; however, a structured questionnaire with multiple options may help bring to the surface the underlying inter- and intrapersonal dynamics associated with the youth's self-injury.

(Clouther and Humphreys 2009: 116)

The authors also highlight the fact that such tools can be a useful means of measuring clinical outcome. Clouther and Humphreys (2009) provide a review of different assessments used to evaluate self-injury. These include self-report measures (i.e. self-injury inventory, Zlotnick et al. 1997; Functional Assessment of Self-Mutilation (FASM), Lloyd et al. 1997) and structured interviews (i.e. Suicide Attempt Self-Injury Interview (SASII), Linehan et al. 2006). They identify that some of the measures can be used as a brief screen, whereas others can be used for a more in-depth assessment.

Response following assessment

During an assessment, when a young person indicates that they have had thoughts of wanting to harm themselves, or they have recently cut themselves, the response of the psychologist is important. It is therefore key for the psychologist to have reflected on how they might respond, well before meeting the young person. The psychologist, or other forensic practitioner, needs to think about how the information will be shared. From the outset, it is important to make sure that the person carrying out the assessment, and the young person themselves, are aware of the limits to confidentiality, and that if the young person is at risk of self-harm then information is highly likely to be shared. The young person's safety is paramount and, despite many practitioners' anxieties in this domain, this takes primacy over keeping information confidential. However, whilst acknowledging this, it is important to be prepared about how to speak to the young person about passing on information. From clinical experience, it appears that it is the *manner* in which this information is shared, rather than the *fact* that the information is shared that is most important. Choice can be given to the young person about whether or not they want to be present when information is shared with a caregiver. The young person needs to be made aware that the practitioner is (likely) working as part of an MDT and that this involves sharing information, but careful thought needs to be given to how best ensure that the young person does not feel embarrassed or betrayed when the information they have disclosed is then passed on to others.

Following an initial assessment, or at subsequent therapy sessions, a young person might disclose that they are at an acute risk of self-harm and an immediate response is required to ensure their safety. Self-harm often serves a function relating to the management of distressing thoughts, feelings and memories.

When the clinician explores the reasons for self-harm, as forms part of any assessment, this can evoke the same upsetting thoughts, feelings and memories that the young person has been successfully avoiding, potentially triggering further self-harm. Within a secure setting, protocols should be in place in relation to immediate risk management. For example, within prison settings the Assessment, Care in Custody and Teamwork (ACCT) system is in place, and immediate action might be taken where the practitioner initiates this process. Within community settings, local procedures should also be followed in relation to risk management. It is important for practitioners, who may be practising within an outreach model of service delivery, to have key emergency numbers to hand and to be aware of local accident and emergency departments.

When working in the community, following the disclosure of self-harm, it is important to develop a safety plan with the young person and their caregiver (or staff if they are in a children's home). Such plans might identify some early initial coping strategies, identifying sources of support, and have key contact numbers available. Such plans need to be carefully thought about and developed in the context of an early understanding of the function of the behaviour.

Case illustration: Assessment and formulation

The following case study is a composite, which reflects clinical work conducted with various different individuals over a period of years. It does not reflect psychological work undertaken with one particular individual.

Initial presentation

Emily is a 15-year-old young woman, admitted to the Psychiatric Intensive Care Unit (PICU) for the management of risk following an increase in her self-harming in the community, culminating in an overdose of 50 paracetamol. Emily was initially admitted to her local adolescent acute unit, but following two attempts to abscond and an increase in her self-harming behaviour she was referred to a PICU.[1] During psychological assessment she made little eye contact, sitting with her legs brought up to her chest and hugging them tightly. She stated that she had been self-harming for a number of years, probably since she was 13. Emily was very clear that she did not think her self-harming behaviour was a problem. She presented as highly ambivalent regarding the intent behind her overdose, stating that she did not really care if she lived or if she died.

Initial assessment

Emily expressed her reluctance to engage in a psychological approach due to her lack of trust in others and her doubt that any positive change could be achieved by this method. For this reason it was agreed that the focus of sessions would initially be to explore Emily's views and provide clarity about what psychological work might involve. It was also agreed that there was no commitment on her part to continue if she was not convinced after three sessions.

Background information

Emily was the eldest of two children born to her parents, Caroline and Steve. Emily had one younger brother, a full sibling, Matthew (aged 12). Caroline suffered from post-natal depression with both children, but this was worse following the birth of her son. Steve had always struggled to control his temper and angry outbursts were not unusual in the family home. However, when Emily was 8, her paternal grandmother died from breast cancer, and her father began to drink heavily and his angry outbursts worsened. He became violent towards Caroline. Over time, Steve became alcohol dependent and the violence increased – often witnessed by both children. Emily felt a strong sense of responsibility for protecting her brother, which was encouraged by her mother. Emily was often tasked with taking her brother upstairs when arguments between her parents started. On a number of occasions, Steve threatened his children with violence and Emily recalled running upstairs with her brother to hide from her father. Sometimes, much later when Emily was alone and in bed, she would scratch the skin on her arms and legs.

When Emily was 12 years old her parents split up. The home environment before the breakdown of her parents' marriage was frequently chaotic and explosive. Afterwards, Caroline and her children moved to a different area of the city, which involved a change of schools for both children. Emily was aware that her mother had been taking anti-depressant medication for a number of years and Caroline would regularly state that she was worried that she 'couldn't cope anymore'. Emily felt worried about her mother's fragility and strove to create as little stress for her as possible by keeping her own feelings to herself. She also tried to look after her brother as best she could, assuming a parenting role towards both him and her mother. Emily had always enjoyed the structure and predictability of school and relished the escape it provided from home, but she struggled to adjust to moving schools part way through Year 7. In addition, she worried about her mother and would sometimes go home from school at lunchtime to check on her, sometimes failing to return to complete the day. Contact with her father was erratic and Emily felt frightened of him, although she again tried to push these feelings down because her mother had asked her to 'be strong for Matthew'. Over a period of six months the contact dwindled until it no longer occurred.

About a year after the move, Caroline met a new partner, Rob, who moved into the family home within a couple of months. Rob had no children of his own and neither Emily nor Matthew got along with him initially. However, he shared an interest in football with Matthew and so gradually they became closer. However, Emily struggled to develop a relationship with Rob and she felt excluded and replaced. The role she had developed as a protector and carer for her mother and brother seemed no longer necessary. Emily struggled to establish a different role within her family unit and often felt distant from her mother, Matthew and Rob, and even a little resentful of their apparent closeness. She began to avoid coming home from school, sometimes hanging out with peers or just sitting in the park. In an effort to fit in with her peers, she started smoking and began to engage in minor anti-social behaviour with a group of girls – including shoplifting on one occasion and minor vandalism. Her mood dipped further and she began cutting on her arms and, on a few occasions, burning her skin with cigarettes.

During the third session of assessment, when the process of formulation was also underway, Emily became very quiet at one particular stage of the life path. Drawing a life path with a young person is a narrative approach used to encourage him or her to tell their story in whatever way they choose. Some young people choose to draw on their life path, whilst others prefer to write or have the practitioner write for them. They may choose to start at the present point and work backwards, or alternatively describe events at the start of their life and move forwards. It is important that any life path work is carried out by a competent clinician and that the pace of the work is reflected upon; it is key that this process does not result in the retraumatisation of the young person. During the life path work it was evident that Emily was not able to discuss a particular stage of her life, and so it was agreed that the session would end early. Later on that day, Emily became distressed and tearful in her bedroom and she disclosed to a member of the nursing team that she had been raped when walking home through the park, a month before she took the overdose leading to her admission.

Formulation

A psychological formulation was developed in collaboration with Emily. Despite her reluctance to engage in a treatment plan, Emily was curious to understand her difficulties better and she was a bright young woman with a good level of psychological mindedness. This made it possible to work on a formulation, and it was agreed that this could be a 'stand-alone' piece of psychological work. Emily seemed to feel more relaxed at the prospect of not being expected to commit to therapy and she proved to be a willing and enthusiastic participant in the process of developing her psychological formulation. Emily readily engaged in a narrative life path approach and information was collected over three sessions using this method. The following formulation emerged.

Emily's childhood was characterised by a chaotic family environment where anger regularly spilled into violence. This was accompanied by an inconsistent degree of care, with her mother being emotionally unavailable at times due to post-natal depression, which then developed into a longer-term difficulty. Emily grew up feeling responsible for others, uncared for herself and not important enough to deserve care. The arrival of her mother's new partner led to feelings of rejection, and Emily's previous role as carer and protector of her family was taken from her.

Emily experienced emotions (both her own and those of others) as overwhelming and uncontrollable states and so, not surprisingly, she sought to avoid them at all costs. As well as her observations that her father's anger was to be feared, she also learned to keep her own feelings held tightly inside so that her younger brother would not sense her fear and would believe her reassurances. Similarly, she felt the need to protect her mother who seemed emotionally fragile. This left Emily experiencing high levels of distress which she tried to keep to herself, struggling to regulate her emotions and having no outlet for them. Her experience of others around her was either as requiring protection or as frightening and unpredictable. This made it highly unlikely that she would approach them for help to manage her emotions, and confirmed to her that keeping her feelings inside was the preferred way of managing. However, as time progressed, this became more difficult as her levels of distress and anxiety escalated and she found them harder to tolerate. It was in this context that her self-harming behaviour started.

Establishing the psychological function of the self-harming behaviour

Emily was able to think about the function of her self-harm, stating that she often felt very quickly overwhelmed by distressing thoughts and feelings, and that when she first started cutting herself, it provided a way of 'getting rid of' these feelings. However, on admission, Emily did not view her self-harming behaviour as something she wanted to change. Assessment revealed that this was for a number of reasons. Emily was confident that hurting herself had proved to be an effective way of coping with distress over a period of years, which did not rely on any support from other people. Secondary to this, but becoming equally important over time, was the function of self-harm as a means of punishment. Since Emily's explanation for her difficulties was that she was to blame, finding a way to punish herself offered her temporary relief from guilty feelings. Emily also revealed that cutting herself had prevented her from trying to end her life, even though she had contemplated suicide at times, because she had felt she could manage her distress.

During assessment, Emily revealed that about 12 months ago her mother had found out about her cutting and had expressed anger and disappointment towards Emily. Since this time, she had developed more intense feelings of guilt around her self-harming behaviour. This set up a vicious cycle whereby she would cut herself to manage overwhelming feelings related to past events, but would quickly feel bad about doing so, with thoughts that she had let herself and her Mum down. These thoughts would trigger another episode of cutting in order to try to get rid of the guilty thoughts and feelings about the first one. Towards the end of the assessment process, Emily acknowledged that self-harm had become less effective over time and often the distressing feelings remained or only reduced for a short period of time.

Impact of sexual trauma

Emily had not disclosed the fact that she had been raped to her family or to professionals. She blamed herself, reasoning that because she had spoken to the man, who was initially friendly towards her, the sexual assault was her fault. Experience had taught her that others could not be relied upon to provide emotional support and that she was not deserving of care, and these beliefs directly influenced her decision to remain silent. She further isolated herself at home and her self-harming behaviour increased, with her cutting become deeper. She experienced nightmares and flashbacks of the rape. It was at this point that thoughts of suicide became more frequent and intense, as Emily struggled to cope with re-experiencing the trauma. She spoke about feeling out of control, expressing the view that the world and those in it were unpredictable and harm could happen to her, or those close to her, at any moment. Emily had long struggled with her inability to protect her mother from her father's violence and she held herself similarly responsible for the sexual assault she experienced. In this way, there was a cumulative impact of traumatic incidents, confirming Emily's view of herself, the world and other people. Emily recognised that feeling out of control with overwhelming levels of distress was a trigger for her cutting behaviour.

Environmental influences

As her admission progressed, the impact of the secure environment became more evident in the changes observed to her method and pattern of self-harm. The secure setting had significantly reduced opportunities for her to use cutting and burning herself as strategies. These long-standing ways of coping with distress were suddenly no longer an option, yet there had not been sufficient time to work therapeutically with her to develop an understanding of the psychological function of self-harm and consider alternative ways of meeting this need. Unfortunately, this led to her using more lethal strategies which she observed in other young people on the ward, for example tying ligatures and inserting objects underneath the skin on her forearm.

Interventions

Self-harm is distinct from other areas identified for intervention in that it represents a way of managing other experiences, such as anxiety, low mood, flashbacks, dissociation and emotional dysregulation, to name but a few.

Self-harm is often the result of a young person with limited coping resources and little support from others, coping in the best way they know how with overwhelming distress. The assessment and formulation process will lead to a detailed understanding of what underlies the self-harming behaviour, and this understanding guides the intervention. Frequently, young people express the view that self-harm is not the problem for them, rather it represents a solution, albeit often a flawed and temporary one, offering less and less relief over time. It is therefore important to be aware of this as interventions are developed. Within any intervention, it is important to understand the function of the behaviour for the young person. Indeed, 'Psychoeducation regarding NSSI in youth is considered an important aspect of treatment during the initial phase as a means to clarify and establish a mutual understanding of this behaviour among treatment participants' (Nixon et al. 2009: 221–222).

NICE (2011) state that the evidence base for self-harm interventions with young people is weak. However, they recommend 3 to 12 sessions of psychological intervention. Given that the evidence base is weak, the competencies of the practitioner psychologist are especially important here, especially the ability to develop a psychological formulation drawing from multiple theoretical frameworks to guide intervention. Moreover, NICE (2011) recommend that care plans are developed and that a risk management plan should form part of this care plan. Such a risk management plan should address each of the immediate and long-term risks, and identify factors that might increase risk, and develop a plan to reduce these risks. They state that a crisis management plan should be included, which includes self-management strategies and also how to access services. These plans should be driven by a multifactorial formulation.

Individual interventions

Hawton and colleagues (2009) carried out a systematic review of the effectiveness of psychological and pharmacological interventions of self-harm. They reviewed 23 studies that met their criteria and included all age ranges as well as both males and females. They found that problem-solving interventions reduced the reported reputation of self-harm compared to after-care treatment as usual (TAU). It was also found that dialectical behavioural therapy (DBT) reduced repetitive self-harm at follow-up. However, Hawton and colleagues (2009: 6) conclude that:

> [T]he results of this updated systematic literature review indicates that there still continues to be insufficient evidence on which to make firm recommendations on the most effective forms of treatment for patients who have recently engaged in DSH.

Additionally, Carr (2009) reviewed interventions that might be promising for adolescents who are suicidal. He states that DBT has been adapted for use with adolescents and there is evidence to support its use from studies with adolescents who have attempted suicide. Carr (2009) also notes that one study has found evidence for the effectiveness of cognitive behavioural therapy (CBT) with adolescents who have attempted suicide.

Less research has examined self-harm interventions specifically with people who have offended. However, Townsend and colleagues (2010), in their systematic review and meta-analysis of interventions relevant for young offenders with a diagnosis of a mood 'disorder', anxiety or self-harm, found preliminary data that CBT might be helpful. More research is needed to evaluate which specific interventions are effective for young people, and to also examine the role of working systemically with young people.

Systemic interventions

It has been recognised that it is important to work with caregivers, whether the young person is in a community or secure setting (Nixon et al. 2009). NICE (2011: 16), within its guidance, puts forward some suggestions in relation to family involvement. It is stated that 'CAMHS professionals who work with young people who self-harm should balance the developing autonomy and capacity of the young person with perceived risks and the responsibilities and views of parents and carers'. Vale and colleagues (2009) outline the fact that is important to promote a predictable family environment, improving interactions and communications, increasing emotional connectedness, and enabling developmental tasks and parental functioning. The family needs 'to validate emotional experiences' (Vale et al. 2009: 241). Finally, Carr (2009), in his review of interventions, found support for the use of a 'youth-nominated support team' (a manualised systemic intervention) and family therapy.

It is evident from the literature that there is a lack of clear evidence on the effectiveness of interventions for self-harming behaviour. Indeed, Ougrin and Latif (2011), in their meta-analysis of self-harm interventions for adolescents, conclude that 'there is no evidence of specific psychotherapeutic treatment leading to a better engagement than TAU in the adolescents who have self-harmed' (Ougrin and Latif 2011: 78). When thinking about carrying out interventions, it is important that the practitioner psychologist draws from multiple theoretical frameworks (e.g. behavioural, cognitive, trauma, attachment, systemic) in order to guide assessment process, interventions and risk management. Moreover, the pace and intensity of the intervention needs to be carefully thought about and monitored on a session by session basis. The young person's behaviour between sessions also needs to be thought about. This would help ensure that the young person is able to tolerate the intervention being offered and is being supported by the system around them.

Case illustration: Intervention

Psychological intervention

The process of working on the formulation was therapeutic in itself in Emily's case. It presented Emily with a normalising and compassionate view of the development of her difficulties, reframing them as a completely understandable response to her experiences and relationships. This was a new way of viewing her difficulties for Emily; she had believed them to be the result of a 'personal' weakness and 'not being good enough' (it is also important for us as practitioners to think about the role of diagnosis in contributing towards young people feeling 'not good enough' and thinking something is 'wrong' with them). This is not to say that Emily was accepting of this alternative viewpoint, rather she was willing to consider it might have merit. The process of formulation and the outcome were presented as merely one way of looking at things using psychological models and theories. It was recognised that there are other ways which also have value and that these could also be examined during the course of therapy – if Emily decided to engage in this next stage. In this way, the dynamic nature of the formulation was highlighted to Emily, which countered her worries about 'signing up to therapy' and her fear that a professional, theoretical understanding of her would be imposed upon her. Emily was invited to be a part of the process of continuing to think about her formulation, alongside what types of intervention might be helpful. She responded very positively to the idea of being an equal partner in her recovery and agreed to engage in therapy.

Emily engaged well in the treatment phase of therapy. A number of 'third-wave' cognitive therapies were used in combination. Throughout therapy there was recognition that Emily had coped in the best way she knew, that self-harm had played a part in helping her to manage her distress and that there was no judgement involved in presenting other ways of thinking about how to cope with her emotions. Using acceptance and commitment therapy (ACT) was central to this work. ACT is a newer from of CBT, which assumes that psychological pain is a normal part of human experience. Psychological distress is caused by upsetting and unwanted thoughts and feelings. The natural instinct of human beings is to struggle with these experiences with the goal of changing how we think and feel. Unfortunately, this doesn't always work. In fact, when we put large amounts of energy into avoiding or changing certain thoughts and feelings, it often increases rather than decreases our distress. ACT shows people how to let go of the struggle with their thoughts and feelings. In summary, ACT promotes psychological flexibility through mindfulness (connecting with yourself and the present moment) and acceptance (letting go of efforts to avoid uncomfortable thoughts and feelings), and values clarification (working out what really matters to you in your life). It is a highly compassionate approach (Harris 2009).

The formulation indicated that Emily was using self-harm as a means of regulating her emotions. This way of coping was rooted in her belief that her emotions were to be feared and avoided lest they prove overwhelming. It was important to target Emily's difficulties in terms of regulating her feelings, and also to target the beliefs supporting her decisions to self-harm. In order to give her a sense of progress it was decided to work on her emotional regulation first, as this was likely to yield positive results more quickly than working on belief change, which is a longer-term commitment. It was hoped that if Emily could learn some new ways of responding to her thoughts then she could experience a sense of being better able to manage them, instead of trying to 'get rid' of them. As PICUs provide relatively short admissions, with the aim of providing containment, the focus tends to be on interventions which support this process and enable the young person to move to a less restrictive environment as quickly as possible.

Alongside the ACT-informed components, a DBT skills approach was also used, with a focus on distress tolerance strategies. DBT combines cognitive and behavioural therapy, incorporating methodologies from various practices, including Eastern mindfulness techniques. Self-soothing is one of four categories of distress tolerance strategies. Emily was receptive to the idea of self-soothing, which was also a good fit with her formulation, because her childhood had provided very few opportunities for her to learn how to soothe herself and she had always focused on the needs of her brother. Self-soothing was explained to Emily as a means of comforting, nurturing and being kind to herself. She was encouraged to think of ways of soothing each of the five senses. This was a challenging exercise in a PICU environment because many items had been removed to reduce risk. Emily was able to identify taking a shower as a soothing experience. She liked to use shower gels and body lotions that were scented, and so the shower helped her to focus on the sense of touch and of smell. The importance of practice was conveyed to Emily and she agreed to try a self-soothing activity once a day. Emily was introduced to the idea of making her own self-soothing box, which she planned in a psychology session and then worked on with the unit's occupational therapist. Emily enjoyed thinking about the items she would like to place in the box and decorating the box itself.

Psychoeducation about emotions was a significant part of the initial intervention. This included the evolutionary origins of emotions and how emotions may be helpful in some situations and troublesome in others. Emily was also introduced to the idea that feelings do not control our actions.

Progress in therapy

Slowly and gradually Emily was able to consider the idea of 'making room' for some of her thoughts and feelings, which she had previously worked hard to avoid. This, together with the acquisition of new skills for managing distressing thoughts, resulted in a decrease in experiential avoidance. Allowing herself to feel her emotions was a very new experience for Emily, which was difficult at first. One benefit that became apparent to Emily was that the large amounts of energy she had previously put into avoidance of her emotions and arguing with her thoughts, could now be directed into new strategies she was starting to practise. She was now able to use self-soothing experiences when distressed, which also helped to reduce her dread of her emotions and increase her confidence in her ability to adjust her emotional temperature.

Mindfulness was introduced as a key idea and skill. Mindfulness is the ability to connect to your experience in the present moment. The rationale provided to Emily was that whilst it is useful that the mind can reflect on the past and imagine the future, this ability can also cause problems. Our minds can pull us back into the past to relive difficult experiences or push us forwards into the future, resulting in us worrying about what might happen at a later date. This means we miss out on appreciating the here and now. When this idea was explored further, Emily easily understood it and agreed to try some mindfulness exercises. This was approached in therapy as an experiment, which would help both her and the practitioner psychologist to learn more about her thoughts. This proved to be successful, with Emily being surprised at the thoughts that popped into her mind when she was engaging in mindfulness. This intervention was useful in two ways: firstly, more information was obtained regarding Emily's thoughts (she had previously experienced her mood as dipping without a trigger, as she had been unaware of what she was thinking). Secondly, Emily was able to learn ways of putting her thoughts to one side and returning the focus of her attention to the present moment.

Working with the nursing team

Emily agreed that her psychological formulation be shared with the nursing team, which was achieved through a formulation meeting. This dissemination of the formulation was vital in order that it become a living document that influenced Emily's care. It also proved useful as a two-way process, with the nursing team contributing to the formulation with information from their interactions with Emily. To further embed the formulation, the psychologist and nursing key worker met to weave the key ideas from the formulation into nursing care plans, which were reviewed with Emily regularly. Emily identified that evenings were particularly difficult for her and so an hour of one-to-one support was scheduled for her, which could be used for her to discuss her feelings with allocated nurse or to engage in a range of coping strategies or activities identified from a list made by Emily and her key worker. In this way, Emily's formulation became a team intervention.

Developing the team's understanding of Emily's self-harming behaviour was an essential part of the care plan. The intervention therefore did not focus solely on providing individual therapy with Emily, but included the system around

Emily. Work with Emily's mother was also indicated in this case. Emily did consent to sharing her formulation with her mother and, although she was nervous about her mother's response, she was also keen to be a part of this process. This occurred towards the end of Emily's stay on PICU and was a highly emotional session. Both Emily and her mother agreed with the team that they would benefit from family therapy when Emily stepped down to her local acute unit. Emily subsequently returned to the acute unit in her local area, which made it possible for her mother to visit more frequently and engage in family therapy, also involving Emily's brother. The psychological formulation was communicated to the new team continuing work with Emily.

Looking after the self

We would like to conclude this chapter by highlighting the need for the practitioner who is working with young people who have self-harmed to look after themselves. Indeed, Heath and Nixon (2009) have noted that 'several studies have demonstrated that even experienced medical and health professionals find self-injuring behaviour one of the most difficult and upsetting behaviors they encounter' (Heath and Nixon 2009: 146). Self-harm generates anxiety among friends, family members and professionals, and it is important for the practitioner working with the young person to be able to be contained, but effective, in managing risk.

The exposure to self-harm behaviour, either directly or indirectly, can be traumatic, and it is essential that support is available for practitioners working with young people who self-harm. Regular clinical supervision is a key component where the psychologist is able to be open and reflective in a contained space, and be held in mind by another. Peer supervision can also be a useful medium to reflect upon practice. Other than supervisory structures, working as part of a cohesive MDT, with clear ethical guidance, is crucial. It is important for the psychologist to have developed a trusted working alliance with team members so that they can work effectively and openly. Moreover, good inter-agency working is central: it allows for effective information sharing and the trust that safety plans will be enacted and that the young person will be worked with in a consistent manner. Professionals working with the young person and their family must attempt to create a professional secure base from which the young person can develop and realise their potential.

Note

1. Adolescent PICUs are few in number and are used as a last resort when a young person's risk to themselves and/or others escalates to the point that it cannot be managed in any other provision. The PICU is designed to provide short-term containment of risk in a secure environment.

References

Abram, K.M., Choe, J.Y., Washburn, J.J., Teplin, L.A., King, D.C., and Dulcan, M.K. (2008) 'Suicidal ideation and behaviours among youths in juvenile detention', *Journal of the American Academy of Child and Adolescent Psychiatry*, 47(3): 291–300.

Alessi, N.E., McManus, M., Brickman, A., and Grapentine, L. (1984) 'Suicidal behaviour among serious juvenile offenders', *American Journal of Psychiatry*, 141: 286–287.

Bennum, I. and Phil, M. (1983) 'Depression and hostility in self-mutilation', *Suicide and Life-Threatening Behavior*, 13: 71–81.

Berman, A.L. and Jobes, D.A. (1999) *Adolescent Suicide Assessment and Intervention*. Washington, DC: American Psychological Association.

Brock, A., Baker, A., Griffiths, C., Jackson, G., Fegan, G., and Marshall, D. (2006) 'Suicide trends and geographical variations in the United Kingdom, 1991–2004', *Health Statistics Quarterly*, 31: 6–22.

Carr, A. (2009) *What Works with Children, Adolescents, and Adults? A Review of Research on the Effectiveness of Psychotherapy*. Hove: Routledge.

Casiano, H., Katz, L.Y., Globerman, D., and Sareen, J. (2013) 'Suicide and deliberate self-injurious behaviour in juvenile correctional facilities: A review', *Journal of the Canadian Academy of Child and Adolescent Psychiatry*, 22(2): 118–124.

Chapman, A.L., Gratz, K., and Brown, M.Z. (2006) 'Solving the puzzle of deliberate self-harm: The experiential avoidance model', *Behaviour Research and Therapy*, 44: 371–394.

Chitsabesan, P., Kroll, L., Bailey, S., Kenning, C., Sneider, S., MacDonald, W., and Theodosiou, L. (2006) 'Mental health needs of young offenders in custody and in the community', *British Journal of Psychiatry*, 188: 534–540.

Clouther, P. and Humphreys, L. (2009) 'Measurement of Nonsuicidal Self-Injury in Adolescent', in M.K. Nixon and N.L. Heath (eds.), *Self-Injury in Youth: The Essential Guide to Assessment and Intervention*. Abingdon: Routledge, 115–142.

Coid, J.W. (1993) 'An affective syndrome in psychopaths with borderline personality disorder?', *British Journal of Psychiatry*, 162: 641–650.

Cooper, J., Kapur, N., Webb, R., Lawlor, M., Guthrie, E., Mackway-Jones, K., and Appleby, L. (2005) 'Suicide after deliberate self-harm: A 4-year cohort study', *American Journal of Psychiatry*, 162(2): 297–303.

Eme, R.F. (2008) 'Attention-deficit/hyperactivity disorder and the juvenile justice system', *Journal of Forensic Psychology Practice*, 8(2): 174–185.

Evans, E., Hawton, K., and Rodham, K. (2005) 'In what ways are adolescents who engage in self-harm or experience thoughts of self-harm different in terms of helpseeking, communication and coping?', *Journal of Adolescence*, 28: 573–587.

Farberow, N.L. (ed.) (1980) *The Many Faces of Suicide: Indirect Self-Destructive Behaviour*. New York: McGraw-Hill.

Fazel, S. and Danesh, J. (2002) 'Serious mental disorder in 23,000 prisoners: A systematic review of 62 surveys', *Lancet*, 359: 545–550.

Ferentz, L. (2014) *Treating Self-Destructive Behaviors in Trauma Survivors: A Clinician's Guide*. Abingdon: Routledge.

Fox, C. and Hawton, K. (2004) *Deliberate Self-Harm in Adolescence*. London: Jessica Kingsley.

Hales, H., Davison, S., Misch, P., and Taylor, P.J. (2003) 'Young male prisoners in a young offenders' institution: Their contact with suicidal behaviour by others', *Journal of Adolescence*, 26: 667–685.

Hall, B. and Place, M. (2010) 'Cutting to cope: A modern adolescent phenomenon', *Child: Care, Health and Development*, 36: 623–629.

Harris, L., Hawton, K., and Zahl, D. (2005) 'Value of measuring suicidal intent in the assessment of people attending hospital following self-poisoning or self-injury', *British Journal of Psychiatry*, 86: 60–66.

Harris, R. (2009) *ACT Made Simple: An Easy-to-Read Primer on Acceptance and Commitment Therapy.* Oakland, CA: New Harbinger Publications, Inc.

Hawton, K. and Harriss, L. (2007) 'Deliberate self-harm in young people: Characteristics and subsequent mortality in a 20-year cohort of patients presenting to hospital', *Journal of Clinical Psychiatry*, 68(10): 1574–1583.

Hawton, K., Rodham, K., Evans, E., and Weatherall, R. (2002) 'Deliberate self-harm in adolescents: Self-report survey in schools in England', *British Medical Journal*, 325: 1207–1211.

Hawton, K., Townsend, E., Arensman, E., Gunnell, D., Hazell, P., House, A., and van Heeringen, K. (2009) *Psychosocial and Pharmacological Treatments for Deliberate Self-Harm*, Cochrane Review. Chichester: Wiley.

Hawton, K., Casey, D., Bale, E., Rutherford, D., Bergen, H., Simkin, S., Brand, F., and Lascelles, K. (2010) *Self-Harm in Oxford 2010.* Oxford: Centre for Suicide Research.

Heath, N.L. and Nixon, M.K.(2009) 'Assessment of Nonsuicidal Self-Injury in Youth', in M.K. Nixon and N.L. Heath (eds.), *Self-Injury in Youth: The Essential Guide to Assessment and Intervention.* Abingdon: Routledge, 143–170.

Howard, J., Lennings, C.J., and Copeland, J. (2003) 'Suicidal behaviour in a young offender population', *Crisis*, 24(3): 98–104.

Hurry, J. and Storey, P. (1998) *Deliberate Self-Harm in Young People: The Hospital Response: Final Report to the Department of Health.* London: HMSO.

Johnstone, L. and Dallos, R. (2006) 'Introduction to Formulation', in L. Johnstone and R. Dallos (eds.), *Formulation in Psychology and Psychotherapy.* London: Routledge, 1–16.

Knowles, S., Townsend, E., and Anderson, M. (2011) 'Factors associated with self-harm in community-based young offenders: The importance of psychological variables', *Journal of Forensic Psychiatry & Psychology*, 22(4): 479–495.

Koplin, B. and Agathen, J. (2002) 'Suicidality in children and adolescents: A review', *Current Opinion in Pediatrics*, 14: 713–717.

Lader, D., Singleton, N., and Meltzer, H. (2000) *Psychiatric Morbidity among Young Offenders in England and Wales*, London: National Statistics.

Lewis, S.P. and Baker, T.G. (2011) 'The possible risks of self-injury web sites: A content analysis', *Archives of Suicide Research*, 15(4): 390–396.

Linehan, M.M., Comtois, K.A., Brown, M.Z., Heard, H.L., and Wagner, A. (2006) 'Suicide-attempt self-injury interview (SASII): Development, reliability and validity of a scale to assess suicide attempts and intentional self-injury', *Psychological Assessment*, 18: 303–312.

Lloyd, E.E., Kelly, M.L., and Hope, T. (1997) 'Self-mutilation in a community sample of adolescents: Descriptive characteristics and provisional prevalence rates'. Poster presentation at the Annual Meeting of the Society of Behavioral Medicine, New Orleans.

Madge, N., Hewitt, A., Hawton, K., de Wilde, E. J., Corcoran, P., Fekete, S., et al. (2008) 'The prevalence of deliberate self-harm within an international community sample of young people: Findings from the Child & Adolescent Selfharm in Europe (CASE) Study,' *Journal of Child Psychology and Psychiatry*, 49 (6): 667–677.

Madge, N., Hawton, K., McMahon, E., Corcoran, P., De Leo, D., de Wilde, E., and Arensman, E. (2011) 'Psychological characteristics, stressful life events and deliberate self-harm: Findings from the child & adolescent self-harm in Europe (CASE) study (2011)', *European Child and Adolescent Psychiatry*, 20: 499–508.

Meltzer, H., Harrington, R., Goodman, R., and Jenkins, R. (2001) *Children and Adolescents who Try to Harm, Hurt or Kill Themselves*. Newport: Office for National Statistics.

Meltzer, H., Jenkins, R., Singleton, N., Charlton, J., and Yar, M. (1997) *Non-Fatal Suicidal Behaviour among Prisoners: Report Based on Secondary Analysis of the ONS Survey of Psychiatric Morbidity among Prisoners in England and Wales Carried Out in 1997 for the Department of Health*. London: Office for National Statistics.

Ministry of Justice (2012a) *Safety in Custody Statistics England and Wales: Update to December 2012*. London: Ministry of Justice.

Ministry of Justice (2012b). 'Self-harm in prison custody 2004–2012', MS Excel Spreadsheet, *GOV.UK*. Available at: https://www.gov.uk/government/publications/safety-in-custody. Accessed 26 January 2015.

Morgan, J. and Hawton, K. (2004) 'Self-reported suicidal behaviour in juvenile offenders in custody', *Crisis*, 25(1): 8–11.

Murray, R. (2012) *Children and Young People in Custody 2011–2012*. London: HM Inspectorate of Prisons and Youth Justice Board.

NICE (National Institute for Health and Care Excellence) (2004) 'Self-harm: The short-term physical and psychological management and secondary prevention of self-harm in primary and secondary care. NICE clinical guidelines 16', *NICE*. Available at: http://www.nice.org.uk/CG16. Accessed on 1 May 2015.

NICE (National Institute for Health and Care Excellence) (2011) 'Self-harm: Long-term management. NICE clinical guidelines 133', *NICE*. Available at: http://www.nice.org.uk/guidance/cg133. Accessed on 1 May 2015.

Nixon, M.K., Aulakh, H., Townsend, L., and Atherton, M. (2009) 'Psychosocial Interventions for Adolescents', in M.K. Nixon and N.L. Heath (eds.), *Self-Injury in Youth: The Essential Guide to Assessment and Intervention*. Abingdon: Routledge, 217–236.

O'Connor, R.C., Rasmussen, S., Miles, J., and Hawton, K. (2009) 'Self-harm in adolescents: Self-report survey in schools in Scotland', *British Journal of Psychiatry*, 194: 68–72.

Ougrin, D. and Latif, S. (2011) 'Specific psychological treatment versus treatment as usual in adolescents with self-harm: Systematic review and meta-analysis', *Crisis: The Journal of Crisis Intervention and Suicide Prevention*, 32(2): 74.

Platt, S., Mclean, J., McCollam, A., Blarney, A., Mackenzie, M., McDaid, D. and Woodhouse, A. (2006) *Evaluation of the First Phase of Choose Life: The National Strategy and Action Plan to Prevent Suicide in Scotland*. Edinburgh: Scottish Executive Social Research.

Plattner, B., The, S.S., Kraemer, H.C., Williams, R.P., Bauer, S.M., Kindler, J, and Steiner, H. (2007) 'Suicidality, psychopathology, and gender in incarcerated adolescents in Austria', *Journal of Clinical Psychiatry*, 68(10): 1593–1600.

Rohde, P., Seeley, J.R., and Mace, D.E. (1997) 'The association of psychiatric disorders with suicide attempts in a juvenile delinquent sample', *Criminal Behavior and Mental Health*, 7: 187–200.

Shaw, J., Baker, D., Hunt, I.M., Moloney, A., and Appleby, L. (2004) 'Suicide by prisoners: National clinical survey', *British Journal of Psychiatry*, 184: 263–267.

Stanford, S. and Jones, M.P. (2011) 'How much detail needs to be elucidated in self-harm research?', *Empirical Research*, 39: 504–513.

Townsend, E., Walker, D., Sargeant, S., Vostanis, P., Hawton, K., Stocker, O., and Sithole, J. (2010) 'Systematic review and meta-analysis of interventions relevant for young offenders with mood disorders, anxiety disorders, or self-harm', *Journal of Adolescence*, 33: 9–20.

Vale, H., Nixon, M.K., and Kucharski, A. (2009) 'Working with Families and Adolescents with NSSI', in M.K. Nixon and N.L. Heath (eds.), *Self-Injury in Youth: The Essential Guide to Assessment and Intervention*. Abingdon: Routledge, 237–256.

Vess, J. and Ward, T. (2011) 'Sexual Offenses against Children', in P. Sturmey and M. McMurran (eds.), *Forensic Case Formulation*. Oxford: Wiley, 175–194.

Walsh, B. (2006) *Treating Self-Injury: A Practical Guide*. London: Guilford Press.

Weierich, M.R. and Nock, M.K. (2008) 'Posttraumatic stress symptoms mediate the relation between childhood sexual abuse and nonsuicidal self-injury', *Journal of Consulting and Clinical Psychology*, 76(1): 39–44.

Zlotnick, C., Shea, M.T., Recupero, P., Bidadi, K., Pearlstein, T., and Brown, P. (1997) 'Trauma, dissociation, impulsivity, and self-mutilation in substance misuse patients', *American Journal of Orthopsychiatry*, 67: 650–654.

11
Substance Misuse

Lisa Shostak and Ben Harper

The association between substance use and criminality is well established (for a meta-analysis see Bennett, Holloway and Farrington 2008). While the association is internationally accepted, the relationship between them is highly complex (e.g. Welte et al. 2005; Seddon 2006). Numerous factors have been evidenced to be associated with both criminality and substance misuse (SM), factors such as: lack of parental monitoring and supervision (e.g. Farrington and Hawkins 1991; Barnes et al. 2000), time spent with anti-social peers (Patterson and Yoerger 1997) and childhood hyperactive behaviour (Eklund and Klinteberg 2003). The presence of multiple overlapping factors highlights the importance of considering the broader picture when addressing SM within the offending population in general, rather than focusing on either SM or offending in isolation.

In terms of the relationship between SM and offending within the youth justice system (YJS) in the UK, the literature is very limited. The majority of work exploring the association between SM and criminality has been undertaken with adult populations and often in the United States of America. Therefore, the exact nature of any pattern and causal pathways are far from clear within the youth offending population. What is clear, however, is that there is a significant proportion of the youth offending population, both within the UK and internationally, for whom SM is both present and problematic (e.g. Dolan et al. 1999; Robertson et al. 2004; Chitsabesan et al. 2006). Studies within the UK have indicated that young people within the YJS are more likely than their peers to have SM difficulties (Hammersley, Marsland and Reid 2003). Regardless of the initial relationship, there is some evidence that engagement with SM intervention can lead to a drop in self-reported criminal activity (Farabee et al. 2001; Henggeler et al. 2002; Jainchill et al. 2005).

The term 'substance misuse' throughout the chapter will be used to describe the use of illegal substances and/or alcohol that is at a level where it has become problematic to the individual involved.

Outline of the chapter

This chapter aims to summarise the type of services in the UK currently offered and/or made mandatory for young people with SM difficulties who are also involved with youth justice services. Prevalence data and the difficulties in establishing this will be discussed, followed by an outline of the legal classification and consequences for engaging with the various illegal substances. The chapter will then move on to explore the current policy guidelines and evidence base with regards assessment and interventions available for this population. Arguments will be made for the importance of basing all treatment plans on thorough multi-systemic formulations in order to drive appropriately individualised treatment and enhance efficacy of any intervention. Finally, an illustrative case study will be provided to reflect on some of the possibilities, but also challenges, when working with young people who engage in SM.

This chapter will attempt to focus on the most common presentations of young people who misuse substances seen within youth justice services in the UK. These common presentations include those who use cannabis, cocaine and alcohol. Individuals who use intravenous drugs such as heroin will not be discussed explicitly. However, the principles of individual formulation of the multiple factors contributing to the behaviour observed, and the subsequent application of evidence-based interventions to address the factors identified, is in every way as valid for this population (the key difference being an acknowledgement of physical addiction as one of the factors and the necessity to seek medical advice when addressing this directly).

The UK context

There is national recognition of the need for specialist SM services for adolescents, both within and outside the YJS (YJB 2008; NTA 2012). The National Treatment Agency (NTA) is the strategic lead of SM treatment and data monitoring in England, and their data indicates that the number of under-18s accessing specialist services for drug and alcohol misuse in 2010–2011 was 21,955. This is thought to be an underestimate as, for example, it excludes young substance users attending other services such as child and adolescent mental health services (CAMHS).

It is also nationally recognised that young people with SM difficulties often have multiple difficulties and their needs fall across a wide range of services (Home Office 2010). Young people with SM difficulties are likely to have complex difficulties which require the input of, and hence the need for, joined-up working between health, social care, education, employment, housing and youth justice services (Home Office 2010). Clinicians may encounter young people with these difficulties in a wide variety of settings. Where young people initially present may depend, in large part, on what need was observed to be most prominent at any given point in time (e.g. local council housing services if the young person is homeless; social care services if there are difficulties within the family home; or CAMHS if the young person has co-morbid mental health concerns and so on).

Within both community and secure settings within the UK, there is government recognition of the need for access to SM services for this population (YJB 2006). Nonetheless, a national audit of services indicated that recognition of drug and alcohol difficulties by staff was variable, and that although there was consistent access to at least some provision, the professional background and training of those employed to provide intervention was also varied (YJB 2006). Current national guidelines provided by the YJB advocate for ensuring that young people have access to a specialist SM worker at all times when within the YJS, and that this person be trained in and have specialist skills in working with SM in this population (YJB 2004, 2006)

Some young people may be 'ordered' to access SM services via formal court proceedings and their engagement may not be voluntary. Whilst clinicians often have concerns that this group of young people appear to experience increased antipathy and ambivalence towards SM intervention, the evidence from adult studies suggests that outcomes for this 'coerced' group are just as positive as those who are 'voluntarily' engaged in treatment (e.g. McSweeney et al. 2007).

At this point, it is perhaps worth noting that being within the YJS should not prohibit young people from also being able to access mainstream CAMHS in the UK, and nor should SM interventions within youth justice settings be withheld due to concerns about co-morbid mental health conditions. It is not unusual for young people who are misusing substances to also be experiencing emotional distress, and indeed it is generally accepted that mental health difficulties are a key factor in increasing the risk of SM and vice versa (e.g. Hawkins et al. 1992; Patton et al. 2002). As such, therefore, the notion of 'dual diagnosis' (and the diagnostic paradigm itself) becomes unhelpful, as it suggests that the two 'diagnoses' are mutually exclusive or separate and therefore need 'separate' services. Given this diagnostic approach, there is commonly some reluctance in CAMHS to see young people with SM difficulties, and similar reluctance within youth justice settings to offer certain interventions to young people with mental health difficulties. This is thought to be, in part, due to a belief that there is not the expertise within these services to adequately address young people with these 'dual-diagnosis' difficulties. In practice, what this often means is that the most vulnerable young people struggle to find a service that can, or will, meet their needs.

It is important that services do not dismiss SM difficulties as something outside of their remit, but understand that SM is just one of a range of complex behaviours, including offending, in which these young people are engaged. Behaviour is inextricably linked with thinking and emotion and, as with any complex behaviour, interventions, regardless of who is offering them and where they are being offered, should then focus on addressing the factors that impact on the likelihood of that behaviour occurring (Henggeler et al. 1998). While the interplay between our emotional experience, distress, mental health and SM can be a complex one, understanding this interplay is a key task for any clinician attempting to assess and offer interventions for young people presenting with SM difficulties, regardless of what additional diagnostic criteria their symptoms might fulfil. As will be discussed in depth in the formulation section of the chapter arguably the most useful way to understand SM and plan for interventions is by developing a psychologically informed individualised formulation with the young person. Such a formulation should incorporate a holistic understanding of the young person in their environmental context, which takes into account their mental health and emotional well-being, as well as their use of substances.

Prevalence

Exact prevalence of SM among the youth offending population of the UK is difficult to establish. Nonetheless, the limited data available indicates a high incidence of problematic substance use within the population. A third of young people referred to community SM services are from youth offending teams (YOTs), and research working directly with young people within the YJS indicated very high levels of SM (NTA 2013). For example, in a survey of 582 young people involved with youth justice services within England, 45 per cent reported that they had a drink or drug problem (User Voice 2011). A study commissioned by the Home Office 2001/02 sampling 293 young people within youth offending services (YOSs), reported that 85 per cent had used cannabis, alcohol and tobacco. Less than 20 per cent had used heroin or crack cocaine, although the rate was still very high for such a young group. Interestingly, this study also demonstrated that alcohol, tobacco and cannabis were more strongly related to offending than the other drugs.

Such data indicates that use among the youth offending population is considerably higher than within the overall youth population in the UK. The Crime Survey for England and Wales is a self-report survey used to collect data on criminal activity in England and Wales. The Crime Survey for the year 2013 indicated that cannabis was the most commonly used drug amongst young adults aged 16–24 years old, with 13.5 per cent of this population using it within the last year. The survey also indicated that cocaine use had increased in 2012–2013, with 3 per cent of young adults aged 16–24 years old reporting that they had used powdered cocaine within the past 12 months (Home Office 2013).

Young people's use of substances and alcohol during adolescence may be developmentally typical for many adolescents. As the Crime Survey indicates, there are large proportions of young people, both within and outside of the criminal justice system (CJS), who recreationally use alcohol and illegal drugs. However, not all young people who use substances go on to develop a problematic relationship with them (Fergusson, Horwood and Nagin 2000; Fergusson, Horwood and Ridder 2007). This presents additional difficulties for trying to define, let alone record, 'problematic' drug use in any youth population. Clinically, it is also important to be mindful of where the young person's use might fall on a continuum of SM. The impact the use is having on the emotional and physical well-being of the young person should be carefully considered, as well as the impact on the systems around the young person; for example, is use putting their school place/job at risk, is there significant parental concern and/or risk to residence in the family home?

The NTA is the strategic lead for SM treatment and data monitoring in England, although, as with the Crime Survey for England and Wales, their data relates to all young people and they report little data related specifically to the population of young people within the YJS. The NTA figures also confirm that the most frequently reported misused drugs are cannabis and alcohol. Opiate use amongst young people is proposed to be significantly lower, with less than 1 per cent of all specialist SM interventions offered for this difficulty. Whilst these figures are low, young people who develop a dependency on opiates may present significant challenges to services. The physical addiction component of any treatment for opiate use is more complex, and individuals usually benefit from medical supervision when withdrawing. These young people also often have additional needs (e.g. homelessness, mental health problems) and require a significantly enhanced intervention package that many local services in the UK are not commissioned to deliver.

When examining the specific population of young people in the YJS, evidence suggests that the pattern of SM is similar, with cannabis and alcohol being the most commonly used substances. However, the numbers involved in using these substances and in using class A drugs is much higher within this group than the general population of young people (Hammersley, Marsland and Reid 2003; NTA 2009).

Young people who develop problematic relationships with substances often use multiple substances (sometimes termed 'poly-drug use') including alcohol, cannabis and cocaine (Wiessing et al. 2009). Indeed, research suggests that multiple drug use in adolescents who are misusing substances is the most frequent presentation (Martin et al. 1996).

Legal status and sentencing

Individuals found in the possession of illegal substances will, in most cases, have the substances confiscated and also be arrested. However, the exact legal consequences of possessing illegal drugs are dependent on a number of factors:

- The class of drugs involved.
- The quantity of drugs involved.
- Where the arrest took place and the details of what was happening at the time.
- The personal history and current personal circumstances of the person handling the drugs, including previous (particularly drug-related) convictions.

If the person is under the age of 18, the police can inform their parent, guardian or carer that they have been caught in possession of drugs. If they are caught in possession of cannabis (a class B drug), the police will confiscate the drug and may place the youth under arrest. In addition, the police may make a referral to a YOS and will likely have a tiered response, dependant on how many previous offences have been committed and the seriousness of the current crime.

The police almost always charge a person who is suspected of supplying or producing illegal drugs. The penalties for the supply or production of drugs are significantly more severe than those for possession. As with possession, the exact penalties are determined by the factors stated in the list.

Table 11.1 provides a summary of which substances fall into which class and the maximum penalties in relation to both the possession and the supply and production of these substances.

The temporary class drug category has notably been used in relation to the emergence of new synthetic drugs (including so-called legal highs), which have become increasingly popular amongst young people (Hillebrand, Olszewski and Sedefov 2010); the legal classification framework within the United Kingdom has attempted to quickly legislate against substances that are known to produce similar effects as illegal drugs. For example, mephedrone (sometimes known as MCAT) was previously within this classification but was reported to produce similar effects as ecstasy. Consequently, it was quickly legislated against in 2010, following widespread concern of its use, and is now a class B drug.

National policies and practice guidelines

There is a range of practice guidelines that should be considered when working with young people who present with SM difficulties. These will not be covered in great depth, as they are all easily and freely accessible online.

The NTA produced 'Exploring the Evidence' (2009) in an attempt to ensure young people had access to interventions that were supported by an evidence base. The NTA document clearly summarises the available evidence and

Table 11.1 The classification of substances and maximum penalties for drug possession, supply (dealing) and production for adults in the UK

Class	Drug	Possession	Supply and production
A	Crack cocaine, cocaine, ecstasy (MDMA), heroin, LSD, magic mushrooms, methadone, methamphetamine (crystal meth)	Up to 7 years in prison, an unlimited fine or both	Up to life in prison, an unlimited fine or both
B	Amphetamines, barbiturates, cannabis, codeine, ketamine, methylphenidate (Ritalin), synthetic cannabinoids, synthetic cathinones (e.g. mephedrone, methoxetamine)	Up to 5 years in prison, an unlimited fine or both	Up to 14 years in prison, an unlimited fine or both
C	Anabolic steroids, benzodiazepines (diazepam), gamma-hydroxybutyrate (GHB), gamma-butyrolactone (GBL), piperazines (BZP), khat	Up to 2 years in prison, an unlimited fine or both (except anabolic steroids – it's not an offence to possess them for personal use)	Up to 14 years in prison, an unlimited fine or both
Temporary class drugs*	e.g. NBOMe and Benzofuran compounds	None, but police can take away a suspected temporary class drug	Up to 14 years in prison, an unlimited fine or both

Source: http://www.gov.uk/penalties-drug-possession-dealing, reproduced under the Open Government Licence v3.0.

outlines numerous good practice points in relation to engagement and retention of young people in services, therapeutic alliance, assessment, interventions and aftercare. It also has a brief section outlining some of the specific issues within the youth offending population, concluding that while there is no irrefutable evidence that intervening to reduce SM reduces offending behaviour in general, there is some evidence relating to self-reported drops in criminal activity among individuals who received SM treatment. Additionally, the known link between criminality and SM is argued to be reason enough to target SM within the youth offending population.

The YJB have historically published *Key Elements of Effective Practice* (KEEP) documents, one of which focuses on SM (YJB 2008). The KEEP documents are described as 'what to do' documents by the YJB, and aim to provide executive summaries of the key evidence available within different areas of youth justice, for example, SM, mental health and so on. One criticism of these documents is that many YOS practitioners have limited access to training to deliver the KEEP-recommended treatments, and those who have had training may often have limited access to ongoing clinical supervision and training.

In 2012, the Royal College of Psychiatrists in the UK published new practice standards on the care of young people with SM difficulties. The standards were developed in partnership with SM organisations, paediatricians, psychologists and nurses. They are aimed at all staff in contact with young people aged 18 and under, across health, social care, education, YJS, and the voluntary and community sector. The standards are collated in a comprehensive document, which offers a great deal of pragmatic and evidence-based guidance regarding the assessment and treatment of young people with SM difficulties.

Finally, the National Institute for Health and Care Excellence (NICE) provides guidance based on the research evidence base for both commissioners of services and individual clinicians, related to reduction and prevention of SM in young people (NICE 2007). Increasingly, CAMHS services are becoming structured to deliver these NICE-recommended treatments (e.g. children and young people's increasing access to psychological therapies, CYP IAPT). However, many CAMHS services in the UK are under-resourced, so are unable to provide the practice recommended by NICE.

Taken together, there are a range of observations and recommendations that are consistent across all documents in relation to treating SM in adolescents (although most of the documents do not specifically refer to adolescents within the YJS):

- That while progress is slowly being made, high-quality evidence for what works in terms of both assessment, and particularly in terms of intervention, with this population, remains very limited.
- That there are, however, a number of psychosocial interventions that have shown some degree of efficacy (these will all be summarised in the intervention: what works and when section of this chapter).
- That these interventions should be offered in preference to non-evidence-based treatments.
- That the exact nature of the intervention needs to be based on individually designed care/treatment plans based on comprehensive multi-systemic assessment and clear formulation of the young person's difficulties.
- That the assessment must include detailed assessment of risk and plans must be made to minimise any risks identified.
- That involving young people's families wherever possible, in both assessment and treatment, is beneficial.

- That multi-professional and multi-agency working is often necessary when working with these young people, and that it is vitally important that this work is as 'joined up' as possible.
- That engagement is difficult, but obviously of vital importance. That services need to be assertive in their methods of engagement, willing to work in a range of locations, including home settings, and to offer multiple opportunities for the young person to engage. Once the young person is in the room, motivational interviewing can be useful in terms of promoting engagement, and that the evidence indicates that even the proper assessment of SM, in and of itself, can be useful.

All of these documents provide very useful reference points for best practice when working with young people with SM difficulties. However, they are, of course, no substitute for comprehensive assessment and evaluation of the individual young person and detailed formulation in order to facilitate targeted intervention. Indeed, the practice standards published by the Royal College of Psychiatrists specifically comments on the need for properly formulated and shared understanding of each young person's needs (Mirza and Mirza 2008).

Assessment

It is well established that a number of factors associated with offending are also associated with SM. Some factors known to be associated with both are: life difficulties and events; disliking and being excluded from school; lack of positive coping mechanisms; and expecting to get into trouble again (NTA 2009). Ultimately, when assessing SM, it is most useful to conceptualise it as a behaviour which, like offending in general, is influenced and maintained by a complex set of determinates (Dishion and Kavanagh 2003). Assessment therefore becomes fundamental to ensuring effective interventions via the process of individualised formulation. As with the understanding of any complex multi-determined behaviour, the more information you can gather in assessment, the more accurate your formulation can be, and, as a result, the more appropriately targeted the intervention.

As a general overarching issue in relation to assessment in this area, it is important to remember that drug use may be part of 'normative' adolescent behaviour. Furthermore, 'community norms' may also influence the likelihood of a young person experimenting with substances. Evidence from longitudinal studies in New Zealand have indicated that nearly 70 per cent of young people used cannabis at some time, but that less than 7 per cent showed signs of abuse (Fergusson, Horwood and Nagin 2000; Fergusson, Horwood and Ridder 2007). This is why it is important that early initial assessment focuses on age of onset, frequency of use and impact of use. This information will help clarify where, on a continuum of abstinence through recreational use to serious substance abuse, the young person's use is.

Many young people who develop problematic relationships with substances have experienced difficult life events, relationship difficulties with their caregivers, have low educational attainment and may be socially excluded (e.g. Lloyd 1998; Swadi 1999). Therefore, it is not surprising that this population, who have experienced significant adversity, may attempt to manage their difficulties through alternative means such as SM and offending behaviour. Viewing SM as a maintaining or compounding factor for life difficulties, rather than causal, is often not only more appropriate, but more clinically helpful (e.g. NTA 2011).

Key areas for consideration in initial assessment

Level and impact of use

The key in assessing a young person's level and impact of use is to get as much information as possible from them and, if appropriate, also the important others in their lives. There is some evidence that just taking a drug history and reflecting on it with the young person/family can be helpful (McArdle and Angom 2012). Therefore, even if this process is initially time-consuming, it is likely to be time well spent.

It can be useful when trying to conceptualise how problematic use is, to be mindful of the continuum of adolescent substance use models and where, given the information you have collected, the young person might fall within these continuums (e.g. Mirza and Mirza 2008; Royal College of Psychiatrists 2012). For some cases it will be very apparent how problematic the use is, in others, it will be a more complex decision regarding whether to move forward to intervention, and may depend more heavily on either the individual's level of motivation to change this behaviour, and/or court order guidance.

Areas for consideration in assessment of level and impact of use:

- *History of and current SM* – This should include the types of substances and how they are used (e.g. inhalation, injection and so on). The assessment would explore the age of onset of the SM and how SM has evolved.
- *Evolution of use and level of dependence* – The young person should be encouraged to chart any changes in patterns or quantities of substance use. This could include making a timeline and/or having a period of either the young person or others in their lives monitoring use. The clinician should enquire if a young person describes minimal drug use on some days, or whether they are replacing this drug with another substance. This aspect of the assessment may also explore wider changes in the young person's life, for example, a

change in education placement or a change in family dynamics. It is also important to ask about whether they use substances alone or with peers. There is some evidence that, when young people actively seek drugs without there being an interaction with their peers, this increases the level of concern (Royal College of Psychiatry 2012).
- *Meaning or functioning of the SM* – This can be difficult for the young person to reflect upon, but it is important to explore what function SM serves for the young person. Many young people progress from recreational to dependent use, and the meaning associated with these different types of use changes (e.g. from pleasure-orientated to relief-orientated use). Furthermore, many young people hold strong beliefs about the drug, for example, 'cocaine makes me confident', or 'cannabis helps me chill'. These beliefs should be elicited and ideally worked with later in treatment, to explore alternative methods of obtaining this goal (e.g. the desire to have increased confidence or relax without substances).
- *Development of SM-related problems* – Some young people who use substances may begin to experience difficulties that have occurred due to their SM. Young people may begin to experience practical difficulties, for example, financial hardship due to drug use, an increase in offending behaviour to fund drug use and/or an increase in sanctions related to SM. There may also be physical or mental health difficulties that develop, either directly or indirectly related to their drug use (Royal College of Psychiatry 2012).
- There are also a number of standardised tools that can be used to screen for problematic alcohol and drug use. Whilst many of the adult measures are yet to be validated for young people, the following measures have been implemented widely:
- Alcohol Use Disorders Identification Test (AUDIT) (Knight et al. 2003) – specifically for screening for problematic alcohol use and can be used with 14–18-year-olds (Royal College of Psychiatry 2012). It is recommended by NICE, but currently only for 16 and 17-year-olds (NICE 2011).
- CRAFFT (Knight et al. 1999) – screens for alcohol and drugs, is developmentally appropriate for adolescents, and has proven validity and reliability (Knight et al. 2003).
- Screening Questionnaire Interview for Adolescents (SQIfA) (YJB 2003) – which is a measure employed by YOSs in the UK and includes questions on SM. It is designed to be completed by any member of the YOS.
- Comprehensive health assessment tool (CHAT) (OHRN 2013) – SM assessment – is an assessment tool developed by the Offender Health Research Network (OHRN) that is being developed for use in the secure estate and YOSs within the UK. While it addresses multiple health needs, there is a specific section that focuses on SM.

Risk and safeguarding concerns

Risk assessment is extremely important within SM services, and regular review of risk is advised. In addition to the likelihood of other risk concerns in the group of young people with SM difficulties (e.g. family breakdown, homelessness), there are significant risks related directly (e.g. possibility of overdoses, the impact of dirty needles) and indirectly to the SM itself (e.g. the increased vulnerability of young people while intoxicated, leading to other high-risk behaviours).

Any risk assessment needs to explore the multi-systemic factors that both maintain and/or can be used to reduce the risk of ongoing use. Risk assessment should not be a separate assessment, but, rather, risk should be a consideration throughout the entire assessment process. It is important to think about what the information you elicit tells you about risk, and how best to manage these, with the formulation informing and guiding risk plans. For example, those with low parental monitoring and/or inconsistent parenting may be more at risk, but if parents are actively willing to engage, this might indicate a clear area for a quick way to reduce risk (Stoker and Swadi 1990; Swadi 2000).

As a result of the wide range of risk issues common within this group, young people within the YJS who are abusing substances often benefit from assessment plans that involve multi-agency partners, for example, education, social care, CAMHS and YOS. These different agencies will have very helpful perspectives on the young person's behaviour and strengths in different settings. All of the best practice guidelines indicate the importance of a multi-professional/multi-agency approach when working with this group (NTA 2009; Home Office 2010; Royal College of Psychiatry 2012).

Multi-agency working can, of course, be challenging, and some services may have inclusion/exclusion criteria that make it difficult for young people to access treatment. For example, a young person with significant SM difficulties and severe anxiety might struggle to access a mainstream CAMHS, due to concerns that the SM would need addressing by specialists before they could usefully offer an intervention. Then the same young person might fail to be able to access a specialist SM service due to concerns that the anxiety is so significant that this needs an intervention from CAMHS before the young person's SM can be addressed. Some teams may have different narratives about risk and may find it difficult to tolerate the potential risk-taking behaviour associated with substance-misusing adolescents. As a result, these young people can be labelled as 'difficult to engage' or 'not ready' for individual therapy, or indeed just outside the remit of the service – which is obviously a clear disservice to them.

It is suggested that individual psychological formulation of young people's difficulties can be highly useful in these situations. If such formulations are shared with other services, and there is, as a result, an increased understanding of the young person's needs, then care plans can be more specifically and clearly defined; which, in turn, improves the management of the risks.

Some of the factors that could indicate young people at particularly high risk are summarised in Box 11.1. This should not be considered a comprehensive list. Indeed, providing a comprehensive list with such a complex group of young people is not possible. However, it is a starting point grounded on the evidence base in terms of things to consider (Swadi 2000; Royal College of Psychiatry 2012).

Box 11.1 Factors indicating high risk

- The young person is using substances very often and not for recreational purposes.
- The young person reports (or appears to be, given information about pattern of use) using substances to manage distressing feelings or make difficult situations more bearable.
- They are using such large qualities there is a risk of overdose.
- They are mixing substances dangerously. Particularly high risk of harm attached to mixing combinations of: alcohol, heroin or benzodiazepines.
- They are putting themselves at risk in order to fund their substance use, e.g. offending or selling sexual favours.
- Their use is causing significant problems in the young person's life, e.g. mental distress, homelessness, loss of job, etc.
- There is use of substance in the family and/or there is a lack of parental monitoring/involvement.

Level of motivation

The initial interview should include an assessment of the young person's motivation to change and their readiness for a SM intervention. This may be assessed by exploring the young person's beliefs about the importance of change and confidence to reduce substance use, as well as thinking about the pros and cons of continued use. It is worth being mindful of the literature and guidance relating to motivational interviewing when trying to elicit beliefs in this area.

Motivational interviewing was developed as an adult intervention for working with ambivalence, and evolved from the treatment of problem drinkers (Miller and Rollnick 1991, 2002). The aim of motivational interviewing is to elicit reasons why the individual should feel motivated to change their behaviour, with the view that this process will increase their motivation to change. Within the interview, the individual is prompted and encouraged to identify what negative consequences they are currently experiencing as a result of their behaviour (within this context, their substance use). They are also encouraged to think about a better future and what the steps might be to achieving this future. It is worth a clinician spending some time familiarising themselves with strategies and techniques proposed by motivational interviewing when working with young people with SM difficulties. Motivational interviewing in general has been evidenced to be effective for young people with SM difficulties (e.g. see Becker and Curry 2008 for a review).

Motivational interview techniques can also be used, as appropriate, to engage and secure the involvement of parents, carers or wider family members in the care and intervention plan. It is important to consider where the greatest motivation for change is located, both in terms of the formulation of the difficulties, but also when planning the most effective intervention plan. Ideally, parents/carers should be actively involved in treatment, as there is strong evidence that family involvement increases the efficacy and long-term sustainability of interventions for SM in adolescents (Velleman, Templeton and Copello 2005).

Other key areas for consideration in comprehensive assessment

Other key areas for consideration when undertaking a comprehensive assessment include:

- *Family history and functioning* – there is extensive literature linking a range of family factors to the likelihood of developing SM and maintaining this behaviour once it is established. For example, low parental monitoring, parental discord, negative communication and inconsistent discipline (Stoker and Swadi 1990; Isohanni, Moilanen and Rantakallio 1991). Both past and current history is important in terms of understanding a young person's relationships, and to inform the formulation regarding how the current difficulties emerged.
- *History in education and/or employment, including any plans for the future* – again there is extensive literature showing clear correlations between difficulties in education and SM (e.g. Lynskey and Hall 2000). Assessing the past and current history of education, as well as plans for the future, helps in terms of being able to aid the young person identify a realistic future plan. Such a plan is likely to enhance their motivation to engage in treatment to overcome their SM. Additionally, detailed information will enable clear planning for the next steps that the young person will need to take to become meaningfully engaged in education and/or employment, which will be important in maintaining any changes (Swadi 2000).
- *Physical health* – SM can have a significant impact on physical health. It is important this is assessed, both to ensure that the young person receives

appropriate care for any physical health difficulties, but also in terms again of helping the young person identify the negative effects the SM is having. Both direct effects, such as abscesses and hepatitis, and indirect effects, such as high-risk sexual activity under the influence, should be considered.

- *Mental health and any difficulties with development or learning* – mental health difficulties and learning disabilities are both very common within the population of young people within the YJS in the UK (Chitsabesan et al. 2006), and hence are also common within the subsection of this population who misuse substances. It is therefore important to ensure assessment of any co-morbid conditions and to be mindful of this when developing the formulations and planning appropriate interventions. Young people should be able to access evidence-based treatments for mental health difficulties, regardless of their SM, and the interaction between the mental health concerns and SM should be considered when deciding where to intervene initially. Many young people who offend and have SM difficulties are given a diagnosis of attention deficit hyperactivity disorder (ADHD) (e.g. Young and Thome 2011) and the complications of medical interventions in this group should be considered when intervening (see Royal College of Psychiatry 2012 for detailed guidance regarding this group of young people).

- *Strengths and resources of the individual* – in assessing and formulating a young person's difficulties, it is always vital to also assess their strengths. Treatment should guide young people to build upon their strengths in order to best facilitate the process of change. Strengths could be things such as: sense of humour, good social skills and 'street smarts' – being able to pick up ideas and concepts quickly. Additionally, it is worth considering what the young person might have managed not to do, rather than focusing entirely on what they have done. For example, if a young person has used substances in order to calm down and thereby avoided violence, it is a skill that they have developed this method and it has worked. Praise in such context can be useful, as it helps young people realise they had the control to do something (e.g. take substances) when they felt at risk of doing something else (e.g. being violent). This level of awareness and control can then be used in formulation and intervention in terms of following the same pattern, but replacing the SM with other more functional/beneficial behaviours.

- *Strengths and resources within the system around the individual* – gaining information about strengths in the system is vital as part of formulating and facilitating effective targeted interventions. Strengths should be considered in all of the various systems the young person exists in: family (a very committed older brother who has experienced similar difficulties), school (a tutor at school who is dedicated to supporting the young person), peers (a group

of old prosocial peers with whom the young person is no longer engaged, but still has access to), community (a football team the young person is interested in being involved in) and so on. Information about strengths in the wider system will help in terms of thinking about how to support the young person in creating and sustaining change.
- *Identification of goals/what the young person would like to be different* – it is important to explore this to increase engagement and motivation with the young person (and/or their family). Awareness of goals allows treatment to be clearly linked and aimed towards meetings these goals, and, from clinical experience, this appears to enhance the likelihood of ongoing engagement. Having clear client-centred goals also allows clinicians to appropriately evaluate their efficacy in intervening.

Confidentiality and assessing drug use

Many young people may not wish to disclose their drug use to adults involved in their care. They may fear reprisal from parents/carers or professionals (e.g. YOS) due to the potentially illegal nature of their drug use.

Professionals working with young people in SM services are guided by the same child protection principles as those in other settings (e.g. CAMHS, school settings and so on). It may be important to establish a clear contract of expectations between the SM worker and the young person about what will and will not remain confidential within the therapeutic relationship. This contracting may be informed by local safeguarding policies and service-specific procedures (e.g. whether substance use that the YOS is unaware of needs to be shared with the rest of the team and/or would need to be shared with court should the need arise for a court report, and so on).

It is very important to consider that many young people who access SM services within YOS may be quite disengaged from other systems (e.g. education, employment and so on), and may have had disappointing or rejecting adult relationships. Therefore, the initial meeting may be extremely important to actively engage the young person and their wider system (e.g. carers/parents) where appropriate.

Some young people may disengage from SM services after the initial appointment, especially if SM intervention is not part of a mandatory YOS order. 'Immediate' interventions may be applied, which could involve simple techniques such as feedback (e.g. completing a SM diary to illustrate the amount/quantity of substances used), decision balance diagrams (e.g. weighing up the pros/cons of attending future appointments) and goal setting and risk-reduction information giving (e.g. avoiding mixing alcohol and drugs and so on). The main therapeutic 'task' within the initial contact with young people is to develop a strong working relationship, which forms a good base for future work.

Summary of assessment

Drug use may be part of many adolescents' 'normative' developmental pathway, but the age of onset and the context in which substances are used are very important to take into consideration. The available evidence indicates that screening for SM for all young people in YOS is very important and may be used as a brief intervention (e.g. psychoeducation). The assessment stage of working with a young person is also very important and is intertwined with intervention. Initial engagement is fundamental in working with this group, who can often be quite ambivalent and disengaged from services. The initial assessment should work towards developing a formulation or 'problem summary', before developing an idiosyncratic treatment plan.

Formulation

Psychological formulation typically involves the application of psychological theory in an attempt to provide a context and understanding for an individual's behaviour. There are multiple approaches to formulation and it should be noted that there is a no 'one' approach. The British Psychological Society Division of Clinical Psychology (DCP 2011) provides an excellent summary of formulation. The NTA and the BPS (NTA 2012) have also produced a proposal to include 'problem summaries' within SM work, which can be used as initial formulations to understand predisposing, precipitating, perpetuating and protective factors.

Young people themselves will often benefit from a basic maintenance formulation – something that makes tentative links between the individual's internal experience (e.g. thoughts/feelings) and their behaviour.

This is outlined in the following example, where a young person who is 'looked after' by the local authority uses cannabis to alleviate their feelings of low mood. The clinician may work alongside the young person to write out a narrative (sometimes in diagrammatic form) that may be something like:

> 'Because I'm in care, I feel fed up and depressed' (feel like I'm stuck and I can't help myself). This feeling might lead the young person to think 'a spliff might make me feel better, I could chill after that'. This thought and permission giving belief could lead the young person to use cannabis, which will temporarily alleviate the initial 'depressed' feeling. However, in the longer term the young person may not be able to develop alternative proactive coping strategies and may feel even more 'stuck' than they initially felt.

The importance of completing a comprehensive and acceptable (to the young person and/or family) formulation cannot be understated. It facilitates a shared understanding of the difficulties and hence rationale for the intervention.

It also, when done effectively, enhances trust in the therapeutic relationship, and engagement and commitment to the treatment plan (BPS 2011). It also, of course, increases the likelihood of the intervention being effective, if it is targeted to the individual strengths and needs of the young person and their ecology. All of the best practice documents highlight (albeit sometimes using different language, such as problem summary) the importance of using formulations when planning interventions with young people who so often display a complex pattern of difficulties and life contexts (NTA 2009; Home Office 2010; Royal College of Psychiatry 2012). It is perhaps also worth noting the increased importance of formulations to provide an anchor in guiding intervention when the evidence base itself is not strong.

Intervention: What works and when?

This section summarises each of the interventions that have been shown to have efficacy for young people with SM difficulties. While it is well acknowledged that the evidence base regarding interventions in this population is still in its infancy, there is sufficient data to conclude that these interventions are the most appropriate place to start when developing a support plan. All of the current best practice guidance supports this view (Royal College of Psychiatry 2012). With the exception of multi-systemic therapy (MST), there is currently no specific literature relating to using these interventions to treat SM difficulties specifically with young people involved with the YJS; and none within this population in the UK (the majority of the studies on MST are US based). The limits of the current evidence base highlight again the importance of comprehensive psychological formulation for each case when making treatment plans, to ensure that intervention targets most effectively the key factors for that individual.

While this section will focus on individual intervention, prevention work is extremely important within this population. It could be argued that, due to the high levels of SM amongst young people within the CJS, all young people who enter the system should receive early intervention work. However, this can be a significant challenge in YOS, where there is often a lack of such resources. Therefore, services are often forced to focus on 'high need' and have limited resources to provide intervention to young people who do not present with such challenges.

A brief overview of the treatment models are outlined below, before a summary of guiding principles is provided.

Cognitive behaviour therapy (CBT)

The evidence base for CBT for young people with SM difficulties is emerging, but there are currently no clear findings that indicate CBT is more effective than other therapies for SM (e.g. Tanner-Smith, Wilson and Lipsey 2013).

Nonetheless, CBT is recommended for young people with SM difficulties and diagnoses of depression and/or anxiety (e.g. NICE 2007).

The CBT model places significant emphasis on making links between thoughts, feelings and behaviour, and focusing on how this 'triad' maintains unhelpful behaviour. CBT could be conceptualised as an empowering therapeutic model, as it places the emphasis of change upon the young person.

Many CBT intervention packages are based on adult treatment models and, as such, they do not fully consider the developmental needs of a young person. CBT often requires young people to have some desire to reduce or completely stop their SM. The approach involves a high level of 'out of session' work, based on self-monitoring through the completion of weekly diaries. This can be a significant challenge for disengaged young people in the CJS and those with limited literacy skills.

In practice, many CBT programmes are often delivered alongside a strong component of motivational enhancement therapy (MET) (e.g. Tevyaw and Monti 2004). From clinical experience, it appears that MET prior to and/or alongside a more 'active' treatment such as CBT can sometimes result in better outcomes for young people who are somewhat ambivalent about their substance use.

Dialectical behaviour therapy (DBT)

This approach has been used extensively within adult services to work with adults who present with unpredictable and highly challenging behaviours, for example, self-harm and/or repeated suicide attempts (e.g. Linehan et al. 1999).

The model's emphasis on emotional regulation skills and interpersonal issues, both of which may be poor with this population, has proved to be effective for some young people (Harned et al. 2008). Within this model, substance use would be conceptualised as a 'quality-of-life interfering behaviour'. Clinicians working within this model would aim to increase the young person's coping skills (e.g. problem solving) and decrease negative behaviours (e.g. SM). There is some evidence that techniques within this model, including self-monitoring, behavioural analysis and problem-solving strategies, are effective in reducing problematic substance use in adults diagnosed with borderline personality disorder (Harned et al. 2008).

Multi-systemic therapy (MST)

MST is an intensive home-based intervention model that aims to eliminate the SM by intervening at multi-levels within the young person's ecology, which may or may not include working individually with the young person. MST starts with a full assessment of the behaviour the young person and/or their family wish to change, which results in a clear formulation of the behaviour, in this case the SM difficulty, in the context of not only individual factors but factors within the wider systemic (e.g. education, family, peers and community)

(Henggeler 1999). This model was effectively used in a large-scale American study (Cannabis Youth Treatment Trial, CYT) and has been implemented as in the UK within some CAMHS and some YOS (Butler et al. 2011).

MST is a 'branded' therapy that requires intensive training and supervision from MST services. However, some of the concepts and techniques for formulation are thought to be helpful clinically when formulating a young person's difficulties, even if the intervention offered is not formal MST.

The model works intensively with the child, their carers and the wider system around the child (e.g. youth justice, education, social care). Therapists within this model have a small caseload (from four to six families) and work with each family up to four to five times per week. MST is therefore often not compatible with the resource limitations of many mainstream service settings. Additionally, MST excludes young people without families around them, and therefore excludes some of the youth at highest risk (those who are functionally homeless or living in low support hostels and so on).

Contingency management programmes (including MST-CM)

The current NICE guidelines suggest that contingency management programmes should be considered with adults, if the offer of incentives can be seen to enhance engagement, behavioural change and willingness to adhere to treatment (NICE 2008: 12–13). There is as yet no guidance regarding the use of such programmes with young people. The majority of evidence regarding the efficacy of contingency management has been with adults (Prendergast et al. 2006), where the financial context is obviously different. Nonetheless, the concept of using rewards to encourage and enhance behaviour change either formally, or more informally within the family setting, should be considered when working with young people with SM.

MST-CM is the contingency management module for MST and so bears significant similarities to standard MST as described. The key difference in MST-CM is that one of its key components and focus of treatment is a contingency management intervention. While MST has become more common in the UK, MST-CM remains in its infancy. It is at present mostly evidenced for young people who have been mandated into treatment, and in the US context, where youth justice services tend to work much more independently than they do in the UK.

Systemic/family-based interventions

Family therapy techniques that focus on engagement with the young person and their family have been shown to increase the likelihood of positive behaviour change occurring in young people with SM (Hogue and Liddle 2009). Additionally, there is consistent evidence that, in general, interventions that are able to involve the wider family in understanding and intervening with the

SM are more likely to result in positive outcomes (Homberger and Smith 2011; Velleman, Templeton and Copello 2005).

Adolescent mentalisation-based integrative therapy (AMBIT)

AMBIT is in the early days of being developed and evaluated. However, there is some data that indicates it may be an effective approach with young people who present with complex co-morbid substance use, mental health, family, educational and offending problems (e.g. Bateman and Fonagy 2008; Bevington et al. 2013). AMBIT is an 'open source' approach to therapy, and there is a web-based platform allowing services/clinicians access to resources and the opportunity to adapt the resources to best fit their local context, while still adhering to evidence-based practice.

Summary of treatment models

There is no clear evidence base to suggest that one specific model or 'brand' of therapy works better than others when providing interventions for SM in adolescence. However, systemic family work has been tentatively shown to be more efficacious than individual work within meta-analysis studies (e.g. Waldron and Turner 2008; Tanner-Smith, Wilson and Lipsey 2013).

However, some, if not all, of the recommended treatments outlined are not routinely applied within standard secure settings or YOS teams within the UK. Therefore, there appears to be somewhat of a gap between best practice research findings and the reality of clinical delivery within 'typical' youth justice services. There is often limited resources to provide these specialist treatments, and local agencies (e.g. CAMHS) are often poorly resourced to work with this population.

Guiding principles to treatment

As outlined, there are no specific treatment models that have been clearly demonstrated to be more effective than others. Therefore, it is proposed that the following guiding principles be considered when working with young people with SM difficulties within the CJS.

Formulation prior to treatment

A meta-analysis indicated that, in addition to good interpersonal skills of the therapist, an accepted rationale for the treatment plan is important (Karver et al. 2006). The formulation is therefore hugely important in providing this rationale, in a form that the young person and the family can understand.

Developing an accurate and young-person and/or family-accepted psychologically informed formulation should be seen as an intervention itself. Following a comprehensive assessment, the clinician should aim to collaboratively develop a formulation or 'problem summary' of the young person's SM difficulties. The formulation, drawing on a broad range of psychological theory, should capture the meaning of the SM and offer 'exits' or suggestions of alternative ways of meeting this need, for example, problem-solving training, emotional regulation skills and so on.

The formulation should ideally explore the links between the young person's SM and any emotional distress or problem-solving deficits they may have. The subsequent treatment should be informed by the idiosyncratic formulation that provides both therapist and client with intervention points that may help to reduce the difficulties that SM is being used to manage.

Systemic involvement

SM can be very difficult for some families to accept and there can be a culture in SM services of working with young people individually, without involving the family. Whilst this may be effective for some young people, in providing them with a confidential service they require, it can place a significant responsibility on a young person to individually manage the challenge of reducing or discontinuing their substance use, without involving those who support them on a daily basis.

As outlined in the section 'Assessment', SM does not occur within a vacuum and is usually linked to other difficulties, which may include behavioural difficulties, family conflict, reduced educational attainment and poor emotional well-being.

Research literature and clinical experience indicates that interventions that involve the wider system (e.g. parents, carers, support workers and so on) are more effective than those that involve isolated one-to-one work with the young person (e.g. Henggeler 1999; Velleman, Templeton and Copello 2005).

Goal focused

SM intervention should aim to be goal focused within a specific, measurable, attainable, relevant and time-bound (SMART) format. Clinically, it seems this is particularly important when working with young people who have multiple difficulties, where small gains may lead to an increase in confidence for the young person, who might otherwise feel overwhelmed.

SMART goals must come from the young person, otherwise they will not engage with the process. The therapist must consider that many young people will not want to discontinue their drug use – something their parents/carers may not be comfortable with.

Integrated therapeutic models

The author recommends that SM treatment involves a 'menu' of psychologically informed treatment options that are integrated and prioritised via an idiosyncratic formulation. Typically, such an intervention might include:

- *Motivational enhancement techniques* – to enhance motivation and decrease ambivalence.
- *Mental health screen* – given the significant numbers of young people who have mental health difficulties.
- *Self-monitoring* – this could take place via diaries, smartphone apps or tally sheets.
- *Harm reduction* – initial treatment goals may aim to reduce high-risk behaviour and reduce any immediate harm the young person may face.
- *Coping mechanisms* – many young people who use substances have poor alternative prosocial coping skills. Problem-solving training may be very effective for this group.
- *Emotional recognition and regulation skills* – linked to the above, some young people have a poor ability to recognise and regulate strong emotions (e.g. anger). These difficulties are often masked and maintained through SM.
- *Relapse prevention* – the majority of young people who use substances will do so again even after they enter treatment, and intervention should specifically address lapses and relapse prevention.
- *Systemic/family work* – there is clear evidence that greater involvement of the systems around the young person results in better outcomes both short term and long term. Wherever possible, families and/or carers should be included. Ideally, psychological formulations should be shared with those around the young person (obviously only if the young person consents to this), so that they can understand the mechanisms of use, and any relapse prevention plan be shared so that families know and can support the plans to sustain the changes the young person has made.

Case study

The following case study will focus on the needs of a 'typical' young person who accesses SM services within the context of a YOS. It is a composite case study, drawing on the experiences of the authors and colleagues.

Background

Eoin, 16, was referred for SM treatment due to concerns about his regular cannabis, cocaine and alcohol use. Eoin was not in education or employment and had been excluded from mainstream school aged 14 years old. He had been educated at a pupil referral unit for the past two years.

Eoin had complex and challenging experiences of family life from a young age, which may have both contributed to and maintained his SM. Eoin was placed on a child protection plan when he was 8 years old, after he was physically abused by his mother's partner, and remained on this for 18 months, until his mother ended the relationship with the man. Eoin had a sister aged 12, who was, at the time of Eoin's referral for SM treatment, on a 'child in need' plan due to concerns about parental neglect by their mother. At this time, the local authority had also requested that Eoin transition into independent living due to the 'risk' that his drug use posed to his younger siblings and mother.

Eoin's mother, Fiona, has a history of using alcohol and cannabis, but she was currently abstaining from substances following input from the local authority. Fiona reported that Eoin's father was a violent man and he had regularly subjected her to domestic violence, something Eoin and his sister had witnessed. Fiona's new partner Saul has a poor relationship with Eoin, and he would like Eoin to move out of the family home.

Eoin experienced low mood, 'flashbacks' in relation to the physical abuse he had been subjected to by mother's partner, and he was very difficult to engage. Eoin had been stabbed 12 months prior to the referral, following a local feud about drug money. Eoin has previously been associating with older male offenders and been involved in supplying drugs. He was placed on an intensive supervision and surveillance plan and required to attend YOS on a daily basis.

Formulation

A psychological formulation was developed collaboratively with Eoin and drawn out pictorially in the assessment session. This was presented as 'what happened in the past', 'how I cope with it', 'what triggers me off' and 'where I might begin to change'. Whilst he minimised the impact of his early experiences, he did accept that he acts in 'survival mode' and he struggled to accept there 'may' be an alternative to this way of being.

Eoin's early exposure to domestic violence may have made it more likely for him to develop subsequent behavioural and emotional difficulties (e.g. Menard 2002; Kitzmann et al. 2003). Furthermore, children who grow up in a violent home may be more likely to present in the CJS for violent crimes (Mitchell and Finkelhor 2001).

The experience of being exposed to violence and an inconsistent caregiver may have made it difficult for Eoin to develop resilience in order to manage emotional difficulties. As a result, he appears to have become heavily reliant on substances to manage emotional distress. Eoin has also been vulnerable to exploitation from older males (e.g. hiding drugs and stolen goods). This behaviour may have been an attempt to seek emotional closeness and validation, which he did not experience from his relationship with his caregivers.

Eoin has been a victim of numerous violent attacks within the community that have significantly impacted on his mood and drug use. His pre-existing experiences of trauma may have predisposed him to more unhelpful coping strategies following the assault he experienced. Furthermore, his high use of substances following the incident may have made it more difficult for Eoin to develop adaptive coping skills. The experience of trauma has also led Eoin

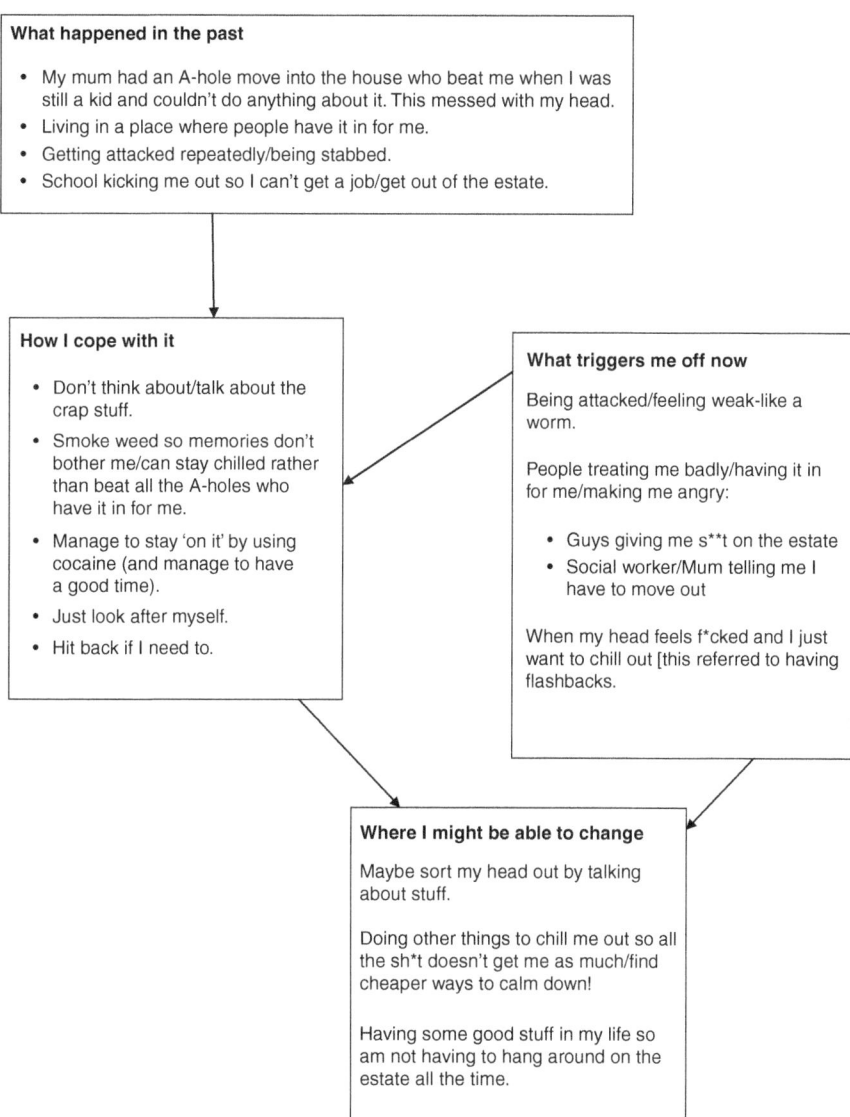

Figure 11.1 Eoin's individual psychologically informed formulation

to become somewhat 'threat focused' or hypervigilant to violence within the community. For example, he was frequently concerned that other young people in YOS may pick fights or attack him.

These beliefs are congruent with a young adult who has been systematically exposed to violence, physically assaulted and humiliated by older males within the community. These experiences have left Eoin feeling 'like a worm, pathetic' and led him to develop the belief that other people cannot be trusted: 'everyone's just out to get you'.

The mental health assessment indicated that the exposure to significant violence has led Eoin to develop experiences associated with high levels of anxiety (e.g. hypervigilance, cognitive rumination and paranoia).

The assessment indicated that Eoin has limited problem-solving skills and is reliant on substance use to manage any emotional distress that he experiences. Reduced problem-solving skills and SM are significant risk factors that could lead to reoffending (Thomas and Penn 2002). As a result, Eoin may be more likely to use substances that would also increase the likelihood of him engaging in offending behaviour. This is evidenced in his history of substance-misuse-related offences.

Eoin continues to hold cognitive distortions (unhelpful beliefs) about his SM that minimise his drug use, and he also has limited insight into his use of substances to manage his mood. The assessment also indicated that Eoin requires further support to develop an awareness of 'high-risk' situations where he is more likely to use substances. For example, he is more likely to use cocaine in social situations and cannabis whilst he is alone and feeling low.

The assessment indicated that Eoin's willingness to reflect on the links between his drug use and low mood may be evidence of protective factors in this case. Furthermore, his engagement with the YOS staff may be indicative of his future ability to form relationships with professionals.

Intervention

The intervention with Eoin initially focused on the 'recognition' of his difficulties, which involved him noticing when he felt that he needed to use drugs, noticing when his flashbacks were at their 'worst' and so on. This recognition stage involved Eoin making entries on his smartphone of significant incidents and exceptions to the problems he was experiencing. The author also completed various maintenance diagrams with Eoin to link internal feelings to external behaviour and vice versa. See Figures 11.2 and 11.3 for two examples of such maintenance diagrams.

The work was completed in consultation with YOS key workers to ensure that Eoin, the key workers and the author had a shared story of his difficulties. This story or formulation was developed alongside Eoin, and provided exit points via a menu of options, many of which were quite basic, for example, talking to a key worker when he felt distressed. These 'mini-exits' proved to be much more effective than formal psychological therapy, and the involvement of the YOS team was very important to avoid Eoin feeling further isolated.

Eoin, like many young people who use high levels of substances, often has associated emotional difficulties, which diagnostically could be labelled

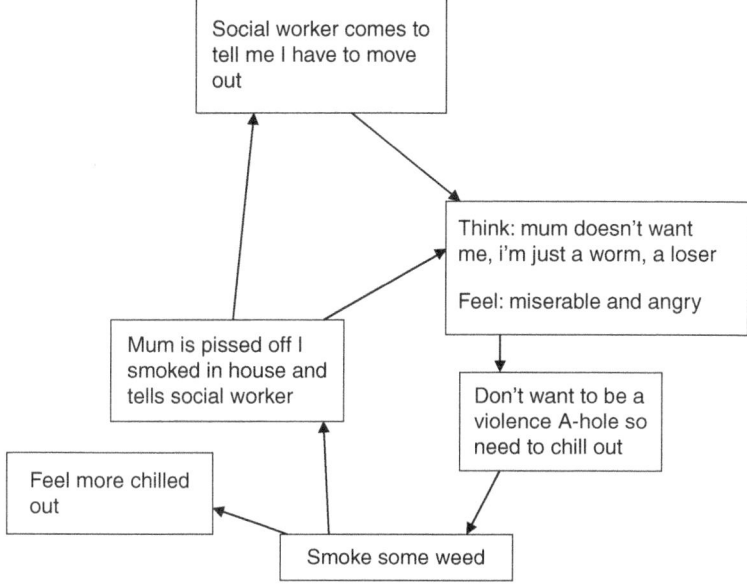

Figure 11.2 Example of Eoin's maintenance cycles for use of cannabis

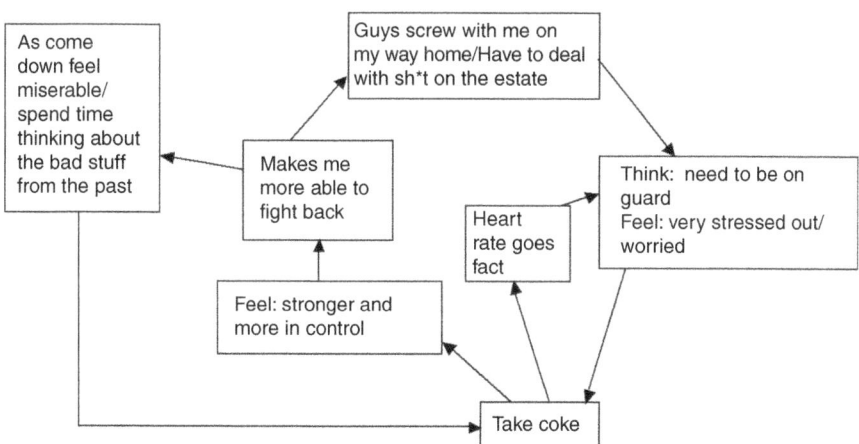

Figure 11.3 Example of Eoin's maintenance cycles for use of cocaine

as 'depression', 'anxiety' and/or 'post-traumatic stress disorder' (PTSD). However, the author framed the difficulties to Eoin and the YOS team within a trauma and SM formulation, rather than a medical illness paradigm. A diagnostic understanding that is based on a model of 'illness' prevented Eoin's difficulties being viewed as something that was outside of the expertise of the team and him being 'sent' to an external team (e.g. CAMHS), where his difficulties may have been further medicalised.

The work within the team enabled Eoin to feel contained by key workers and helped him generalise the skills he developed in his individual work within the multiple contacts he had with the YOS team on a near daily basis. The case study highlights the importance of assessing and formulating systemic factors. Eoin, like many young people who access SM services within YOS, has been exposed to trauma and loss and may use substances to help manage his mood or regulate his emotions.

The case study also highlights the role of traumatic experiences impacting upon young people who use substances. Substances can make it difficult for young people to develop more adaptive methods of processing difficult life events, for example, talking to family/friends, engaging in sports/hobbies and so on. SM problems within adolescence (and indeed within adulthood) are best conceptualised within the context of wider family and systemic dynamics.

Conclusions

Many young people, especially those involved within the YJS, use legal and illegal substances at some point during adolescence. While, for the majority, this is a developmental stage that does not impact detrimentally, a significant proportion of these young people develop SM difficulties that necessitate intervention. Many of the factors that place young people at increased risk of being involved in the YJS also increase their risk of developing SM difficulties. As a result, it is not surprising that SM is relatively common within the population of young people who offend, and that this group of young people often have complex lives and multiple vulnerabilities.

Supporting young people with SM difficulties to access and engage with appropriate interventions is the responsibility of all professionals involved with the young person's care. Joined-up working across services and among professionals is essential. While the literature base at present is limited, this should not negate the need to ensure that any interventions offered are as evidence based as possible and systemic in their approach. Evidence base and national guidelines should be born in mind at all times. These, however, should be no substitute for an adequate individualised understanding of the young person's needs. Care plans should be set out clearly and guided by a comprehensive and holistic understanding of the young person's difficulties. We argue this is most effectively done via the use of individualised psychologically informed formulation. Such formulations should be devised in collaboration with young people, and should be the cornerstone of offering effective and targeted interventions for this vulnerable group of young people.

References

Barnes, G.M., Reifman, A.S., Farrell, M.P., and Dintcheff, B.A. (2000) 'The effects of parenting on the development of adolescent misuse: A six wave latent growth model', *Journal of Marriage and Family*, 62: 175–186.

Bateman, A. and Fonagy, P. (2008) '8-year-follow-up of patients treated for borderline personality disorder: mentalisation-based treatment versus treatment as usual', *The American Journal of Psychiatry*, 165(5): 631–638.

Becker, S.J. and Curry, J.F. (2008) 'Outpatient interventions for adolescent substance abuse: A quality of evidence review', *Journal of Consulting and Clinical Psychology*, 76(4): 531.

Bennett, T., Holloway, K., and Farrington, D. (2008) 'The statistical association between drug misuse and crime: A meta analysis', *Aggressive and Violent Behaviour*, 13: 107–118.

Bevington, D., Fuggle, P., Fonagy, P., Target, M., and Asen, E. (2013) 'Innovations in practice: Adolescent mentalization-based integrative therapy (AMBIT) – a new integrated approach to working with the most hard to reach adolescents with severe complex mental health needs', *Child and Adolescent Mental Health*, 18(1): 46–51.

Butler, S., Baruch, G., Hickey, N., and Fonagy, P. (2011) 'A randomized controlled trial of multisystemic therapy and a statutory therapeutic intervention for young offenders', *Journal of the American Academy of Child & Adolescent Psychiatry*, 50(12): 1220–1235.

Chitsabesan, P., Kroll, L., Bailey, S., Kenning, C., Sneider, S., MacDonald, W., and Theodosiou, L. (2006) 'Mental health needs of young offenders in custody and in the community', *British Journal of Psychiatry*, 188(6): 534–540.

Dishion, T.J. and Kavanagh, K. (2003) *Intervening in Adolescent Problem Behavior: A Family-Centered Approach*. New York: Guilford Press.

Division of Clinical Psychology (2011). *Good Practice Guidelines on the Use of Psychological Formulation*. Leicester: British Psychological Society.

Dolan, M., Holloway, J., Bailey, S., and Smith, C. (1999) 'Health status of juvenile offenders: A survey of young offenders appearing before the juvenile courts', *Journal of Adolescence*, 22(1): 137–144.

Eklund, J.M. and Klinteberg, B.A.F. (2003) 'Childhood behavior as related to subsequent drinking offences and violent offending: A prospective study of 11- to 14-year-old youth into their fourth decade', *Criminal Behaviour and Mental Health*, 13: 294–309.

Farabee, D., Shen, H., Hser, Y.I., Grella, C.E., and Anglin, M.D. (2001) 'The effect of drug treatment on criminal behavior among adolescents in DATOS-A', *Journal of Adolescent Research*, 16(6): 679–696.

Farrington, D.P. and Hawkins, J.D. (1991) 'Predicting participation, early onset and later persistence in officially recorded offending', *Criminal Behaviour and Mental Health*, 1: 1–33.

Fergusson, D.M., Horwood, L., and Nagin, D.S. (2000) 'Offending trajectories in a New Zealand birth cohort', *Criminology*, 38(2): 525–552.

Fergusson, D.M., Horwood, L.J., and Ridder, E.M. (2007) 'Conduct and attentional problems in childhood and adolescence and later substance use, abuse and dependence: Results of a 25-year longitudinal study', *Drug and Alcohol Dependence*, 88: S14–S26.

Gilvarry, E., McArdle, P., O'Herlihy, A., Mirza, K.A.H., Bevington, D., and Malcolm, N. (eds.) (2012) *Practice Standards for Young People with Substance Misuse Problems*. London: Royal College of Psychiatry.

Hammersley, R., Marsland, L., and Reid, M. (2003) *Substance Use by Young Offenders: The Impact of the Normalisation of Drug Use in the Early Years of the 21st Century*. London: Home Office.

Harned, M.S., Chapman, A.L., Dexter-Mazza, E.T., Murray, A., Comtois, K.A., and Linehan, M.M. (2008) 'Treating co-occurring Axis I disorders in recurrently suicidal women with borderline personality disorder: A 2-year randomized trial of dialectical behavior therapy', *Journal of Consulting and Clinical Psychology*, 76: 1068–1075.

Hawkins, J.D., Catalano, R.F., and Miller, J.Y. (1992) 'Risk and protective factors for alcohol and other drug problems in adolescence and early adulthood: Implications for substance abuse prevention', *Psychological Bulletin*, 112(1): 64.

Henggeler, S.W. (1999) 'Multisystemic therapy: An overview of clinical procedures, outcomes, and policy implications', *Child and Adolescent Mental Health*, 4(1): 2–10.

Henggeler, S.W., Clingempeel, W.G., Brondino, M.J., and Pickrel, S.G. (2002) 'Four-year follow-up of multisystemic therapy with substance-abusing and substance-dependent juvenile offenders', *Journal of the American Academy of Child & Adolescent Psychiatry*, 41(7): 868–874.

Henggeler, S., Schoenwald, S.K., Borduin, C.M., Rowland, M.D., and Cunningham, P.B. (1998) *Multisystemic Treatment of Antisocial Behavior in Children and Adolescents: Treatment Manuals for Practioners*. New York: Guildford Press.

Hillebrand, J., Olszewski, D., and Sedefov, R. (2010) 'Legal highs on the Internet', *Substance Use & Misuse*, 45(3): 330–340.

Homberger, S. and Smith, S.L. (2011) 'Family involvement in adolescent substance abuse treatment and recovery: What do we know? What lies ahead?', *Children and Youth Services Review*, 33: 70–76.

Home Office UK (2010) 'Reducing demand, restricting supply, building recovery: Supporting people to live a drug-free life', *The 2010 Drug Strategy*. London: Home Office, https://www.gov.uk/government/uploads/systems/uploads/attachment_data/file/118336/drug-strategy-2010.pdf.

Home Office (2013) 'Drug misuse: Findings from the 2012 to 2013 crime survey for England and Wales'. Available at: https://www.gov.uk/government/publications/drug-misuse-findings-from-the-2012-to-2013-csew/drug-misuse-findings-from-the-2012-2013-crime-survey-for-england-and-wales, accessed 08 May 2015.

Houge, A. and Liddle, H. (2009) 'Family-based treatment for adolescent substance abuse: Controlled trials and new horizons in services research', *Journal of Family Therapy*, 31(1): 126–154.

Isohanni, M., Moilanen, I., and Rantakallio, P. (1991) 'Determinants of teenage smoking, with special reference to non-standard family background', *British Journal of Addiction*, 86: 391–398.

Jainchill, N., Hawke, J., and Messina, M. (2005) 'Post-treatment outcomes among adjudicated adolescent males and females in modified therapeutic community treatment', *Substance Use & Misuse*, 40(7): 975–996.

Karver, M.S., Handelsman, J.B., Fields, S., and Bickman, L. (2006) 'Meta-analysis of therapeutic relationship variables in youth and family therapy: The evidence for different relationship variables in the child and adolescent treatment outcome literature', *Clinical Psychology Review*, 26(1): 50–65.

Kitzmann, K.M., Gaylord, N.K., Holt, A.R., and Kenny, E.D. (2003) 'Child witnesses to domestic violence: A meta-analytical review', *Journal of Consulting and Clinical Psychology*, 71: 339–352.

Knight, J.R., Sherritt, L., Harris, S.K., Gates, E.C., and Chang, G. (2003) 'Validity of brief alcohol screening tests among adolescents: A comparison of the AUDIT, POSIT, CAGE, and CRAFFT', *Alcoholism: Clinical and Experimental Research*, 27(1): 67–73.

Knight, J.R., Sherritt, R., Harris, L., Sion, K. and Grace, C. (2002) 'Validity of the CRAFFT substance abuse screening test among adolescent clinic patients', *Archives of Pediatrics & Adolescent Medicine*, 156: 607–614.

Knight, J.R., Shrier, L.A., Bravender, T.D., Farrell, M., Vander Bilt, J., and Shaffer, H.J. (1999) 'A new brief screen for adolescent substance abuse', *Archives of Pediatrics & Adolescent Medicine*, 153(6): 591–596.

Linehan, M.M., Schmidt, H., Dimeff, L.A., Craft, J.C., Kanter, J., and Comtois, K.A. (1999) 'Dialectical behavior therapy for patients with borderline personality disorder and drug dependence', *American Journal on Addictions*, 8: 279–292.

Lloyd, C. (1998) 'Risk factors for problem drug use: Identifying vulnerable groups', *Drugs: Education, Prevention, and Policy*, 5(3): 217–232.

Lynskey, M. and Hall, W. (2000) 'The effects of adolescent cannabis use on educational attainment: A review', *Addiction*, 95(11): 1621–1630.

McArdle, P. and Angom, B. (2012) 'Adolescent substance misuse: An update on behaviours and treatments', *Advances in Psychiatric Treatment*, 18(4): 299–307.

McSweeney, T., Stevens, A., Hunt, N., and Turnbull, P.J. (2007) 'Twisting arms or a helping hand? Assessing the impact of "coerced" and comparable "voluntary" drug treatment options', *British Journal of Criminology*, 47(3): 470–490.

Martin, C.S., Kaczynski, N.A., Maisto, S.A., and Tarter, R.E. (1996) 'Polydrug use in adolescent drinkers with and without DSM–IV alcohol abuse and dependence', *Alcoholism: Clinical and Experimental Research*, 20: 1099–1108.

Menard, S. (2002) 'Short and long-term consequences of adolescent victimization', *Office of Juvenile Justice and Delinquency Prevention*, 19: 121–125.

Miller, W.R. and Rollnick, S. (1991) *Motivational Interviewing: Preparing People to Change Addictive Behavior*. New York: Guilford Press.

Miller, W.R. and Rollnick, S. (2002) *Motivational Interviewing (Second Edition): Preparing people for change* New York. Guildford Press

Mirza, K.A.H. and Mirza, S. (2008) 'Adolescent substance misuse', *Psychiatry*, 7(8): 357–362.

Mitchell, K.J. and Finkelhor, D. (2001) 'Risk of crime victimization among youth exposed to violence', *Journal of Interpersonal Violence*, 16(9): 944–964.

NICE (National Institute of for Health and Care Excellence) (2007) 'Interventions to reduce substance misuse among vulnerable young people'. Available at: http://www.nice.org.uk/guidance/ph4, accessed 08 May 2015.

NICE (National Institute for Health and Care Excellence) (2007) 'Drug misuse-psychosocial interventions' Available at: https://www.nice.org.uk/guidance/CG51, accessed 08 May 2015

NICE (National Institute for Health and Care Excellence) (2011) 'Alcohol-use disorders: diagnosis, assessment and management of harmful drinking and alcohol dependence' Available at: http://www.nice.org.uk/guidance/cg115

NTA (National Treatment Agency) (2011) *Substance Misuse among Young People 2010–2011*. London: National Treatment Agency.

NTA (National Treatment Agency) (2012) *Psychosocial Interventions in Drug Misuse: A Framework and Toolkit for Implementing NICE-Recommended Treatment Interventions*. London: National Treatment Agency.

NTA (National Treatment Agency) (2013) *Substance Misuse among Young People in England 2012–2013*. London: National Treatment Agency.

NTA (National Treatment Agency) for Substance Misuse (2009) *Young People's Specialist Substance Misuse Treatment: Exploring the Evidence*. United Kingdom: National Treatment Agency.

OHRN (Offender Health Research Network) (2013) 'Comprehensive health assessment tool'. Available at: http://www.ohrn.nhs.uk/OHRNResearch/CHAT, accessed 08 May 2015.

Patterson, G.R. and Yoerger, K. (1997) 'A Developmental Model for Late-Onset Delinquency', in R. Dienstbier and D.W. Osgood (eds.), *The Nebraska Symposium on Motivation*. Lincoln, NE: University of Nebraska Press, 119–177.

Patton, G.C., Coffey, C., Carlin, J.B., Degenhardt, L., Lynskey, M., and Hall, W. (2002) 'Cannabis use and mental health in young people: Cohort study', *BMJ*, 325(7374): 1195–1198.

Prendergast, M., Podus, D., Finney, J., Greenwell, L., and Roll, J. (2006) 'Contingency management for treatment of substance use disorders: A meta-analysis', *Addiction*, 101(11): 1546–1560.

Robertson, A.A., Dill, P.L., Husain, J., and Undesser, C. (2004) 'Prevalence of mental illness and substance abuse disorders among incarcerated juvenile offenders in Mississippi', *Child Psychiatry and Human Development*, 35(1): 55–74.

Seddon, T. (2006) 'Drugs, crime and social exclusion social context and social theory in British drugs: Crime research', *British Journal of Criminology*, 46(4): 680–703.

Stoker, A. and Swadi, H. (1990) 'Perceived family relationships in drug-abusing adolescents', *Drug and Alcohol Dependence*, 25: 293–297.

Swadi, H. (1999) 'Individual risk factors for adolescent substance use', *Drug and Alcohol Dependence*, 55(3): 209–224.

Swadi, H. (2000) 'Substance misuse in adolescents', *Advances in Psychiatric Treatment*, 6(3): 201–210.

Tanner-Smith, E.E., Wilson, S.J., and Lipsey, M.W. (2013) 'The comparative effectiveness of outpatient treatment for adolescent substance abuse: A meta analysis', *Journal of Substance Abuse Treatment*, 44: 145–158.

Tapert, S.F., Caldwell, L., and Burke, C. (2004) 'Alcohol and the adolescent brain', *Alcohol Research & Health*, 28: 205–212.

Tevyaw, T.O.L. and Monti, P.M. (2004) 'Motivational enhancement and other brief interventions for adolescent substance abuse: Foundations, applications and evaluations', *Addiction*, 99(2): 63–75.

Thomas, C.R. and Penn, J.V. (2002) 'Juvenile justice mental health services', *Child & Adolescent Psychiatry Clinics North America*, 11: 731.

UK Government (2014) 'Drug penalties'. Available at: https://www.gov.uk/penalties-drug-possession-dealing. Accessed 28 January 2015.

User Voice (2011) 'What's Your Story? Young Offenders' Insights into Tackling Youth Crime and its Causes'. Available at: http://www.uservoice.org, accessed 08 May 2015.

Velleman, R.D., Templeton, L.J., and Copello, A.G. (2005) 'The role of the family in preventing and intervening with substance use and misuse: A comprehensive review of family interventions, with a focus on young people', *Drug and Alcohol Review*, 24(2): 93–109.

Waldron, H.B. and Turner, C.W. (2008) 'Evidence-based psychosocial treatments for adolescent substance abuse', *Journal of Clinical Child & Adolescent Psychology*, 37(1): 238–261.

Welte, J.W., Barnes, G.M., Hoffman, J.H., Wieczorek, W.F., and Zhang, L. (2005) 'Substance involvement and the trajectory of criminal offending in young males', *American Journal of Drug and Alcohol Abuse*, 31: 267–284.

Wiessing, L., Olszewski, D., Klempová, D., Vicente, J., and Griffiths, P. (2009) 'EMCDDA annual report 2009: Cocaine and heroin maintain firm hold on Europe's drug scene', *Euro Surveill*, 14: 46.

YJB (Youth Justice Board) (2003) 'The mental health screening questionnaire interview for adolescents'. Available at: https://www.gov.uk/government/uploads/system/uploads/attachment_data/file/377538/SQUIFA.pdf, accessed 08 May 2015

YJB (Youth Justice Board) (2004) 'Substance misuse and the juvenile secure estate'. Available at: http://yjbpublications.justice.gov.uk/en-gb/Resources/Downloads/SubstanceMisuseJSEsummary.pdf, accessed 08 May 2015

YJB (Youth Justice Board) (2006) 'YOT substance misuse worker: Integrating youth justice provision and substance misuse treatment (B271)'. Available at: http://www.dldocs.stir.ac.uk/documents/youthguide.pdf or for download at http://yjbpublications.justice.gov.uk/en-gb/scripts/prodView.asp?idProduct=298&eP=, accessed 08 May 2015

YJB (Youth Justice Board) (2008) *Key Elements of Effective Practice: Substance Misuse*. London: Youth Justice Board.Young, S. and Thome, J. (2011) 'ADHD and offenders', *World Journal of Biological Psychiatry*, 12(1): 124–128.

12
Intellectual Disabilities

Charlotte Staniforth and Yve Griffin

Introduction

Over recent years the interest in young people with an intellectual disability (ID) within forensic settings has increased. There is growing awareness of the vulnerability factors that could increase the likelihood of contact with forensic services and affect ability to fully comprehend and participate in the criminal justice process.

This chapter will commence by defining ID, as well as outlining the co-morbidities associated with this diagnostic label. It will also discuss the reasons why those with an ID come into contact with services, along with issues to consider when assessing, formulating and providing interventions for this population. To demonstrate how this translates into practice, a case study will be presented.

The language used when talking about the high-risk behaviours of young people with ID can be hard to navigate when terms such as challenging behaviour, risk behaviour and offending behaviour are used interchangeably. For continuity, the term 'high-risk behaviour' will be used in this section to refer to any behaviour that can put the young person or members of the public at risk of significant psychological or physical harm, whether or not this behaviour has resulted in a conviction. Examples of high-risk behaviours include: physical aggression, sexually harmful behaviour, fire-setting, substance abuse and acquisitive offending.

Definition

Although a variety of terms, including learning disabilities and mental retardation, have been used when referring to people who have impairments that impact on their cognitive and adaptive functioning, this chapter will use the term 'intellectual disabilities' to refer to this population. ID refers to the onset of delayed developmental milestones, which impacts on intellectual and functional development, hence independent functioning is likely to be significantly lower than that of the average person during their lifetime (WHO 2001). The British Psychological Society (BPS 2000) stress that, for a person to have an ID, they must have significant impairment in both intellectual functioning and social/adaptive functioning, with these impairments present since childhood.

Although diagnostic systems can be useful in terms of aetiology and as taxonomies that can aid research and intervention guidelines, there are significant limitations to the diagnostic approach, highlighted in ongoing debates about the most helpful way to understand and help people with mental health difficulties (BPS-DCP 2011). There are two main classification systems used to diagnose mental disorder: the International Classification of Diseases (Version 10, ICD-10; WHO 1992) and the *Diagnostic and Statistical Manual of Mental Disorders*, which has recently published its fifth version (DSM-5; American Psychiatric Association (APA) 2013b).

DSM-5 now uses the term intellectual disability (intellectual developmental disorder), moving away from the mental retardation label and bringing DSM-5 in line with ICD-10. Intellectual developmental disorder has three domains: conceptual, social and practical, with the emphasis being on the exploration of how cognitive deficits impact adaptive functioning in all three domains. DSM-5 also highlights the importance of not overemphasising cognitive ability without adequately considering functioning levels, which can be especially important for forensic cases. Further details on the changes in DSM-5 can be found in the guidelines published by the APA (2013).

Young people with an ID represent a heterogeneous group in terms of the extent and nature of their strengths and impairments (WHO 2001) (see Table 12.1).

Prevalence

Current estimates suggest that 2 per cent of people meet the criteria for ID in the UK (Emerson et al. 2012). Studies of young offender populations report varying ID prevalence rates, although all studies report that the prevalence is higher than in the general population. For example, Kazdin (2000) cited prevalence rates between 7 and 15 per cent for delinquent youth populations. However, more recent studies found the prevalence of ID in young offenders in custody and in the community to be much higher (between 20 and 32 per cent) (Chitsabesan et al. 2007; Hughes et al. 2012). If young people with below average IQ scores (rather than a diagnosis of a formal ID) are considered, the rates are higher still (Chitsabesan et al. 2007).

Young people with an ID are over-represented in the use of community-based sanctions such as Antisocial Behaviour Orders (ASBOs; Fyson and Yates 2011).

Table 12.1 Table of impairments associated with ID

Domain	How impairment may present
Cognitive abilities including executive functioning	• Concrete thinking • Planning and organisation • Problem solving • Consequential thinking • Emotional regulation • Impulsivity • Frustration tolerance • Disinhibition
Social abilities	• Overfamiliarity • Discrimination with regards to the recipient of their interactions • Social comments and actions related to context and recipient • Understanding of social rules and norms
Adaptive behaviours	• Expressive and receptive communication • Awareness of safety and risk • Academic functioning (literacy, numeracy and so on) • Activities of daily living (self-care and home living)
Physical health	• Predisposition to genetic disorders or health conditions • Awareness of good physical health and recognising symptoms of ill health and how to manage these • May be linked with other health complications from birth trauma and/or syndromes
Sensory	• Over- or undersensitive to pain, noise, touch, taste, texture of foods, visual stimuli, vestibular and proprioceptive stimuli

In a British study, Campbell (2002) found that 9 per cent of young people receiving an ASBO had an ID. The British Institute for Brain Injured Children (2005) compared data from antisocial behaviour co-ordinators (ASBs) and youth offending teams (YOTs). The ASBs reported that 5 per cent of ASBOs were given to children with an ID or mental health disorder, but they did not identify any cases of autism spectrum disorder (ASD). YOTs reported a much higher rate of 37 per cent for ID and mental health problems, and 20 per cent for ASD.

In summary, prevalence studies suggest disproportionally high rates of ID across a range of forensic settings for young people. Studies highlight issues around poor recognition and identification of ID in young offenders, and the disparity between prevalence rates across settings and services may reflect this. Mild ID and significant learning difficulties may be missed in mainstream schools due to attention being paid to the more salient externalising problems presented (behavioural overshadowing). This means that any impact ID has on the behaviour of young people may be underestimated. This is despite the fact that cognitive ability is likely to have a major role to play in a variety of factors related to prosocial behaviour, such as decision-making (Kazdin 2000), impulsivity, problem solving and social vulnerability (including suggestibility and compliance). The relevance for forensic practice is that young people with an ID may get involved with the criminal justice system (CJS) more than their peers without an ID, not because they are more predisposed to antisocial behaviour, but due to factors linked to their ID that may not have been appropriately identified or managed previously. This could lead to the criminalisation of behaviour that can also be influenced by attributions held by others. Once within the CJS, young people with an ID face a range of further disadvantages, which will be explored later in the chapter.

Co-morbidity

Young people with an ID have been found to be at least six times more likely to have a co-morbid psychiatric diagnosis or neurodevelopmental disorder than their non-ID peers, including being 33 per cent more likely to have a diagnosis of ASD, eight times more likely to have a diagnosis of attention deficit hyperactivity disorder (ADHD) and four times more likely to have a diagnosis of emotional disorder (Emerson and Hatton 2007). The same authors highlighted the fact that 3 per cent of British children with an ID accounted for 14 per cent of the total psychiatric morbidity. A systematic review of co-morbidity of ID and a mental health diagnosis in children found co-morbidity to be between 30 and 50 per cent (Einfeld, Ellis and Emerson 2011). The authors state that only age, gender and severity of the ID have been investigated with any degree of regularity, and the results regarding these potential risk factors are inconclusive. In another UK study, 50.7 per cent of a sample of adolescents with an ID screened positive for a mental health diagnosis, mainly in the disruptive and antisocial domains. Almost all of those were found to have an identifiable ICD-10 diagnosis of mental disorder. The most common diagnoses included pervasive developmental disorders, hyperkinetic disorder and emotional disorders, with males and those with autism being more likely to be reported as cases. Co-morbidity can also be an important issue for families, as the mental well-being of parents with children with ID is more strongly influenced by the severity of the child's mental disorder than the severity of their ID (Tonge and Einfeld 2003).

Reasons for referral to adolescent forensic services

Young people with an ID are referred to community and secure forensic services for a range of high-risk behaviours, including sexually harmful behaviour, aggression, self-injurious behaviour and fire-setting. As these high-risk behaviours are discussed in detail in other chapters, this section will focus on specific overarching issues relating to working with high-risk behaviours with ID populations.

There is a dearth of literature exploring the prevalence of the types of high-risk behaviour displayed by young people with an ID. There is a wider literature base relating to adults, although studies are fraught with methodological difficulties, including whether behaviour has been considered to be an offence or 'challenging behaviour', locating the sample (whether people with borderline intellectual disabilities are included in ID registers) and having a valid control group. People with an ID are not more predisposed to crime, but they are more likely to experience risk factors associated with criminal behaviour (Dickson, Emerson and Hatton 2005).

For adolescents with an ID, aggression is one of the strongest predictors of crisis intervention referrals and admission/readmission to residential facilities (Lakin 1983; Shoham-Vardi et al. 1996). Aggressive and disruptive behaviours are also one of the strongest predictors of parental stress for families caring for a young person with an ID (Baker et al. 2002). Although aggressive behaviour appears to be relatively common in people with an ID, McClintock, Hall and Oliver (2003) found, in their meta-analysis, that the prevalence of aggression is increased in young people with both ASD and ID, and is higher in this group than for those who have an ID alone.

A well-cited systematic review conducted in 2001 (Simpson and Hogg 2001a, 2001b) concluded that there was no convincing evidence that people with ID had higher prevalence rates of forensic activity when compared to those without an ID. The same review found that sexual offending, criminal damage and burglary were possibly over-represented in people that had a 'borderline' ID, whereas murder and armed robbery were under-represented. Rose and colleagues (2008) completed an audit of people with an ID who were 16 years or over, who were using services in a single urban district in the UK and who had been in contact with the CJS. They found that sexual assaults against adults and children and physical violence were the most common type of forensic behaviour identified from file review and staff interview. Physical violence and property destruction frequently co-occurred.

In a Dutch study using a sample of young people from ID and mainstream school, Douma and colleagues (2007) found that 10–20 per cent of young people with an ID engaged in antisocial or delinquent behaviours. In terms of the type of antisocial behaviour, young males with an ID were significantly more likely to engage in being mean to others, physical aggression, theft or arson and property destruction. No difference was observed in girls with or without an ID. In terms of persistence of antisocial behaviour, the authors found that behaviour at the time of initial assessment time one predicted behaviour five years later.

Dickson, Emerson and Hatton (2005) compared the self-reported antisocial behaviour of young people with and without ID in the UK. They found that those with an ID reported more antisocial behaviours over one year, including stealing valuable items, using weapons, arson, destroying property, stealing in the street, bullying and threatening behaviours, and being in trouble with the police, with the latter two being the most commonly reported. Young people with an ID also reported being involved in more physical violence and forced sexual acts. However, the difference did not reach statistical significance. The authors concluded that these differences could be accounted for by the higher prevalence of mental health problems and social deprivation in the ID sample.

Despite the relative lack of research relating to young people, there is evidence that neurodisability may put young people 'at risk' of offending due to hyperactivity and impulsivity, poor emotional regulation, cognitive and language impairment and alienation (Hughes et al. 2012), making it crucial to assess young people's strengths and deficits. The impact of abuse is also important to consider, given that children who have been mistreated are at a higher risk of delinquency (Maxfield and Widom 1996), and given that many juveniles in the legal system have a history of abuse (Widom 1989). This may be particularly relevant for ID offender populations when considering that children with an ID are at higher risk of maltreatment (Westcott and Jones 1999).

Assessment and formulation

Due to the complex needs of this population, assessments from a variety of professionals are necessary to ensure all areas of functioning are assessed, including mental state, physical health and development, social and daily living skills, intellectual and academic abilities, family make-up and dynamics and communication skills. Information gleaned from these assessments can help practitioner psychologists and others to formulate difficulties and to adapt their approach to aid assessment. A team approach can also encourage debates and ensure that information is considered from a variety of different perspectives, potentially challenging any bias. Good communication between professionals can aid the streamlining of care and ensure priority needs are met in a co-ordinated fashion without unnecessary duplication of intervention.

Consideration should be given to the assessment *process* to ensure that it is developmentally appropriate and not overly aversive, which can be distressing and impact on the outcomes of the assessment. One such consideration is to break down larger assessments into achievable 'chunks' to improve the validity of the outcomes. If these amendments are required, it is important to document them appropriately. For further information on methodological issues, including the role of acquiescence when assessing people with an ID, please refer to Finlay and Lyons (2002).

Assessment of ID

It is important to assess all areas highlighted in Table 12.1 of this chapter. A description of all relevant assessments is beyond the scope of this chapter, (see Carr et al. 2007 for a review).

Internationally, three criteria need to be met before an ID can be identified: intellectual impairment, social or adaptive dysfunction and early onset (developmental history in line with developmental delay) (Holland 2011). A comprehensive assessment of this type can be time-consuming and requires a certain level of psychological expertise, particularly in administering and interpreting cognitive assessments, such as the Wechsler Intelligence Scale for Children (4th Edition, WISC-IV) (Wechsler 2003). This can be administered to children aged between 6 years and 16 years and 11 months of age, while the Wechsler Adult Intelligence Scale (4th Edition, WAIS-IV) (Wechsler 2008) can be administered to individuals aged 16 years to 90 years 11 months of age.

There is no agreed systematic approach to identifying young offenders with an ID. Screening tools are not sufficient and staff have little training in this area (Chitsabesan et al. 2007). From clinical experience, it has been noted that if cognitive assessments are administered early in admission, the scores can be affected by a number of factors, including poor mental state and a lack of engagement and/or motivation. Some services, including youth offending institutions (YOIs) or secure training centres (STCs) may not have the resources in terms of staff expertise to administer more reliable neuropsychological assessments. Noble and Conley (1992) found that IQ scores tended to be lower when people were tested shortly after entering prison. Scores may be difficult to interpret as young people with an ID and co-morbid diagnoses may have uneven cognitive profiles, or discrepancies between their cognitive and adaptive abilities. Again, co-morbidity can create a complicated picture, as many young people may have a history of head injury, significant substance misuse (SM), epilepsy or developmental trauma for example, all of which may influence a cognitive profile. Chitsabesan and colleagues (2007) found that many young offenders had a significant discrepancy between verbal and performance IQ, with performance IQ generally being the higher score and difficulties with verbal reasoning being common. These deficits are important to assess, as verbal reasoning has been linked to antisocial risk factors such as hostile attributional bias (Crick and Dodge 1994; Wong and Cornell 1999). Understanding a young person's individual cognitive profile can also aid the tailoring of interventions and the consideration of future risks of reoffending.

Measures of adaptive functioning such as the Vinelands Adaptive Behaviour Scale: Version 2 (Sparrow, Chiccetti and Balla 2005) and the Adaptive Behaviour Assessment System: Version 2 (ABAS-II; Harrison and Oakland 2003) can be used to assess areas such as conceptual, practical and social ability: the three areas of assessment recommended in DSM-5.

It is also important to assess the physical health of young people with an ID, as they are more prone to experience health difficulties such as dysphasia, epilepsy, bowel problems and conditions relating to the aetiology of their ID, such as birth complications (Royal College of General Practitioners 2012). Sometimes, challenging behaviour is linked to discomfort associated with these health conditions or feeling physically unwell, something which the young person may not be able to communicate effectively. Furthermore, there are certain behaviour phenotypes that are related to ID such as fragile X, XYY syndrome, and foetal alcohol syndrome (Cassidy and Allanson 2010). If possible, genetic testing is recommended if these syndromes are suspected.

Assessment of psychosocial functioning

It is important not to assume that a young person's high-risk behaviour is due to their ID alone, and key to assess psychological functioning, including the presence of any emotional or mental health difficulties. Many assessments rely on the individual reporting their internal state, which is often difficult for young people with an ID if they are unaware of, or have difficulty labelling, their experiences. Initial psychological assessment should therefore consider the emotional and social understanding of the self and others. There are tools that can help professionals with this task, such as The Awareness of Social Inference Test (TASIT) (McDonald et al. 2003) which uses video vignettes to explore social perception, and the Mind Reading Programme (Baron-Cohen 2006), which is a computerised programme that can be used to both assess and develop awareness of emotions in the self and others based on facial and voice cues.

There are few psychometrics that have been specifically designed for an adolescent ID population, and psychometrics that are used to assess typically developing adolescents may not be valid or appropriate. Psychometrics that have been developed for use with people with an ID are usually designed for adults. This means that the clinician working with the adolescent has a choice of using either a measure designed for adults, or designed for adolescents without an ID. Even with these hurdles, it may be possible to use some psychometrics if any questionable validity is explicitly stated in reports and certain adaptations are made. For example, it may be possible to use some of the most widely used psychometrics such as the Beck Youth Inventories: Version 2 (BYI-II; Beck et al. 2005) and Strength and Difficulties Questionnaire (SDQ) (Goodman, Meltzer and Bailey 1998) if the language is slightly adapted and the young person is supported with visual aids such as Likert scales. This may also be the case for psychometrics that aim to capture offence-related and specific factors; for example, the Fire Attitude Scale (Muckley 1997), the How I Think Questionnaire (Gibbs, Barriga and Potter 2001), the Victim Empathy Scales (Beckett and Fisher 1994) and the Maudsley Violence Questionnaire

(Walker 2005). Any adaptations in the use of psychometrics and, consequently, the potential impact on validity need to be explicitly stated in reports.

Although no comprehensive assessment should rely too heavily on psychometrics, this is especially the case for young people with ID, where assessments need to be multimodal. Interviewing the young person is usually recommended, although the format this takes may vary depending on the young person's presentation. Awareness of the approach needed in interacting with a person with an ID is very important. Leading questions should be avoided, due to the increased chance of a young person with an ID being acquiescent and compliant (Finlay and Lyons 2001). Adaptations are wide ranging, but may include assessments occurring over a shorter time frame or with breaks. The context or setting may be adjusted, for example talking to the young person whilst going out for a walk, sitting on the sofa or playing a game. The means of communication may be adapted or varied depending on the young person's favoured mode of communication. An example would be using picture cards showing choices, such as a low stimulus room or a sensory activity. When communicating verbally, concrete examples may need to be used by saying, for example, 'have you tried the weighted blanket, that worked really well yesterday' rather than 'use your coping skills'.

Information from third parties such as families, previous carers, and the observations and feedback from staff currently caring for the young person can be invaluable, especially if the young person's difficulties are such that they cannot report their internal states or they are currently refusing to engage in the assessment process. Indeed, due to cognitive and social difficulties, challenging behaviour may in fact represent the young person's way of communicating their internal world. For this reason, functional analysis of behaviour will often be useful in identifying the functions of behaviour and helping staff teams understand what may be maintaining unhelpful behaviours. Antecedent, behaviour and consequence charts are often a useful tool for identifying triggers and functions of problem behaviour, although at times more complex observation methods may be required, due to the fact that a behaviour may have more than one function. For example, the same behaviour may be used to communicate and to avoid demands (see Sturmey 2008 for a review).

The assessment and treatment of people with an ID who have experienced trauma is an under-researched area, which is problematic considering people with ID have higher than average rates of emotional trauma, abuse and neglect (Yates 2009b). Young people should be asked about their negative life experiences at initial interview. There are tools available to aid professionals with this task, which, from clinical experience, are useful with an ID group. These questionnaires include the Trauma Symptom Checklist for Children (TSCC; Briere 1996) and the Impact of Events Scale (IES; Weiss and Marmar 1997). The TSCC is used to assess indicators of trauma, including those arising from sexual abuse, whereas the IES looks at a wider range of traumatic stressors. Although these types of psychometrics may be useful in highlighting areas for further assessment and treatment for specific traumatic experiences, they have limited utility in assessing developmental trauma. There is increasing awareness that early chronic developmental trauma has a different presentation, which can mirror and overlap deficits present in ID, such as difficulties with self-regulation, social skills and empathy (Schore 2013).

Repeating psychometric assessments post-intervention can provide useful outcome data. However, self-report psychometrics often focus on problems and should not be the sole measure of outcome. Carer reports regarding the young person's functioning and skill development should be sought, whether in questionnaire or interview format. A more holistic approach means that much richer information about skill development can be sought, including: changes in the young person's ability to relate, acquisition of hobbies and preferred activities, and development of coping skills, for example. Observable changes in behavioural presentations, including positive behaviours engaged in, and attendance and engagement in interventions offered, also provide useful information about therapeutic progress. Although this approach to measuring outcome requires more subjective feedback from those involved in the young person's care, it is more person centred, with a positive skill-based focus.

Risk assessment

It is important that young people with an ID with forensic needs have an appropriate assessment of risk undertaken, so that professionals can develop an in-depth understanding of the risks presented, giving the best opportunity for effective risk management. Structured professional judgement (SPJ) tools are considered the most effective approach to violence risk management (DH 2007). SPJ tools aim to use structured assessment approaches (based on research) to inform rather than replace clinical decision-making. A comprehensive risk assessment should always lead to a risk formulation. A risk formulation provides an explanation of the historical and current, individual and contextual factors specific to the risks in question, which can then inform intervention planning. Risk assessment can identify specific risk factors and how these can be managed by avoidance of trigger situations and the development of improved coping strategies with appropriate supervision (Murphy 2010). However, the risk assessment is only as good as the communication of the summary and scenarios that follow. A key role of the practitioner psychologist within adolescent forensic settings is to ensure that other members of the team have an understanding of the risks a young person may present, situations in which they are most likely to occur, and the best way to monitor and manage the risk.

There are no tools specifically designed to assess risk in relation to adolescents with ID, although there have been risk assessment tools designed for adult ID populations. These include the Assessment of Risk and Manageability of Individuals with Developmental and Intellectual Limitations who Offend (ARMADILO; Blacker et al. 2011), the ARMADILO-S, specifically for adults with an ID who sexually offend (Boer et al. 2012), and the Dynamic Risk Assessment and Management System (Lindsay et al. 2004). However, the predictive validity of these measures should be approached with some caution. Additionally, the STATIC-99 (Hanson and Thornton 2000) and the Violence Risk Appraisal Guide (Quinsey et al. 2006) have good predictive validity for violence and sexual offending respectively with adults who have an ID (Lindsay et al. 2008).

Common risk tools used with adolescents include the Structured Assessment of Violence Risk in Youth (SAVRY Version 1.1; Borum, Bartel and Forth 2003) and the Estimate of Risk of Adolescent Sexual Offence Recidivism (ERASOR Version 2.0; Worling and Curwen 2001). Although these were not designed with an ID population in mind, there is a growing evidence base that they may have predictive utility with this group (Adamson, McLean and Sher 2011). The authors have found that using the 'additional items' section to consider factors potentially implicated in the risk of offending in people with ID is helpful. These factors often include specific cognitive impairments, empathy, social and emotional recognition and understanding, emotional regulation and patterns of arousal levels. In terms of the developmental delay experienced by people with ID and the fact that they are often cared by for others, it is recommended that the young people with ID continue to be assessed using the SAVRY and ERASOR until the age of 21, rather than 18 (Boer et al. 2010). A detailed discussion of this topic is beyond the scope of this chapter; see Adamson, McLean and Sher (2011) for a review.

Assessing fitness to plead and supporting vulnerable witnesses

People with an ID may be disadvantaged in the criminal justice process. They may struggle to understand the legal processes and be more likely to make false allegations/confessions (Drizin and Leo 2004). Gudjonsson and Henry (2003) have investigated the importance of suggestibility as it applies to child and adult witnesses with ID. They found that children and adults with an ID have poorer memories and are more suggestible than those without an ID, with the children being more susceptible than the adults to altering their responses under pressure. Furthermore, the authors' discovered that young people with an ID are more vulnerable to subtle psychological influences such as persuasion, deception and coercion (Gudjonsson and Henry 2003).

The attributions of others may also influence a young person's experience and outcome in the CJS. For example, a study using a mock trial found that jurors favoured a young person with an ID as a victim of, or witness to, an offence, more so than those without an ID, although this was not the case in more serious offences (Najdowski, Bottoms and Vargas 2009). Also, jurors' attributions can be that young people with an ID are more likely to commit crimes such as vandalism, rather than offences that require planning, such as burglary (Gibbons, Gibbons and Cissin 1981). Jurors are also more likely to make external attributions regarding the motivations of young people with an ID. For example, being more likely to believe that the young person has been coerced, rather than engaging in the crime for financial gain (Gibbons, Sawin and Gibbons 1979).

As a result of these factors, people with an ID often require special legal provision. Practitioner psychologists have an important role to play in aiding the court to ensure that young people with an ID are treated fairly and appropriately in the judicial system. Assessments may include whether young people can understand the court proceedings and what role, if any, their ID had in their victimisation or offending. As well as cognitive and adaptive functioning, suggestibility, acquiescence and compliance may be important areas to assess. Some young people are also diverted to hospital under the Mental Health Act, without the facts of the case being heard and guilt established. Specialist assessments can be extremely important in informing the court about the nature of the young person's disability and may provide some insight into the offence committed. Furthermore, these assessments can also inform any specialist support that the young person may require through the legal process.

In terms of fitness to plead, young people must be assessed on the written or oral evidence of two or more registered medical practitioners, at least one of whom must be duly approved under Section 12 of the Mental Health Act (1983). Although it is not mandatory at present, the authors would recommend that the assessing psychiatrist has expertise in either, but preferably both, adolescent forensic and ID psychiatry. To aid in this process, someone may be transferred to a hospital setting for assessment. If it is ascertained that the offending occurred in the context of a diagnosed mental health disorder, the forensic mental health assessment can be invaluable, as treatment of the mental illness can reduce the likelihood of future offending (WHO 2001).

There are drives to increase the awareness of ID amongst professionals involved in the legal system, such as court officials, the police and solicitors. This is important, as it means that young people are supported from the earliest opportunity by, for example, the provision of the appropriate adult and a videotaped interview. In a study conducted by Medford, Gudjonsson and Pearse (2003), the presence of an appropriate adult at police interview increased the likelihood that legal representation will be present, was associated with less interrogative pressure and indicated that the legal representative would take a more active role.

Psychological formulation

Information from a range of assessments, including the risk assessment, are used to come to a tentative understanding (formulation) of how the young person's difficulties have developed, how they are currently manifesting and what is maintaining them. A good formulation should guide intervention planning, consider systemic factors and also identify the young person's strengths. It may be that a number of areas for intervention have been highlighted, and thought needs to be given in terms of prioritising and then sequencing interventions. For example, a young person may need to develop social skills and emotional understanding and regulation skills before it is appropriate for them to take part in an adapted sex offender treatment programme.

Young people with an ID are a very heterogeneous group and specific diagnostic labels rarely inform formulation directly. Formulating the needs of young people with an ID should be undertaken using the same guiding principles as a young person without an ID (for guidance on best practice in formulation see BPS-DCP 2011). However, there may be certain aspects of a formulation to which the clinician working with an adolescent with an ID may pay particular attention. An individualised assessment of the specific deficits associated with the ID is really important, for example, cognitive, social, behavioural, sensory (Murphy 2010). Any identified deficits can then be explored, and any strengths can be built upon and used to aid intervention. Gralton, Staniforth and Griffin (2011) have suggested certain key aspects of cognitive and social functioning that may need specific consideration, including: social skills and understanding, attention and concentration, communication skills, memory, problem-solving deficits, reduced ability to understand abstract concepts and language, suggestibility, compliance, empathy and theory of mind.

Formulations are most useful when they are shared, which means that the clinician may need to be creative and flexible regarding how this is achieved. Young people with an ID may benefit from a more visual and structured approach that considers one aspect at a time. The authors' experience is that formulation meetings with staff and families often work best when the participants generate the information and the clinician develops the formulation 'in the moment'. This guided discovery approach to exploring what the function of behaviour may be, or which responses from carers are maintaining behaviour, can be very powerful. For example, through discussion of behaviours, staff may have entered a formulation meeting with the assumption that the young person's aggression is unpredictable. However, during the course of discussions about the context of the behaviour, it is discovered that there are usually a number of other people present at the time, leading to the environment being noisy and chaotic. Considering that the behaviour is usually managed through isolating the young person in a low stimulus environment, staff begin to hypothesise whether the function of the behaviour is avoidance of noise/chaotic environments. If people looking after the young person can develop a shared understanding, this can help with increasing consistency in the way any problem behaviour is managed. This understanding can then challenge attributions about risk behaviours which may be misinformed.

Intervention

There is very little research in the area of psychological treatments for adolescents with an ID who display high-risk behaviours. Therefore, professionals tend to rely on the literature for interventions for adolescents without an ID. The focus in this section of the chapter will be on considerations required when working with a young person with an ID, including treatment adaptations.

A multidisciplinary approach is crucial when working with young people with an ID as it enables interventions offered to be co-ordinated and complimentary. Professional groups such as occupational therapists and speech and language therapists can provide crucial information and interventions for social communication impairments, sensory needs, optimal communication strategies and life skill development. The information gained from these assessments can also be used to facilitate psychological interventions by, for example, using sensory strategies at the beginning and end of sessions to encourage optimal engagement.

Individual and group work

Although it is known that people with an ID are likely to experience a number of psychosocial risk factors associated with high-risk behaviour, there is little specific research examining psychosocial interventions (Dagnan 2007; Brown et al. 2011). The most common approaches to address mental health needs and high-risk behaviours use both cognitive and behavioural strategies on both an individual and group basis (Willner 2005; Taylor, Lindsay and Willner 2008; Brown et al. 2011). Although it is reported that these approaches can be effective for issues such as anxiety and anger, as well as sexually harmful behaviours (Lindsay 1999), there are a number of methodological problems with the studies. Many of researched interventions have a number of intervention components, hence it is difficult to ascertain the effectiveness of each component (Bhaumik et al. 2011). In addition, the authors highlight that many of these trials have small numbers of participants, poor designs, lack control groups and use different measurements (Bhaumik et al. 2011).

Prior to considering the use of cognitive behavioural therapy (CBT), professionals must challenge their own perspectives and focus on the feelings and motives behind behaviours, rather than focusing on the behaviours themselves, as well as being prepared to work with the individual in a collaborative manner (Stenfert-Kroese 1997). Binnie and Blainey (2013) extend this view further and suggest that high-quality CBT should be formulation driven, and if the client's specific difficulties are incorporated and understood, therapy can be individualised to suit the client. Awareness of cognitive strengths and weaknesses is crucial for appropriately designing interventions, ensuring there is a good fit between the young person's understanding and communication abilities. For example, less focus on verbal delivery for a young person with poor verbal comprehension abilities. Adaptations made to the method of delivery of CBT for children and young people with an ID may include emotion recognition training, greater use of written and visual information, a more concrete and structured approach with greater repetition of topics, simplified cognitive activities and maintaining attention by offering regular breaks, for example. For further information see Stenfert-Kroese, Dagnan and Loumidis (1997). It is important to recognise the sequencing of interventions and the fact that, before embarking on specific diagnosis-driven or behaviour-specific work, young people may need to complete preparatory work which targets emotional regulation, coping skills and social skills.

If risk behaviour is related to co-morbid mental health needs, then the mental health needs will need to be addressed before focusing on the high-risk behaviour, as the latter may not be required or the focus may change following symptom reduction. If no coexisting mental health difficulties, physical disorder or environmental problem has been identified as triggering, or maintaining the behaviour that challenges, the young person should be offered a psychosocial intervention (informed by a functional behavioural analysis) as a first-line treatment. NICE guidelines (2011) would recommend that antipsychotic medication should be considered for challenging behaviours when psychosocial or other interventions are insufficient or could not be delivered because of the severity of the behaviour (NICE 2011).

If high-risk behaviour continues, despite more generic interventions being offered (such as emotional regulation and social skills work) and the co-morbid mental health condition has been addressed, the young person may benefit from evidence-informed offence-specific treatments such as fire-setting programmes and sex offender programmes. Given the paucity of research, it is recommended that practitioners use the same interventions as evidenced for those without ID, but with adaptations as discussed in the section 'Adaptations for treatment'. Some programmes have already been designed with young people with ID in mind, for example, the Adapted Sex Offender Treatment Programme (O'Callaghan 2005). Furthermore, interventions should adopt a 'Good Lives Model' (GLM) (Ward 2002) to encourage a more positive, integrated approach to reducing high-risk behaviour. The GLM holds the assumption that, while people who engage in high-risk behaviours have obligations to respect other people's entitlements to well-being and freedom, they are also entitled to the same considerations. According to the GLM, increasing well-being and reducing risk are inextricably linked, and the model considers the best way to create a safer society is to assist those who engage in high-risk behaviours to adopt more fulfilling and socially integrated lifestyles.

From clinical experience, offering interventions in a group setting (with individual support if required) can be helpful in demonstrating to the young people that there are others who experience similar difficulties, particularly if they feel alienated from their peers due to an increased awareness and perception of the self as being different.

Although there is quite an extensive literature on offence-specific treatments for adults with ID (Lindsay and Taylor 2005), there is a dearth of literature evaluating offence-specific treatments for young people with an ID and co-morbid mental health needs. This is most probably a reflection of the lack of specialised services that exist for adolescents with an ID, which means difficulties in gaining adequate samples with whom to conduct research. With this in mind, the most common approach seems to be the same as for any co-morbid mental health difficulties; use the same intervention as for those without an ID and make adaptations. This is an area that requires collaboration between services to increase the evidence base.

Furthermore, concerns have been raised that the skills learnt are often not generalised, as the individuals with an ID are often unaware that they have learnt a new skill. However, it has been suggested that this can be overcome through the use of meta-cognition training (Williams and Jones 1997). Williams and Jones suggest that people with an ID are dependent on external cues and guidance, a hypothesis which they tested. The results indicated that if participants were encouraged to ask themselves questions about new tasks they are learning and engage in verbal rehearsal whilst completing the task, they were more likely to consolidate new learning.

Adaptations for treatment

Special consideration will need to be given to the materials used in groups and group membership. Although the interventions offered to young people with an ID are commonly the same as those for the general population, to be effective, certain adaptations are suggested (see Box 12.1). To increase engagement and support the young person's processing of the information provided, these adaptations should take into account the young person's particular strengths and weaknesses.

> **Box 12.1 Suggested adaptations of interventions for young people with an ID**
>
> - Use a similar format across the different treatments offered (CBT structure is a good starting point). This will ensure the young people know what to expect each week, which will reduce anxiety.
> - Reduce the amount of change that occurs by having the same facilitators, and ensuring sessions occur at the same time and in the same place.
> - Visual material should be provided wherever possible, including the session structure and content.
> - Use simplified language and ensure the young person knows what the words used mean.
> - Use concrete examples and be mindful of the young person's tendency to take language literally.
> - Sessions should be multimodal to enable the young people to practise the skills using different methods, e.g. written, role play and discussion.
> - Make the sessions as fun and engaging as possible, ideally using the young person's special interest where possible.
> - Reduce distractions as much as possible.
> - Develop clear rules and expectations for sessions, ideally with the young person's involvement.
> - Encourage social interactions by asking group members to evaluate each other's behaviour.
> - Use positive reinforcement as much as possible, e.g. use of stars and fun review sessions for positive engagement.

Systemic and environmental factors

It is important to understand the social and environmental factors that may influence young people with an ID who offend. As discussed, young people with an ID may not have had their early developmental needs met due to a number of issues, such as lack of recognition, behavioural overshadowing, inappropriate educational provision and a lack of specialist community services. Impairments in social, communication and intellectual abilities can impair a young person's ability to understand expectations. Across a range of service provision, abnormal sensory sensitivities can lead to young people being distressed by the environment, resulting in an increase in risk behaviours with typical verbal interventions (de-escalation) being unlikely to be effective (Gabriels et al. 2012). People with an ID can be vulnerable to victimisation and assault from more able peers when placed in non-specialised forensic settings (Talbot 2008). Young people with an ID have additional needs to their peers without an ID, meaning that staff, carers or family members looking after them require specialist skills and training. If in a specialist setting, higher carer to service user ratios may be required.

When young people who cannot be managed at home transition to an appropriate and robust specialist placement, their behaviour may improve due to the high levels of structure, containment and other environmental factors provided by the service. This does not necessarily mean that any risk has reduced when the young person transitions to another service, especially as times of transition can be particularly stressful and destabilising for a young person with an ID. This means that additional support is required at times of transition to prepare the young person and limit distress. The topic of transition is covered in more detail in Chapter 13.

In addition to the physical environment, how staff approach, interact and manage young people with an ID can greatly impact on the behaviour displayed. This is particularly important as many interventions are offered indirectly through families or staff working with young people, for example, by using behaviour management plans. It can also be helpful to consider other environmental and systemic factors that may be at play, such as institutional disempowerment and attributions of others about the young person's difficulties.

Behavioural interventions, often provided indirectly through nursing or care staff, are the most common forms of interventions provided to people with an ID. Using these principles, functional assessment aims to understand the motivation for the behaviour displayed. Once ascertained, an individually tailored intervention can be developed and implemented, which will strengthen the adaptive behaviours that can serve the same function as the high-risk behaviour (Sturmey 2008). For example, following a functional analysis it may be identified that a young person is being aggressive in order to be secluded, due to a desire for a low stimulus environment. This knowledge can be used to generate a replacement behaviour that serves the same function. For example, the young person can be provided with a flash card communicating the need to use the quiet room or have some room time, through the use of functional communication training. It is important to remember that the replacement behaviour should take less effort than the current behaviour, if it is going to be successfully adopted by the individual (see Sturmey 2008 for a review of the behavioural approaches used with people with an ID).

For the reasons stated, staff training in working with young people with ID is crucial. Suggested themes for training include: at least an introduction and basic awareness of mental health, a basic awareness and understanding of child and adolescent development, understanding ID, applied behaviour principles and communication strategies. However, there can be numerous difficulties in training staff in terms of releasing them from duty, getting appropriate trainers and funding. The Bradley Report (DH 2009) indicates that attempts to train prison staff on ID awareness have been ineffective. It may not be the training per se that is ineffective, rather it may be that staff can find it difficult to apply the theory they have learnt to practice, particularly as no two individuals presenting with an ID are the same. In order to enhance the skills of the workforce in supporting young people with ID, ongoing support could be offered, such as using formulation meetings, offering consultation, supervision, modelling and encouraging staff to engage in reflective practice.

Ethical considerations

Professionals working with young people with an ID need to be particularly mindful when they are working with a potentially disempowered group of people. Every effort should be made to involve the young person in their own care as much as possible, even when this means changing the format that staff and external professionals are used to. This point was highlighted nationally following the exposure of physical and psychological abuse directed towards service users with intellectual disabilities and challenging behaviour, who were admitted to a private hospital in South West England, Winterbourne View. In the wake of the Winterbourne View Report, there are a number of findings and recommendations (DH 2012). In terms of outcomes, the report advised that those who use services for people with an ID and behaviour that challenges should be able to say:

> I am safe, I am treated with compassion, dignity and respect, I am involved in decisions about my care, I am protected from avoidable harm, but also have my own freedom to take risks, I am helped to keep in touch with my family and friends, those around me and looking after me are well supported, I am supported to make choices in my daily life, I get the right treatment and medication for my condition, I get good quality general healthcare, I am supported to live safely in the community, where I have additional care needs, I get the support I need in the most appropriate setting, my care is regularly reviewed to see if I should be moving on.
>
> (DH 2012: 51)

As with all client groups, confidentiality principles should be adhered to. It should not be assumed that information about treatment can be shared with the mother of an 18-year-old service user without asking them first. Often, staff may need to check that any consent given is informed consent and that the young person has the capacity to consent. To have capacity to consent, the young person must be able to understand the decision, weigh up the consequences of the decision, retain the information and be able to communicate the decision (Mental Capacity Act 2005). It cannot be assumed that a person does not have capacity (unless they are under 16); it must be assumed they do unless there is evidence otherwise. Assuming capacity needs to be carefully balanced with protecting young people from victimisation due to compliance and suggestibility. Capacity to consent is an area which needs to be revisited regularly, depending on the decision the young person needs to make. However, consent can often be raised as an issue in relation to sexual relationships, particularly in inpatient services where there can be a tendency to desexualise young people with an ID. This can highlight conflicting attitudes of staff towards the sexuality of people with an ID. There may also be specific issues that need consideration when conducting research with young people with an ID. These include each person's capacity to provide informed consent, and adapting materials and methodology to enable their participation as much as possible.

Practitioner psychologists have an important role to play in multidisciplinary team (MDT) decisions that may include consideration of potential issues such as care plans for restraint and seclusion (particularly restraint belts), behaviour programmes and isolation in extra care facilities. It is important that applied psychologists comply with good practice guidelines and use their knowledge regarding the young person to ensure that care and behaviour plans are individualised and consider the preferences of the young person (Royal College of Psychiatrists 2007). For example, if it is known that verbally communicating with the young person when they are aroused increases their arousal levels, then this should not be engaged in. It is important this is achieved to prevent over-restrictive or punitive practice, bearing in mind the vulnerability of this client group. This is especially pertinent currently, as there have been a number of recent high-profile reviews of the use of restrictive practices, which have been critical in terms of the overuse of these practices, leading to the development of guidelines for services (MIND 2013; DH 2014).

Professionals need to be aware of the legal frameworks and best practice guidelines linked to managing extreme risk behaviours, including safeguarding children and vulnerable adults, deprivation of liberty issues, the Children's Act (2004), the Mental Health Act (1983) and the Mental Capacity Act (2005). The abuse uncovered at Winterbourne View also highlighted the responsibility of professionals to report any practice they think is unethical. One of the recommendations from the Winterbourne View Report was that the National Institute for Clinical Excellence (NICE) will publish quality standards and clinical guidelines on challenging behaviour and ID in 2015 and quality standards and clinical guidelines on mental health and ID in 2016 (DH 2012).

Case study

The following composite case study attempts to highlight the complexities of psychological assessment and intervention with a young person with ID.

Background

Johnny is a 15-year-old male who has been referred to the Youth Offending Service (YOS) after he was convicted of robbery and assault with a weapon, which he had committed with an older peer. During the robbery Johnny had threatened the victim with a knife and punched him several times in the head and body.

Johnny is the middle child of seven born to his parents, who are now separated. Johnny grew up in an environment characterised by domestic violence and neglect. His father and older brothers had a history of antisocial behaviour and the area he grew up in was very deprived.

Johnny displayed challenging behaviour at home and at school in the form of oppositional behaviour, truancy and aggression towards peers. Due to this behaviour at school, the special educational needs teacher identified that he had learning difficulties and referred him to Child and Adolescent Mental Health Services (CAMHS) when he was 6 years old. However, Johnny's family refused to engage with services. Johnny's behaviour escalated and his mother struggled to manage him, leading to another referral to CAMHS after social services became involved when he was 10. At this point, Johnny received a diagnosis of ADHD and conduct disorder. He was then prescribed medication; however, this had little effect on his behaviours as Johnny often refused take this. Due to the escalation in his behaviours, Johnny was permanently excluded from school and, following a serious assault on a teacher, Johnny was referred to a school for young people with emotional and behavioural problems.

In the couple of years prior to his index offence, Johnny truanted from school more frequently and would spend his time mixing with older peers in his area.

Assessment

Prior to meeting Johnny, the practitioner psychologist reviewed the collateral information gathered from school, CAMHS and social services. From this it was noted that Johnny had a history of victimisation from peers in a variety of different settings. Also, most of Johnny's high-risk behaviours had generally occurred in the presence of older and more able antisocial peers, with various professionals commenting on Johnny's level of vulnerability.

From this collateral information, the psychologist identified areas to be assessed, such as Johnny's mental health, cognitive abilities and antisocial beliefs. Johnny was able to complete the BYI-II (scoring highly on anxiety, anger and disruptive behaviours), but struggled with assessments that contained longer statements and a wider number of response options.

After spending some time with Johnny, it was clear that Johnny had a rigid thinking style a concrete understanding and difficulty expressing himself clearly, which often led to him displaying frustrations. Therefore, Johnny was asked to complete a cognitive assessment using the WISC-IV. The results from the WISC-IV indicated that Johnny had a full-scale IQ of 64, with an even profile across the indexes. His level of adaptive functioning as assessed using the ABAS was consistent with this, showing a composite score of 62.

To assess his emotional and social functioning, the practitioner psychologist used various activities, such as playing cards and board games, as well as asking general questions and listening to comments Johnny made. Whilst Johnny was in a relaxed state, the psychologist was able to assess skills such as turn taking, frustration tolerance, ability to initiate and maintain conversation, and nonverbal communication skills. To assess his offending behaviour, Johnny was shown various DVDs of TV programmes or films depicting antisocial behaviour, and encouraged to share his views about what he had seen and relate it to his own experiences.

Using this approach, Johnny engaged in the sessions and the psychologist was able to ascertain some additional factors that were thought to be linked to his offending behaviour. Johnny spoke about how he looked up to his older brothers, who had spent brief spells in prison, but also had the latest clothing and gadgets and were respected by people in the local community.

During the assessments, Johnny engaged better than expected. The psychologist had spent a few sessions prior to completing the assessments getting to know Johnny's likes and interests and building engagement. One of these interests was football, hence the psychologist took Johnny to the park on a couple of occasions to kick a ball around. This continued during future assessment sessions, which were completed over several shorter periods. The psychologist used reinforcement strategies, such as taking Johnny to the park or to buy a drink from a cafe once he completed the work. In addition, Johnny was also referred to other services in order to have a full MDT assessment. Due to concerns regarding Johnny's communication, it was recommended that a speech and language therapist provide an assessment. Johnny was also assessed by an occupational therapist, to investigate his adaptive behaviours and sensory profile. Information gathered from the assessments were used to inform a SAVRY, with the risk formulation indicating that there was a significant risk of Johnny engaging in violent behaviour should individual and environmental factors remain unaddressed.

Formulation

Information from the assessment was used to develop a psychological understanding of how Johnny's difficulties had developed and were being maintained, so that an intervention plan could be devised. Johnny had been exposed to early trauma in the form of witnessing domestic violence and being a victim of neglect. These experiences were likely to have affected Johnny's attachment relationship with his primary caregiver, his ability to self-regulate and sooth, and his ability to reflect on his own feelings and the feelings of others. His difficulties with concentration and hyperactivity, were hypothesised to be influenced by a sense of hypervigilance to threat, which had developed as a result of his traumatic experiences. The result of Johnny's early life experiences were likely to be exacerbated by having ID. Johnny's level of ID highlighted poor social skills, verbal comprehension deficits and poor problem-solving abilities, making him even more vulnerable to the negative impact of developmental trauma. As Johnny grew up, he was exposed to the antisocial attitudes and behaviour of his father and brother. Johnny learnt that aggression and intimidation were effective ways to get needs met, avoid things he did not want to do and feel powerful. At school, Johnny repeated behaviour he had seen at home, which led to him not doing well in class, the other children not wanting to be around him and frequent exclusions. Johnny lacked alternative ways to cope with his feelings and therefore aggression became an entrenched strategy for coping. Johnny started to hang around with older young people who were also antisocial, as this made Johnny feel accepted, which enhanced his self-esteem. High levels of suggestibility meant that Johnny did whatever the older boys asked him to do. Although the school noticed Johnny's difficulties, he did not receive appropriate help due to a lack of engagement from both Johnny and his family. His difficulties were then exacerbated further by permanent exclusion from school, and poor parental supervision and management. Johnny started to spend increasing amounts of time with antisocial peers in the local community, where his antisocial behaviour began to escalate up to the point where he committed the index offence. For a diagrammatic formulation, see Figure 12.1.

Intervention plan

Information from assessment and formulation led to the psychologist prioritising interventions addressing emotional regulation and coping skills. For targeting antisocial attitudes, the practitioner psychologist recommended cognitive behavioural interventions addressing problem-solving and moral-reasoning work. In terms of influencing the wider system, social inclusion was felt to be important. Due to a lack of previous prosocial role models, it was decided that a mentoring project may support Johnny to become involved in prosocial activities, for example, a local football club project for excluded youth. Re-engaging Johnny with vocational skills was also recommended as crucial in developing self-esteem and giving a sense of meaningful activity. Johnny was also referred for a speech and language therapy assessment for advice on additional strategies to help in terms of his communication. Furthermore, an opinion was sought from a psychiatrist within CAMHS in relation to the validity of a diagnosis of ADHD in the context of an ID, and possible medication interventions in

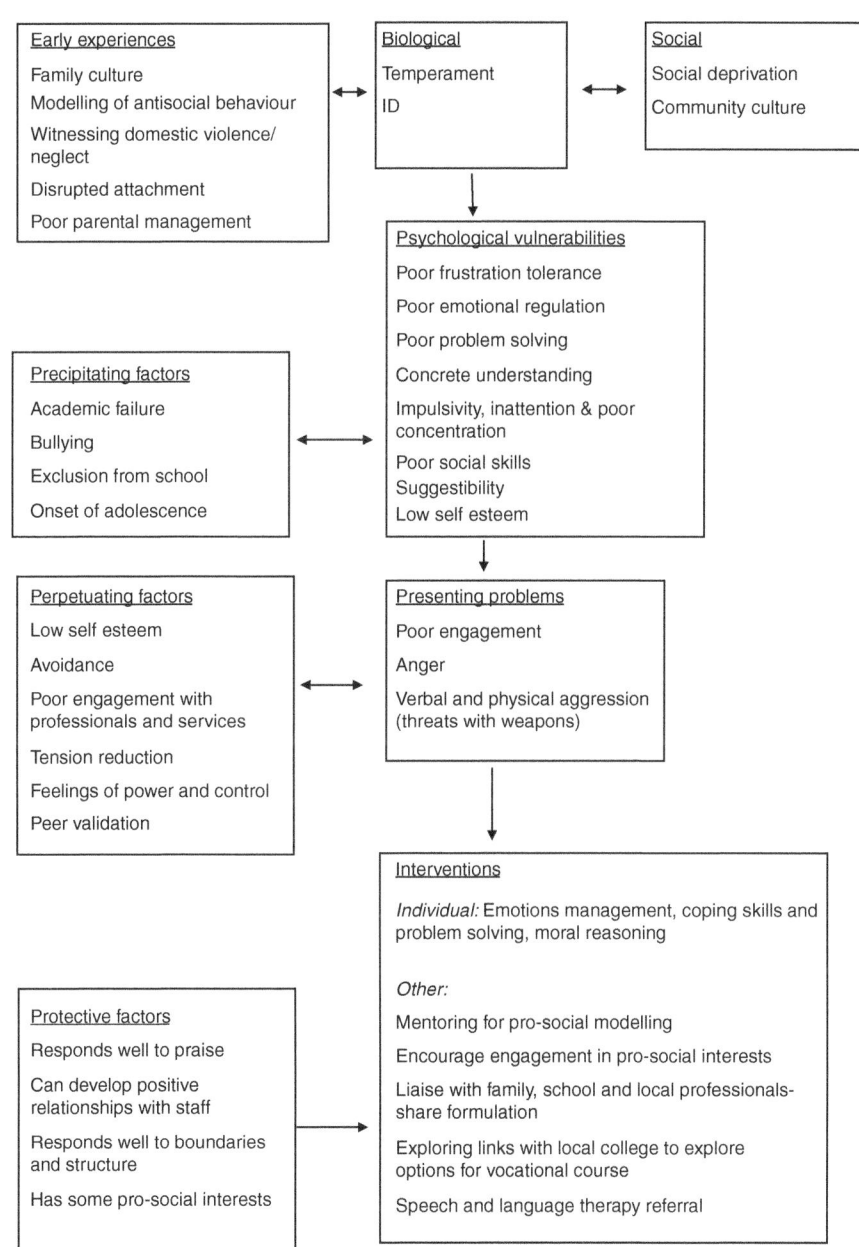

Figure 12.1 Psychological formulation

relation to aspects of concentration and hyperactivity. For these interventions to occur, communication between various professionals and the family was key, and therefore a care co-ordinator from CAMHS was identified to support this process and monitor progress.

Conclusions

This chapter has provided an overview of some of the main issues to consider when working with young people with an ID who display high-risk behaviours. In summary, the prevalence of young people with ID in the CJS is high. They experience a higher number of risk factors for both offending and poor mental health, and therefore the early identification of such young people, and ensuring appropriate support, management and intervention, is crucial to prevent them being disadvantaged, alienated and criminalised unnecessarily. Practitioner psychologists have an important role to play in understanding the individual differences among young people with an ID, what has contributed to their high-risk behaviour and the best way to support them, particularly in terms of considering the environmental factors and through multifactorial formulation, helping teams to develop a shared understanding of the young person and their needs. This is an area that requires further research, which could aid service and policy development.

References

Adamson, L., McLean, A., and Sher, M. (2011) 'Risk Assessment in Adolescents with Developmental Disabilities', in G. Gralton (ed.), *Forensic Issues in Adolescents with Developmental Disabilities*. London: Jessica Kingsley Publishers, 142–154.

APA (American Psychiatric Association) (2013a) 'DSM-5 intellectual disability fact sheet', *American Psychiatric Association*. Available at: http://www.dsm5.org/Documents/Intellectual%20Disability%20Fact%20Sheet.pdf. Accessed 16 June 2014.

APA (American Psychiatric Association) (2013b) *Diagnostic and Statistical Manual of Mental Disorders*. 5th edn. Arlington, VA: American Psychiatric Publishing.

Baker, B.L., Blacher, J., Crnic, K.A., and Edelbrock, C. (2002) 'Behavior problems and parenting stress in families of three-year-old children with and without developmental delays', *American Journal of Mental Retardation*, 107: 433–444.

Baron-Cohen, S. (2006) *Mindreading Programme*. London: Jessica Kingsley Publishers.

Beck, A.T., Beck, J.S., Jolly, J., and Steer, R. (2005) *The Beck Youth Inventories, Second Edition for Children and Adolescents; BYI-II*. Oxford: Pearson Assessments.

Beckett, R.C. and Fisher, D. (1994) 'Assessing Victim Empathy: A New Measure'. Paper presented to the 13th annual conference of the Association for the Treatment of Sexual Abusers, San Francisco.

Bhaumik, S., Gangadharan, S., Hiremath, A., and Russell, P.S.S. (2011) 'Psychological treatments in intellectual disability: The challenges of building a good evidence base', *British Journal of Psychiatry*, 198: 428–430.

Binnie, J. and Blainey, S. (2013) 'The use of cognitive behavioural therapy for adults with autism spectrum disorders: A review of the evidence', *Mental Health Review Journal*, 18: 93–104.

Blacker, J., Beech, A.R., Wilcox, D.T., and Boer, D.P. (2011) 'The assessment of dynamic risk and recidivism in a sample of special needs sex offenders', *Psychology, Crime and the Law*, 17: 75–92.

Boer, D.P., Frize, M., Pappas, R., Morrissey, C., and Lindsay, W.R. (2010) 'Suggested Adaptations to the HCR-20 for Offenders with Intellectual Disabilities', in L.A. Craig, W.R. Lindsay, and K.D. Browne (eds.), *Assessment and Treatment of Sexual Offenders with Intellectual Disabilities: A Handbook*. Chichester: John Wiley and Sons, 177–192.

Boer, D.P., Haaven, J., Lambrick, F., Lindsay, W., McVilly, K., Sakdaln, J., and Frize, M. (2012) *ARMADILO-S*. Available at: http://www.armidilo.net. Accessed 15 September 2014.

Borum, R., Bartel, P., and Forth, A. (2003) *Manual for the Structured Assessment of Violence Risk in Youth*. Odessa, FL: Psychological Assessment Resources.

BPS (British Psychological Society) (Professional Affairs Board of the British Psychological Society) (2000) *Learning Disability; Definitions and Context*. Leicester: British Psychological Society.

BPS-DCP (British Psychological Society – Division of Clinical Psychology) (2011) *Good Practice Guidelines on the Use of Psychological Formulation*. Leicester: British Psychological Society.

Briere, J. (1996) *Trauma Symptom Checklist for Children: Professional Manual*. Florida: Psychological Assessment Resources Inc.

British Institute for Brain Injured Children (2005) *Young People with Learning Disabilities and Antisocial Behaviour*. Available at: http://www.bibic.org.uk. Accessed 20 June 2014. http://www.scie-socialcareonline.org.uk/search?q=subject_terms%3A%22court+orders%22&page=1&f_author_editor_name_facet=BRITISH+INSTITUTE+FOR+BRAIN+INJURED+CHILDREN

Brown, M., Duff, H., Karatzias, T., and Horsburgh, D. (2011) 'A review of the literature relating to psychological interventions and people with intellectual disabilities: Issues for research, policy, education and clinical practice', *Journal of Intellectual Disabilities*, 15: 31–45.

Campbell, S. (2002) *A Review of Anti-Social Behaviour Orders: Home Office Research Study 236*. London: Home Office.

Carr, A., O'Reilly, G., Noonan Walsh, P., and McEvoy, J. (2007) *The Handbook of Intellectual Disability and Clinical Psychology Practice*. London: Routledge.

Cassidy, S.B. and Allanson, J.E. (2010) *Management of Genetic Syndromes*. 3rd edn. London: Wiley-Blackwell.

Chitsabesan, P., Bailey, S., Williams, R., Kroll, L., Kenning, C., and Talbot, L. (2007) 'Learning disabilities and educational needs of juvenile offenders', *Journal of Children's Services*, 2: 4–17.

Crick, N.R. and Dodge, K.A. (1994) 'A review and reformulation of social information-processing mechanisms in children's social adjustment', *Psychological Bulletin*, 115: 74–101.

Dagnan, D. (2007) 'Psychosocial interventions for people with intellectual disabilities and mental ill-health', *Current Opinion in Psychiatry*, 20: 456–460.

DH (Department of Health) (2007) *Best Practice in Managing Risk: Principles and Evidence for Best Practice in the Assessment and Management of Risk to Self and Others in Mental Health Services*. London: Department of Health.

DH (Department of Health) (2009) *The Bradley Report: Lord Bradley's Review of People with Mental Health Problems or Learning Disabilities in the Criminal Justice System*. London: Department of Health.

DH (Department of Health) (2012) *Transforming Care: A National Response to Winterbourne View Hospital*. London: Department of Health.

DH (Department of Health) (2014) *Positive and Proactive Care: Reducing the Need for Restrictive Interventions*. London: Department of Health.

Dickson, K., Emerson, E., and Hatton, C. (2005) 'Self-reported anti-social behaviour: prevalence and risk factors amongst adolescents with and without intellectual disability', *Journal of Intellectual Disability Research*, 49: 820–826.

Douma, J.C.H., Dekker, M.C., de Ruiter, K.P., Tick, N.T., and Koot, H.M. (2007) 'Antisocial and delinquent behaviours in youths with mild or borderline disabilities', *American Journal on Mental Retardation*, 112: 207–220.

Drizin, S.A. and Leo, R.A. (2004) 'The problem of false confessions in the post-DNA world', *North Carolina Law Review*, 82: 891–1007.

Einfeld, S.L., Ellis, L.A., and Emerson, E. (2011) 'Comorbidity of intellectual disability and mental disorder in children and adolescents: A systematic review', *Journal of Intellectual and Developmental Disability*, 36: 137–143.

Emerson, E. and Hatton, C. (2007) *The Mental Health of Children and Adults with Learning Disabilities in Britain: Institute of Health Research*. Lancashire: University of Lancashire.

Emerson, E., Hatton, C., Robertson, J., Baines, S., Christie, A., and Glover, G. (2012) *People with Learning Disabilities in England, 2012: Easy Read*. London: Improving Health and Lives: Learning Disability Observatory, supported by Department of Health.

Finlay, W.M.L. and Lyons, E. (2001) 'Methodological issues in interviewing and using self-report questionnaires with people with mental retardation', *Psychological Assessment*, 13: 319–335.

Finlay, W.M.L. and Lyons, E. (2002) 'Acquiescence in interviews with people who have mental retardation', *Mental Retardation*, 40: 14–29.

Fyson, R. and Yates, J. (2011) 'Anti-social behaviour orders and young people with learning disabilities', *Critical Social Policy*, 31: 102–125.

Gabriels, R.L., Agnew, J.A., Beresford, C., Morrow, M.A., Mesibov, G., and Wamboldt, M. (2012) 'Improving psychiatric hospital care for pediatric patients with autism spectrum disorders and intellectual disabilities', *Autism Research and Treatment*, 12: 1–7

Gibbons, F.X., Gibbons, B.N., and Cissin, S.M. (1981) 'Reactions to the criminal behaviour of intellectually disabled and non-disabled offenders', *American Journal of Mental Deficiency*, 86: 235–242.

Gibbons, F.X., Sawin, L.L.C., and Gibbons, B.N. (1979) 'Evaluations of mentally retarded persons: "sympathy" or patronization?' *American Journal of Mental Deficiency*, 84: 124–131.

Gibbs, J.C., Barriga, A.Q., and Potter, G.B. (2001) *The How I Think Questionnaire: HIT*. Illinois: Research Press Publishers.

Goodman, R., Meltzer, H., and Bailey, V. (1998) 'The strengths and difficulties questionnaire: A pilot study on the validity of the self-report version', *European Child and Adolescent Psychiatry*, 7: 125–130.

Gralton. E., Staniforth, C., and Griffin, Y. (2011) 'Care Pathways and Models of Secure Inpatient Care for Adolescents with Developmental Disabilities', in E. Gralton (ed.), *Forensic Issues in Adolescents with Developmental Disabilities*. London: Jessica Kinsley Publishers, 247–268.

Gudjuonsson, G.H. and Henry, L. (2003) 'Child and adult witnesses with intellectual disability: The importance of suggestibility' *Legal and Criminological Psychology*, 8: 241–242.

Hanson, K. and Thornton, D. (2000) 'Improving risk assessments for sex offenders: A comparison of three actuarial scales', *Law and Human Behavior*, 24: 119–136.

Harrison, P. and Oakland, T. (2003) *Adaptive Behavior Assessment System (ABAS-II)*, 2nd edn. New York: The Psychological Corporation.

Holland, K. (2011) *Factsheet: Learning Disability*. Worcestershire: British Institute for Learning Disability (BILD).

Hughes, N., Williams, H., Chitsabesan, P., Davies, R., and Mounce, L. (2012) *Nobody Made the Connection: The Prevalence of Neurodisability in Young People Who Offend*. London: Children's Commissioner.

Kazdin, A.E. (2000) 'Adolescent Development, Mental Disorders, and Decision Making of Delinquent Youths', in T. Grisso and R.G. Schwartz (eds.), *Youth on Trial: A Developmental Perspective on Juvenile Justice*. Chicago: University of Chicago Press, 33–65.

Lakin, K.C. (1983) 'New admissions and readmission to a national sample of public residential facilities', *American Journal of Mental Deficiency*, 88: 13–20.

Lindsay, W.R. (1999) 'Cognitive therapy', *Psychologist*, 12: 238–241.

Lindsay, W.R. and Taylor, J.L. (2005) 'A selective review of research on offenders with developmental disabilities: Assessment and treatment', *Clinical Psychology and Psychotherapy*, 12: 201–214.

Lindsay, W.R., Hogue, T., Taylor, J.L., Steptoe, L., Mooney, P., Johnstone, S., and Smith, A.H. (2008) 'Risk assessment in offender with intellectual disabilities: A comparison across three levels of security', *International Journal of Offender Therapy and Comparative Criminology*, 52: 90–111.

Lindsay, W.R., Murphy, L., Smith, G., Murphy, D., Edwards, Z., Chittock, C., Grieve, A., and Young, S.J. (2004) 'The Dynamic Risk Assessment and Management System: An assessment of immediate risk of violence for individuals with offending and challenging behaviour', *Journal of Applied Research in Intellectual Disabilities*, 17(4): 267–274.

McClintock, K., Hall, S., and Oliver, C. (2003) 'Risk markers associated with challenging behaviours in people with intellectual disabilities: A meta-analytic study', *Journal of Intellectual Disability Research*, 47: 405–416.

McDonald, S., Flanagan, S., Rollins, J., and Kinch, J. (2003) 'TASIT: A new clinical tool for assessing social perception after traumatic brain injury', *Journal of Head Trauma Rehabilitation*, 18: 219–238.

Maxfield, M.G. and Widom C.S. (1996) 'The cycle of violence: Revisited six years later', *Archives of Pediatric and Adolescent Medicine*, 150: 390–395.

Medford, S., Gudjonsson, G.H., and Pearse, J. (2003) 'Efficacy of the appropriate adult safeguard during police interviewing', *Legal and Criminological Psychology*, 8: 253–266.

Mental Capacity Act (2005). London: Her Majesty's Stationery Office and Queen's Printer of Acts of Parliament.

MIND (2013) *Mental Health Crisis Care: Physical Restraint in Crisis: A Report on Physical Restraint in Hospital Settings in England*. London: MIND.

Muckley, A. (1997) *Addressing Fire-Setting Behaviour with Children, Young People and Adults: A Resource and Training Manual*. Redcar and Cleveland Psychological Service.

Murphy, D. (2010) 'Understanding offenders with autism-spectrum disorders: What can forensic services do?' *Advances in Psychiatric Treatment*, 16: 44–46.

Najdowski, C.J., Bottoms, B.L., and Vargas, M.C. (2009) 'Jurors' perceptions of juvenile defendants: The influence of intellectual disability, abuse history and confession evidence', *Behavioral Sciences and the Law*, 27: 401–430.

NICE (National Institute for Health and Care Excellence) (2011) *Autism: Recognition, Referral and Diagnosis of Children and Young People on the Autism Spectrum*. Clinical guidelines CG128 (September).

Noble, J.H. and Conley, R.W. (1992) 'Toward an Epidemiology of Relevant Attributes', in R.W. Conley, R. Luckasson, and G.N. Bouthilet (eds.), *The Criminal Justice System and Mental Retardation*. Baltimore, MD: Paul H. Brookes, 17–53.

O'Callaghan, D. (2005) 'Group Treatment of Young People with Intellectual Impairment Who Sexually Harm', in R. Longo and D. Prescott (eds.), *Current Perspectives: Working with Sexually Aggressive Youth and Youth with Sexual Behavior Problems*. Massachusetts: Neari Press, 325–348.

Quinsey, V.L., Harris, G.T., Rice, M.E., and Cormier, C.A. (2006) *Violent Offenders: Appraising and Managing Risk*, 2nd edn. Washington, DC: American Psychological Association.

Rose, J., Cutler, C., Tresize, K., Novak, D., and Rose, D. (2008) 'Individuals with an intellectual disability who offend', *British Journal of Developmental Disabilities*, 54: 19–30.

Royal College of General Practitioners and the Royal College of Psychiatrists (2012) *Improving the Health and Wellbeing of People with Learning Disabilities: An Evidence-Based Commissioning Guide for Clinical Commissioning Groups (CCGs)*, Improving Health and Lives, Learning Disability Observatory. London: Public Health England.

Royal College of Psychiatrists, British Psychological Society, Royal College of Speech and Language Therapist (2007) *Challenging Behaviour: A Unified Approach*. London: Royal College of Psychiatrists.

Schore, A.N. (2013) *Affect Dysregulation and Disorders of the Self: Norton Series on Interpersonal Neurobiology*. London: W.W. Norton & Company.

Shoham-Vardi, I., Davidson, P.W., Cain, N.N., Sloane-Reeves, J.E., Giesow, V.E., and Quijano, L.E. (1996) 'Factors predicting re-referral following crisis intervention for community-based persons with developmental disabilities and behavioural and psychiatric disorders', *American Journal of Mental Retardation*, 101: 109–117.

Simpson, M.K. and Hogg, J. (2001a) 'Patterns of offending among people with intellectual disability: A systematic review. Part 1: Methodology and prevalence data', *Journal of Intellectual Disability Research*, 45: 384–396.

Simpson, M.K. and Hogg, J. (2001b) 'Patterns of offending among people with intellectual disability: A systematic review. Part II: Predisposing factors', *Journal of Intellectual Disability Research*, 45: 397–406.

Sparrow, S.S., Chiccetti, D.V., and Balla, D.A. (2005) *Vineland Adaptive Behavior Scales, Second Edition (Vineland-II)*. San Antonia, TX: Pearson.

Stenfert-Kroese, B. (1997) 'Cognitive-Behaviour Therapy for People with Learning Disabilities: Conceptual and Contextual Issues', in B. Stenfert-Kroese, D. Dagnan, and K. Loumidis (eds.), *Cognitive-Behaviour Therapy for People with Learning Disabilities*. London: Routledge, 1–15.

Stenfert-Kroese, B., Dagnan, D., and Loumidis, K. (eds.) (1997) *Cognitive-Behaviour Therapy for People with Learning Disabilities*. London: Routledge.

Sturmey, P. (2008) *Behavioral Case Formulation and Intervention: A Functional Analytic Approach*. Chichester: Wiley-Blackwell.

Talbot, J. (2008) *No One Knows; Report and Final Recommendations. Prisoners' Voices: Experiences of the Criminal Justice System by Prisoners with Learning Disabilities and Difficulties*. London: Prison Reform Trust.

Taylor, J., Lindsay, W., and Willner, P. (2008) 'CBT for people with intellectual disabilities: Emerging evidence, cognitive ability and IQ effects', *Behavioural and Cognitive Psychotherapy*, 36: 723–733.

Tonge, B.J. and Einfeld, S.L. (2003) 'Psychopathology and intellectual disability: The Australian Child to Adult Longitudinal Study', *International Review of Research in Mental Retardation*, 26: 61–91.

Walker, J.S. (2005) 'The Maudsley Violence Questionnaire: Initial validation and reliability', *Personality and Individual Differences*, 38: 187–201.
Ward, T. (2002) 'Good lives and the rehabilitation of sexual offenders: Promises and problems', *Aggression and Violent Behavior*, 7: 513–528.
Wechsler, D. (2003) *Wechsler Intelligence Scale for Children: Fourth Edition (WISC-IV)*. San Antonio, TX: The Psychological Corporation.
Wechsler, D. (2008) *Wechsler Adult Intelligence Scale: Fourth Edition (WAIS-IV)*. San Antonio, TX: The Psychological Corporation.
Weiss, D.S. and Marmar, C.R. (1997) 'The Impact of Events Scale Revised', in J.P. Wilson and T.M. Keane (eds.), *Assessing Psychological Trauma and PTSD*. New York: Guilford Press, 399–441.
Westcott, H.L. and Jones, D.P.H. (1999) 'Annotation: The abuse of disabled children', *Journal of Child Psychology and Psychiatry*, 40: 497–506.
WHO (World Health Organization) (1992) *ICD-10 Classifications of Mental and Behavioural Disorder: Clinical Descriptions and Diagnostic Guidelines*. Geneva: World Health Organization.
WHO (World Health Organization) (2001) *Mental Health and Intellectual Disabilities: Addressing the Mental Health Needs of People with Intellectual Disabilities, Report by the Mental Health Special Interest Group of the International Association for the Scientific Study of Intellectual Disabilities to the World Health Organization*. Geneva: World Health Organization.
Widom, C.S. (1989) 'The cycle of violence', *Science*, 244: 160–166.
Williams, H. and Jones, R.S.P. (1997) 'Teaching Cognitive Self-Regulation of Independence and Emotional Control Skills', in B. Stenfert-Kroese, D. Dagnan, and K. Loumidis (eds.), *Cognitive-Behaviour Therapy for People with Learning Disabilities*. London: Routledge, 63–85.
Willner, P. (2005) 'The effectiveness of psychotherapeutic interventions for people with learning disabilities: A critical overview', *Journal of Intellectual Disability Research*, 49: 73–85.
Wilner, P. and Smith, M. (2008) 'Attribution theory applied to helping behaviour towards people with intellectual disabilities who challenge', *Journal of Applied Research in Intellectual Disabilities*, 21: 150–155.
Wong, W. and Cornell, G. (1999) 'PIQ > VIQ discrepancy as a correlate of social information processing and aggression in delinquent adolescent males', *Journal of Psychoeducational Assessment*, 17: 104–112.
Worling, J.R. and Curwen, T. (2001) 'Estimate of Risk of Adolescent Sexual Offense Recidivism (Version 2.0: The "ERASOR")', in M.C. Calder (ed.), *Juveniles and Children Who Sexually Abuse: Frameworks for Assessment*. Lyme Regis: Russell House Publishing, 372–397.
Yates, J. (2009b) 'Structural Disadvantage: Youth, Class, Crime and Poverty', in W. Taylor, R. Hester, and R. Earle (eds.), *Youth Justice Handbook: Theory, Policy and Practice*. Cullompton: Willan Publishing, 5–22.

13
Autism Spectrum Disorder

Yve Griffin and Charlotte Staniforth

Introduction

There is increasing awareness of the prevalence of young people with autism spectrum disorder (ASD) within forensic settings and the specific issues these young people may present to services. Furthermore, the difficulties young people with a diagnosis of ASD experience often impacts on their ability to fully comprehend and participate in the criminal justice process. As a result, it is becoming increasingly common for professionals working within the criminal justice system (CJS) to seek training to increase their awareness of ASD and how it may impact on the young person.

Young people with a diagnosis of ASD represent a heterogeneous group in terms of how the difficulties are experienced and expressed (WHO 2001). A common analogy used is that of a graphic equaliser to represent those skill strengths and difficulties in each of the areas listed in Table 13.1. These strengths and difficulties can be experienced at different levels of severity within and across individuals. For example, one individual with ASD may have a reasonable level of communication skills, but experience a range of social difficulties, whereas another person with ASD may have a higher degree of difficulties in both areas.

This chapter will commence by defining ASD, as well as outlining the co-morbidities associated with this diagnosis. It will also discuss some of the reasons why those with ASD come into contact with forensic services, along with issues to consider when assessing, formulating and providing interventions.

The language used when talking about the high-risk behaviours of young people with ASD can be hard to navigate when terms such as challenging behaviour, risk behaviour and offending behaviour are used interchangeably. For continuity, the term high-risk behaviour will be used to refer to any behaviour that can put the young person or members of the public at risk of significant psychological or physical harm, whether or not this behaviour

Table 13.1 Difficulties associated with ASD

Area of difficulty	How it may present
Cognitive skills, including executive functioning	Concrete thinking, difficulties in planning and organisation, poor problem solving, difficulties in consequential thinking, low emotional regulation, high impulsivity, low frustration tolerance, disinhibition
Social skills	Overfamiliarity, difficulty adapting social behaviours to context or recipient, difficulty reading social situations, difficulties in understanding social rules and norms
Adaptive behaviours	Poor expressive and receptive communication, low awareness of safety and risk, low academic functioning (literacy, numeracy, etc.), difficulties in activities of daily living (self-care and home living)
Physical health	Predisposition to genetic disorders or health conditions, low awareness of good physical health and recognising symptoms of ill health and how to manage these. May be linked with other health complications from birth trauma and/or syndromes
Restricted interests	Obsession-like quality to specific area or behaviours, these can be linked directly to high-risk behaviours (interest in violence) or indirectly (can lead to violence if prevented from engaging in them or pursuit of them can lead to high-risk behaviours)
Sensory	Hypo or hypersensitivity to pain, noise, touch, taste, texture of foods, visual stimuli, vestibular and proprioceptive stimuli

has resulted in a conviction. Examples of high-risk behaviours include: physical aggression, sexually harmful behaviour, fire-setting, substance abuse and acquisitive offending. At the end of the chapter a case study will be presented to encourage theory–practice links and to bring the material to life.

Definitions

The National Autistic Society (NAS 2013) describes ASD as a lifelong developmental disability that affects how a person communicates with, and relates to, other people. ASD also affects how people make sense of the world around them. Within the literature, this is frequently referred to as the triad of impairments (Wing and Gould 1979), with the difficulties experienced being within the domains of communication, social understanding and flexibility of thought. However, current thinking also considers additional difficulties that are likely to be experienced by those with ASD, such as sensory processing, unusual cognitive profiles and impairments in adaptive behaviours.

Within the International Classification of Diseases: Version 10 (ICD-10) (WHO 1992), ASD is one of a number of diagnoses which fall under the umbrella term of pervasive developmental disorder, and these terms are often used synonymously. However, with the introduction of the *Diagnostic and Statistical Manual: Version 5* (DSM-5; APA 2013), all of these diagnoses have been collapsed into two conditions: ASD, for those who present with the full range of autistic symptoms, and a new category, social communication disorder for those who would have been previously considered to have an atypical presentation (Wilson et al. 2013). The aim of this new approach is to reduce the variability within the diagnostic category of ASD. It is hoped that this will improve service provision, as it can be more tailored to meet the needs of the individuals. Given the use of two diagnostic systems, however, there still remains a significant variability in those who may be given a diagnosis of ASD. If the stricter DSM-5 criteria are applied, it could be argued that less people would meet thresholds for diagnosis and, as a result, receive specialist support (Sturmey and Dalfern 2014). This is likely to impact further on young people with ASD in forensic settings, who are less likely to have their individual needs appropriately assessed and treated. One implication is that, without appropriate identification of need and intervention, these young people are more likely to continue to engage in high-risk behaviour.

Prevalence

Current estimates suggest that one in a hundred people meet the diagnostic criteria for ASD (Chakrabarti and Fombonne 2005; Mattila et al. 2007; NAS 2011), but with the proposed changes to the diagnostic criteria this number is thought likely to reduce (Wilson et al. 2013). There are few UK prevalence studies of young people with ASD in youth custody: the majority have been conducted with adults (Scragg and Shah 1994; Hare et al. 1999; Långström et al. 2008) or with young people in forensic psychiatry settings (Williams et al. 2012). Interestingly, there has been a historical assumption that the prevalence of ASD in young offenders is low; however, there is increasing evidence that the prevalence of ASD is higher than anticipated. For example, in Sweden it has been found that the rates of ASD in both 'special institution' for adolescents and youth custody was at 15 per cent, compared to 0.6–1.2 per cent in the general population (Siponmaa et al. 2001; Anckarsater et al. 2007). A Dutch study of children at first arrest found that autistic symptoms (not diagnosis) were more prevalent in this sample than a control group representing the general population (Geluk et al. 2012).

Sverd and colleagues (1995) found ASD prevalence rates of 2 per cent in psychiatrically hospitalised children, which increased to 3.2 per cent when just considering boys. ASD was under-recognised and associated with a wide array of psychiatric and behavioural disturbance, including affective and psychotic disorders. In a study exploring the prevalence of young people with ASD in a UK medium secure mental health hospital, a high prevalence of ASD was identified in the developmental disability division, as would be expected (64 per cent). However, there was also a prevalence of 20 per cent in the mental health division (Staniforth and Griffin 2013). Sutton and colleagues (2013) found that 60 per cent of young people aged between 14 and 20 placed in American state facilities for adolescent sexual offenders met the criteria for ASD.

Co-morbidity

In addition to the possible difficulties presented in Table 13.1, it is estimated that approximately 70–75 per cent of children with ASD have IQ scores of 70 or below (Kaplan and Saddock 1998; Croen, Grether and Selvin 2002). Therefore, a large proportion of those with ASD have additional difficulties associated with having an intellectual disability (ID), and are often more impaired, particularly in relation to self-injurious behaviour and disruptive behaviours than those with either ID or ASD alone (Smith and Matson 2010). Due to the high co-occurrence of ID and ASD, many of the issues discussed in Chapter 12 (this volume) will also be relevant for young people with ASD.

Understanding co-morbidity is particularly important in terms of ASD forensic populations, as co-morbid psychiatric diagnoses may be important risk factors for offending in people with ASD (Palermo 2004; Mouridsen 2012). Newman and Ghaziuddin's (2008) literature review suggested that an overwhelming number of cases reviewed had coexisting psychiatric diagnoses at the time of committing the offence.

Mental health

The presence of difficulties associated with ASD, and commonly ID, increase the likelihood that young people with this diagnosis will experience mental health difficulties. For example, social skills difficulties can lead to experiencing high levels of anxiety. Prevalence rates of children and adolescents with an ID or ASD attracting a diagnosis of a mental disorder vary widely (10–60 per cent for ID and 9–89 per cent for ASD) (Howlin 2000; de Bruin et al. 2006; Lecavalier 2006; Leyfer et al. 2006), and some have suggested up to four times the prevalence rates of those without a diagnosis of ASD (Bradley et al. 2004). However, there is little specific research into the mental health risk and protective factors of young people with a diagnosis of ASD compared to those without.

The wide prevalence range of mental health difficulties in ASD populations can perhaps be best explained by a range of methodological issues, including sample bias such as how groups are categorised (i.e. high-functioning ASD, Asperger's syndrome or basing group membership on IQ alone). Young people with ASD may have extremely varied cognitive strengths and weaknesses which are not fully captured by an IQ score. Another confounding issue is that studies tend to use diagnostic assessments that have not been validated on an ASD population, which means the assessment may fail to take into account different presentations of mental health difficulties in this group. Despite the methodological concerns, co-morbidity is the rule rather than the exception for young people with ASD (Anckarsater et al. 2007).

Within adolescent inpatient units, it is suggested that the prevalence rates of ASD is higher than the general population, supporting the findings that there is a high rate of psychiatric co-morbidity in this population (Sverd et al. 1995; Wozniak et al. 1997; Wolff 1998). This is further supported by Joshi and colleagues (2010) who have reported that not only are the rates of psychiatric co-morbidity in young people with ASD significantly higher than those in mental health settings without ASD, but that young people with ASD often have more than one co-morbid condition, with most having three or more co-morbid conditions – the symptoms presenting in a similar manner to those without ASD (Sverd, Dubey, Schweiter and Ninan 2003). When looking more closely at the co-morbid conditions of those with ASD, the most common diagnoses are depression and bipolar affective disorder (Morgan, Roy and Chance 2003) social anxiety disorder (29.2 per cent), attention deficit hyperactivity disorder (ADHD) (28.2 per cent), and oppositional defiant disorder (28.1 per cent) (Siminoff et al. 2008). Other diagnostic labels and symptoms associated with a diagnosis of ASD include obsessive-compulsive disorder (OCD) and psychotic symptoms, such as paranoia and hallucinations (Sverd 2003; Matson and Nebel-Schwalm 2005; Tiffin and Le Couteur 2005).

High rates of mental illness in those with ASD are not just restricted to persons in inpatient mental health settings (Brereton 2006), with community mental health samples often displaying similar co-morbid conditions and risk behaviours as those in the inpatient service (Sverd et al. 1995; Siminoff et al. 2008).

Impact on diagnosis

Identifying young people with ASD is made more complicated by high rates of co-morbidity in relation to ID and other mental health presentations. These co-morbidities can obscure core features of ASD and lead to difficulties in developing clarity regarding diagnosis (Sverd et al. 1995) due to behavioural overshadowing. For example, where young people may display behaviour consistent with a diagnosis of ADHD it is recommended that they are assessed for ASD before considering a diagnosis of ADHD with co-morbid conduct disorder (Harada et al. 2009). Assessing the presence of additional mental health needs for people with a diagnosis of ASD is complex due to a number of factors, including distinguishing between mental health symptoms indicative of alternative diagnoses and factors inherent to ASD, and the lack of validated measures to assess co-morbidity in ASD.

It is also important to note that young people may also appear to present with needs consistent with a diagnosis of ASD, but, from clinical experience, this is often a misdiagnosis. Young people presenting with a history of complex developmental trauma and attachment disruption are commonly referred to forensic mental health services. If working within a diagnostic paradigm, without an adequate diagnostic category (or often system understanding) that captures and explains the complexity of the impact of early and chronic trauma, clinicians are left with the complex task of trying to disentangle core ASD symptoms from any effects of complex trauma and attachment disruption. NICE guidelines (2012) advise professionals to be aware that, for some children and young people, there may be uncertainty about the diagnosis of ASD, particularly for young people where there is little information about their early life, such as those who are looked after or adopted, older teenagers or those attracting a diagnosis of coexisting mental health disorder (such as ADHD, conduct disorder or attachment disorder). In an attempt to highlight some of the difficulties of distinguishing between a diagnosis of ASD and attachment disorder, Moran (2010) has developed the Coventry Grid. This aims to distinguish between characteristics of ASD and attachment difficulties by exploring the subtleties of how social, communication and behavioural difficulties are expressed. Reaching the appropriate diagnosis for young people with ASD in combination with histories of developmental trauma can be extremely challenging. Using psychological formulation that aims to describe the development of the particular needs and the interactions between the specific difficulties, rather than trying to identify symptom cluster to support a diagnosis, can help overcome these issues.

Reasons for referral to adolescent forensic services

Violence is not one of the most common offences associated with ASD in the research literature, although aggression is a common reason for referral to mental health services. Aggression is not a core feature of an ASD diagnosis, yet research suggests there is an association between a diagnosis of ASD and increased risk of aggression. Kanne and Mazurek (2011) used parents' reports to look at rates of aggression in young people with ASD aged 4 to 17. The parents reported higher rates of aggression towards a caregiver (68 per cent) than to others (49 per cent). They also found that self-injurious behaviour, ritualistic behaviours and resistance to change were predictors for aggression. Several factors that predicted aggression in typically developing children, such as level of parental education, gender, level of ID and language ability, did not predict aggression in those with ASD. Consistent with the literature on typically developing children, age was related to aggression, with younger children displaying higher levels of aggression. ASD-related severity, as assessed by clinicians, did not predict aggression, but parent-rated social communication difficulties and repetitive behaviours did.

Children with ASD may be more at risk of hospitalisation than children attracting diagnoses of other disorders. A quarter of children with a diagnosis of ASD receiving support in community mental health settings in America have been hospitalised, with aggression and self-injurious behaviours increasing this risk (Mandell et al. 2005). However, it was noted that sometimes hospitalisation may represent a failure of adequate community services for children with ASD. In another American data sample of 760 carers of children with ASD, 10.8 per cent of the children had been hospitalised (Mandell 2008). Predictors of hospitalisation included: self-injury, aggression, depression, OCD, use of psychotropic medication and a high level of clinical complexity. Risk of hospitalisation increased with age and over time.

Typically, forensic services, including both mental health services and criminal justice provisions such as youth offending services (YOSs), fail to provide adequate services for people with ASD (Murphy 2010). There is an understandable, but maybe a misinformed, reluctance to admit young people with ASD who present high-risk behaviours to hospital settings. Instead, there is the option of managing such behaviours with community orders, but this runs the risk of criminalising young people with ASD who may not have the ability to understand and therefore abide by the order. Similarly, the orders themselves may be trying to target a behaviour that is inherently linked to a core difficulty experienced by a young person with ASD, for example, obsessionality or staring. Such behaviours can be addressed through interventions, such as anxiety management and social skills training. There is a clear need for specific specialist forensic services at all levels, such as community mental health, hospital and criminal justice services, and better communication between them (Murphy 2010).

It is important to bear in mind that, for young people to access specialist ASD services, they first need to be identified. Generally, in mainstream forensic mental health services within the UK, there is poor recognition and understanding of ASD. This suggestion is supported by prevalence studies in UK high secure hospitals, where many of the cases of ASD that were identified had not previously been diagnosed or had been misdiagnosed, often as mental health disorders such as schizophrenia or personality disorder (Scragg and Shah 1994; Hare et al. 1999). Misdiagnosis may be especially prevalent in adolescents and young adults, or for those with higher functioning or atypical ASD. A presentation consistent with a diagnosis of ASD symptoms can often be misdiagnosed as depression, adjustment disorder, schizophrenia or emerging Cluster A personality disorder (Haskins and Arturo Silva 2006).

The clinical experience of the authors suggests that whether or not a young person is considered an offender (whether they are convicted of an offence), is influenced by factors such as: who the victim was, where the young person was residing at the time and by whom the young person was convicted (i.e. the presiding magistrate or jury members). The latter is important, as it depends on the level of understanding these people have of ASD and the attributions they make regarding the behaviour (i.e. was the person in control of their behaviour, were they encouraged to behave in such a manner and so on). For these reasons, there is huge variability in the way young people with ASD who display risk behaviours are labelled, where they reside and the treatment, if any, they receive. The variability of opinion in relation to the seriousness of behaviour, culpability, appropriate consequences and rehabilitative strategies for young people with ASD who engage in high-risk behaviours is no doubt influenced by the attributions of the public, professionals, the law and society in general. Although some professionals may be ambivalent about involving the police, it has been suggested that reporting to the police can be a useful intervention with people with ASD and ID who present with challenging behaviour, when used as part of a comprehensive, multi-professional therapeutic process (Raggi et al. 2013). This can enable staff to feel legally supported, and can promote learning of social rules, with respect to young people's rights and responsibilities, and promote rehabilitation rather than incarceration.

Association between ASD and offending

The literature exploring possible links between ASD and offending is complex, and most studies are usually small case studies using adults (Cashin and Newman 2009). The research on adolescents presenting with ASD and high-risk behaviours is minimal, and therefore clinicians often rely on the adult literature as a starting point. Adults with ASD have been found to be overrepresented in secure hospitals, with studies finding prevalence rates of between 2 and 2.4 per cent (Scragg and Shah 1994; Hare et al. 1999; Långström et al. 2008). This is a larger magnitude than would be found in the general population (one in a 100; NAS 2011).

In a recent audit of the characteristics of young people (n = 85) diagnosed with ASD admitted to a secure psychiatric unit within the UK, the sample came from a variety of previous placements including home, residential units and schools, mental health settings, bespoke placements and secure settings, including secure children's homes (SCHs), children's secure units and young offender institutions (YOIs) (Staniforth and Griffin 2013). In terms of reason for referral, 35 per cent of the sample had an index offence, and there was consistency with the adult research in that sexual offences (17.6 per cent) and arson (11.8 per cent) were most prevalent, with violent offences (Actual Bodily Harm) being lower (2.9 per cent). Young people were detained under a range of sections under the Mental Health Act (DoH 1983) including: Section 37 (disposal via court to hospital for treatment), Section 38 (interim hospital order whilst awaiting sentencing), Section 37/41 (as above for S37 but with restrictions monitored by the Home Office) and Sections 47–49 (transfer of a sentenced prisoner to hospital for treatment). The majority of the sample (68 per cent), were detained under Section 3 (admission for treatment) of the Mental Health Act, and a third (32 per cent) were on hospital orders (were directed by a court to be detained in a mental health setting under the Mental Health Act to receive treatment). Being held under a Section 3 did not necessarily mean that the young person had not accrued previous convictions, or that their behaviour was less serious than that of a young person on a Section 37/41. For those admitted on Section 3, the most common reasons for admission in order of prevalence were: aggression (87 per cent), sexually harmful behaviour (29 per cent) and self-harm (25 per cent). Other reasons were repeated absconding and fire-setting. Often, young people had presented with a range of high-risk behaviours prior to admission. Although there was a broad range of behaviours displayed on the units, the predominant behaviour displayed since admission was aggression (physical, verbal and against property), followed by sexually inappropriate behaviour.

There remains conflicting opinions about any associations between those diagnosed with ASD and offending, and there is a lack of a robust evidence of a direct association between a diagnosis of ASD and criminal offending (Ghaziuddin, Tsai and Ghaziuddin 1991; Mouridsen 2012). In fact, due to the rigid way many people diagnosed with ASD keep to rules and regulations, it has been suggested that they may be more law-abiding than the general population and, in fact, may be more at risk as victims of crime rather than as offenders (NAS 2011). There tends to be two main schools of thought regarding why people with a diagnosis of ASD may offend; one that offending is related to the core features of ASD, and the other that offending is linked to the same risk factors as found in the general offending population.

In terms of the 'core features' argument, some of the core features of a diagnosis of ASD that may be associated with offending include: theory of mind deficits, intense narrow interests, deficient social awareness of interpersonal and social constraints on behaviour, and the triad of deficits (social, communication and flexibility of thought) (Haskins and Arturo Silva 2006). Weak central coherence theory has also been suggested as a way ASD can lead to offending behaviour, through excessive preoccupations and rigid routines which impact on behaviour via disconnection with the social environment (Barry-Walsh and Mullen 2004; Haskins and Arturo Silva 2006). Research has found that people with ASD who offend have a lack of empathy and impaired social development

(Realmuto and Ruble 1999; Sutton et al. 2013) in the form of an inability to read social situations (Palermo 2004) and misinterpretation of facial expressions and non-verbal cues (Schwartz-Watts 2005; de la Cuesta 2010). Allen and colleagues (2008) found that classical traits associated with ASD such as lack of concern, social naivety, impulsivity and misinterpretation of rules, and overriding obsessions, influenced engagement in offending behaviour. Many people with ASD have what is commonly known as 'special interests'. These are interests that the individual is obsessed with, to the point where such interests interfere with adaptive functioning, as the individual focuses incessantly on the interest to the point where they know all they can about it. Special interests have also been linked to offending; in one study up to 84 per cent of the sample had special interests, a quarter of which were related to violent themes (Hare et al. 1999).

Despite this, Mouridsen (2012) completed a review of the adult literature and concluded that having a diagnosis of ASD does not increase the overall likelihood of offending. There were, however, links indicated between ASD and certain types of serious offences, with ASD typically being associated with sexual abuse and arson (Mouridsen 2012). Mouridsen and colleagues (2008) completed the first controlled case study to examine the relationship between ASD and all types of offending, finding that only arson had increased prevalence in the ASD group. This supports previous findings that arson is overrepresented in ASD populations (Hare et al. 1999; Siponmaa et al. 2001; Mouridsen 2012). Furthermore, Woodbury-Smith and colleagues (2006) explored whether the cognitive impairments observed in people with a diagnosis of ASD are associated with vulnerability to offending. Compared with comparison groups, offenders with ASD showed greater impairment in recognising emotional expressions of fear. However, those diagnosed with ASD who did not offend showed impaired theory of mind and executive functioning, and those with ASD who offended did not. This finding contradicts the 'core features' argument to some degree, in that there may be particular features of ASD that are associated with offending more than others.

Another theory is that any link that exists between ASD and offending may be explained by the same factors associated with offending in the general population, such as: being male, having higher functioning ASD (such as those diagnosed with Asperger's syndrome rather than autistic disorder) and having co-morbid psychosis and/or substance use disorders (Woodbury-Smith et al. 2006; Långström et al. 2008). This argument is also relevant for those with broader IDs (Winter, Holland and Collins 1997; Simpson and Hogg 2001).

In terms of sexual behaviour, two important findings have been reported in the literature. The first is that children with a diagnosis of ASD experience typical physical development and sexual drives, and, secondly, the potential impairments people with ASD experience may impede their acquisition of sexual knowledge and development. People with ASD are less likely to have exposure to complex social experiences, have more limited access to erotic material and often do not encounter appropriate potential sexual partners (Sutton et al. 2012). All of this may result in unacceptable or deviant sexual behaviours. Furthermore, poor emotional regulation may lead to improper management of sexual interest and arousal (Sutton et al. 2013). As such, sexually inappropriate behaviours that adolescents with ASD may engage in range from kissing strangers, intruding on personal space of those they are infatuated with and inappropriate masturbation, to sexual violence (Sutton et al. 2013). In the same study, young people with a diagnosis of ASD reported engaging in a variety of criminal acts, most prominently under the influence of alcohol. Furthermore, most of the participants reported negative mood or low levels of enjoyment. Ruble and Dalrymple (1993) surveyed 100 caregivers exploring the sexual knowledge and behaviours of children they cared for. The carers reported that 23 per cent of the children masturbated in public, 18 per cent touched the opposite sex inappropriately, 14 per cent masturbated with unusual objects and 65 per cent touched their genitalia in public. Ruble and Dalrymple (1993) suggest that delayed social functioning, associated with theory of mind deficits, may lead to expression of inappropriate sexual behaviour.

It is often the case that there has been an escalation in the frequency or severity of behaviours prior to admission to a forensic unit. The young people may present significant challenges to community services that do not have the resources or physical environment to manage their behaviour or provide appropriate interventions. The relative lack of specialist mental health or forensic community services for young people with ASD within the UK means, therefore, that the support the young person and their family would have received may not have been adequate. It is not unusual to find that young people have been managed in isolation before coming to secure services (Paterson 2007).

Assessment and formulation

Prior to any treatment being offered, it is important that a full psychologically informed assessment is undertaken. Assessments from other members of the multidisciplinary team (MDT), such as occupational therapists and speech and language therapists, can also be invaluable. All professionals have a role in assessing the areas highlighted in Table 13.1. Information gleaned from these assessments can help practitioner psychologists to formulate difficulties and to adapt their approach to aid assessment. This section will discuss assessments specifically relating to ASD, in terms of identifying needs and assessing risk.

Assessment of psychosocial functioning

The methods used to support a diagnosis of ASD can vary, and have in the past often been based on clinical opinion rather than the use of ASD-specific tools, although this has changed over recent years. There are no specific physical or psychological tests for ASD. In order to identify the key impairments associated with a diagnosis of ASD, information must be collected in a systematic way. It is clearly recognised by experts within the field that one of the most important parts of the assessment process is the gathering of a comprehensive developmental history. In the UK, the recently published National Institute for Health and Care Excellence (NICE) guidelines for ASD diagnosis in young people (NICE 2011), recommend that the following areas are assessed: young person's experiences across a variety of settings, developmental history, behavioural features, neurodevelopmental factors, mental disorders, medical history, physical examination, communication, strengths and skills. The guidelines recommend using an autism-specific tool for assessment and that differential diagnosis is considered. There are semi-structured interviews available to aid this process, one of which is the Diagnostic Interview for Social and Communication Disorders (Wing et al. 2002). The NAS state that its special value is that it collects information concerning all aspects of each individual's skills, deficits and untypical behaviour, not just the core features of ASD. The NICE guidelines on autism in children and young people (NICE 2011) and the NICE guidelines for adults with autism (NICE 2012) set out clear guidelines for recognising and diagnosing ASD. The Autism Diagnostic Interview – Revised (ADI-R; Lord, Rutter and Le Couteur 1994) is considered the 'gold standard' for gathering a detailed developmental history, and the Autism Diagnostic Observation Schedule: Version 2 (ADOS-2; Lord et al. 2008) is the equivalent for the observed assessment of social and communication difficulties. For more detailed information on the tools used to assess ASD in children and adolescents refer to NICE guidelines (2011).

The information gathered during assessment can be used to create a needs-based management plan, taking into account family and educational context. As with most NICE guidance relating to the mental health of children, the importance of family involvement and the timely sharing of information are stressed.

Diagnosing ASD can be a complex business. It has been proposed that many individuals with ASD are undetected or misdiagnosed with mental health problems (Schwartz-Watts 2005; Allen et al. 2008). The scope for misdiagnosis may be particularly likely in 'non-classical' cases (Sverd et al. 1995), particularly those who are higher functioning, due to clinical unfamiliarity with the presentation (Haskins and Arturo Silva 2006). Sometimes the difficulties associated with ASD have been noticed, but the young person has not been diagnosed until mid-childhood (Sverd et al. 1995). Providing a diagnosis of ASD is made more complicated by high rates of co-morbidity in relation to ID and mental health difficulties.

In addition to mental health needs, individuals with ASD are also prone to co-morbid physical health conditions. Treating Autism and Autism Treatment Trust (2013) have developed a booklet providing an overview of the medical co-morbidities that could be present in this population, to guide professionals in their assessments and treatments. It states that these health conditions include: 'eczema, allergies, asthma, ear and respiratory problems, gastrointestinal problems severe headaches, migraines and seizures' (Schieve et al. 2012: 1). It is important that any underlying physical health issue is identified and treated, as these in themselves can be the trigger to some of the high-risk behaviours engaged in (Buie et al. 2010).

Risk assessment

Although there is not a specific structured professional judgement (SPJ) tool to assess risk in individuals with ASD, factors related specifically to ASD, such as the role of special interests, should be considered. Furthermore, certain items considered in SPJ tools may be relevant to an ASD population, but for potentially different reasons than the sample on which the research was conducted. For example, a lack of empathy is usually included when assessing risk in consideration of the presence of callous and unemotional traits, common in individuals who engage in antisocial behaviour (Dadds, Whiting and Hawes 2006; Fite, Stoppelbein and Greening 2009).

However, in those with ASD, the absence of empathy is more likely to be due to theory of mind deficits (Baron-Cohen 2001). It also needs to be remembered that there are different forms of empathy and not all may be impaired in ASD. For example, many young people with ASD have cognitive empathy in that they are aware logically of how behaviours may impact on others, but they often lack emotional empathy in that they find it difficult to emotionally connect with others and 'step into another's shoes'. Similarly, not all individuals with ASD experience complete deficits in their theory of mind (Baron-Cohen 1998). Peer rejection is also considered as a particular risk factor for young people in the general population, as many individuals who engage in high-risk behaviours have been rejected by prosocial peers, leading them to be more likely to engage with delinquent peers. However, many individuals with ASD are either unaware of the peer rejection, or are not overly concerned that they have been rejected as they lack the desire to socialise. On the other hand, some individuals with ASD do desire social interactions, but lack the skills to achieve this appropriately and are often more vulnerable and able to be taken advantage of by more able, antisocial peers. Hence, when assessing risk in individuals with ASD, the risk items need to be considered in a different manner, always considering factors associated with ASD (Gunasekaran 2012). This information should be incorporated into the formulation, if using a psychological approach, and used to inform areas for intervention.

Interventions

Psychosocial

Information gathered during the assessment process will be used to develop a psychological formulation of the young person's presentation. The formulation should identify factors linked to the needs and high-risk behaviour that will be targeted for intervention. These factors may be linked to the core features of ASD, or they may be a result of trauma or previous life experiences, or a combination of the two. The factors that may need targeting can be wide ranging. However, common targets for intervention will include: enhancing social skills and understanding of relationships, improving the young person's ability to recognise, understand and manage emotions, and replacing maladaptive coping skills with more prosocial alternatives (problem solving) to enhance communication skills and cognitive empathy.

A key initial goal will often be to reduce the arousal levels of the young person, as this is likely to heighten the probability of them engaging in high-risk behaviours. Many young people with ASD often find it difficult to recognise this heightened arousal and, even if acknowledged, struggle to reduce it appropriately (Chalfant 2011). Not being in a state of heightened arousal can often feel alien for a variety of reasons, including a particular sensory profile, difficulties adapting to change and feeling out of control. This means that a relaxed state may be experienced as anxiety provoking initially, hence the need to prepare the young person for this and to introduce change in small steps.

Some interventions may be contraindicated due to the core features of ASD, for example empathy-focused interventions (Wong 2000). Due to poor theory of mind, interventions exploring the effect any risk behaviour has on preferred activity may be more effective than relying on exploration of moral empathic understanding. Emphasis should also be placed on managing dysfunctional and restricted coping strategies (Murphy 2010). Comic strips and visual aids can be used to describe situations as they occurred, including the impact on the individual and others, as well as prosocial alternatives which can be helpful in developing theory of mind and empathy, and in developing the young person's coping strategies.

Young people may also have little or no understanding of their diagnosis, which may lead to intense feelings of being different or 'defective' in some way. For this reason, psychoeducation about what autism is and the unique way that the young person is affected by it, can be really helpful, both to gather information on the strengths and deficits of each individual, and for the young person's self-awareness.

In terms of interventions for the core features of ASD, many focus on social-communication deficits. Two such interventions are Socialeyes (NAS 2010) and the Programme for the Education and Enrichment of Relational Skills (PEERS; Laugeson and Frankel 2010). Socialeyes is a resource to facilitate social skills and social understanding, not by changing inappropriate behaviours, but by providing alternative skills and strategies that could be used. PEERS is a manualised social skills programme, with a good evidence base. Laugeson and colleagues (2009) conducted a randomised controlled trial (RCT) with 17 adolescents (13–17 years) receiving PEERS, compared to a matched control group. They found those who received PEERS showed a significant improvement in their social knowledge, participated in more social situations and showed improved overall social skills when compared to the control group.

Co-morbid mental health problems

NICE guidelines (2012) state that any co-morbid mental health condition present in combination with ASD should be treated in line with NICE guidance for the co-morbid condition, with adaptations made to the method of delivery. For example, it can be helpful to incorporate the child or young person's special interests into therapy, to increase their motivation to engage. Involving a parent or carer to support the implementation of the intervention can also be helpful, and any adaptations need to be done collaboratively with the young person and families/carers (NICE 2011). This is important, as generalisation of skill development is an area with which young people with ASD often have difficulty. For example, they may consider that social skills only occur during a social skills group and struggle to comprehend that these skills should be used continuously. By including families or staff in the interventions, these people can aid in supporting the young person to use the skills learnt outside of the group session and aid generalisation.

Cognitive behaviour therapy

Cognitive behavioural therapy (CBT) is often the evidence-based treatment recommended for many mental health problems that may be co-morbid with ASD (e.g. diagnoses of depression and anxiety disorder). It could be assumed, therefore, that CBT could help people with ASD and decrease co-morbid psychiatric symptomatology. In terms of the adult literature for those with ASD, a recent systematic review concluded that individually delivered CBT (there was only one study exploring group CBT) shows promise in decreasing co-morbid psychiatric symptomatology, but there is little evidence that CBT can increase social and communicative functioning (Binnie and Blainey 2013). This research highlighted the lack of good-quality evidence for the effectiveness of CBT for ASD populations. Evidence suggests that, for children and adolescents with ASD, interventions focusing on providing parent training and CBT for anxiety (Sopronoff, Attwood and Hinton 2005; Chalfant, Rapee and Carroll 2007), social skills and managing challenging behaviours may be useful to improve social communication, language use and, potentially, symptom severity (Warren et al. 2011). There is a dearth of good-quality studies that assess psychological interventions other than CBT, and there is a lack of information on modifiers of effectiveness, generalisation of effects outside the treatment context, components of multicomponent therapies that drive effectiveness and predictors of treatment success (AHRQ 2011).

Systemic and environment interventions

High-risk behaviours may be reduced in certain environments due to adaptations to the physical environment that minimise anxiety. These adaptations may include the amount and type of personal space given, size of rooms, number of staff and other service users, visual supports (e.g. words, pictures or symbols), the colour of walls and furnishings, lighting, noise levels, and processes of health or social care (e.g. arranging appointments at the beginning or end of the day to minimise waiting time, or providing single rooms for children and young people admitted to hospital). Some of these factors are considered in the Structure, Positive, Empathy, Low Arousal, Links (SPELL) framework (NAS). The SPELL framework recognises the individual and unique needs of each child and emphasises that planning and intervention be organised on this basis by building on strengths and reducing the disabling effects of ASD, so that progress can be made in personal growth and development, and the promotion of opportunity and as full a life as possible (http://www.nas.org.uk). This approach can also be used in conjunction with a Treatment and Education of Autistic and Related Communication Handicapped Children approach (TEACCH; Mesibov, Shea and Schopler 2004), which uses cognitive, behavioural and social learning principles to meet the learning styles and needs of young people with ASD. The primary aim of the TEACCH programme is to help to prepare people with autism to live or work more effectively by reducing or removing 'autistic behaviours' (see Mesibov, Shea and Schopler 2004).Young people with ASD often require highly structured interventions, environments and support for learning and, consequently, any treatment for high-risk behaviour may need to be fundamentally different for an adolescent who has an ASD than for an adolescent without ASD.

Transitions

A number of recently published reports and studies have highlighted the difficulties that can occur when young people transition to adult mental health services (AMHS) (Barnard, Prior and Potter 2000; Barnard et al. 2001; Lavis and Hewson 2011). These reports have concluded that young people in hospital can become invisible if their placement is stable, or out of area, and that transitions are often not well planned and young people are not kept informed or involved. In the UK it has been highlighted that transitioning between adolescent and AMHS can be particularly difficult for those with ASD or ADHD and those without an agreed diagnosis, such as young people with conduct disorder or emerging personality disorder (Lavis and Hewson 2011). The clinical experience of the authors is that transitions are not always well managed and young people with developmental disabilities may not be given enough time, or the correct forum, to communicate their hopes and fears about leaving and going somewhere new.

From clinical experience, funding decisions can mean that a young person may be required to transition to another service quickly (within weeks), or they may be waiting to move for over a year. This can lead to significant anxiety and associated deteriorations in mental state and behaviour. Anxieties may be expressed through behaviour (acting out), including attempting to sabotage the transition: 'If I'm risky I'll stay here'. Sudden high levels of stress and anxiety can also trigger a relapse of symptoms associated with diagnoses of mental illness. This can have profound effects on the young person's future placement and cause conflict between the service and families, who lose faith in the 'system'. In terms of good practice, transition planning should start at least six months in advance, with a consistent proactive lead professional coordinating. Discharge planning should be considered as early as possible after the young person's admission to an inpatient setting. Structured peer support can be very helpful in supporting young people, and consideration should be given to facilitating a group for those who may be shortly making a transition. Outcomes should be monitored and feedback should be sought from the young people, so that services can make improvements to the transition process (Brodie, Goldman and Clapton 2011). Barriers to successful, well-managed transitions may include the 'invisibility' issue, funding difficulties or meeting stringent referral criteria (particularly for those with borderline ID or less obvious ASD and a lack of clarity of needs, or those with complex or unusual presentations). For young people with ASD in the UK, there may be a lack of specialised services to which they can transition. This means they may fall between a gap in ID and mental health services. There continue to be very few ASD-specific forensic services in the UK; although, over recent years, a few ASD-specific secure services have emerged. However, with a lack of appropriate community services, many young people with ASD may be admitted to secure services unnecessarily.

NICE guidelines for young people aged 16 or older, whose needs are complex or severe, suggest the use of the Care Programme Approach (CPA) (DH 2008) in England, or care and treatment plans in Wales, as an aid to transfer between services. Children and young people with high-risk behaviours can face particular difficulties and crises as they move from child to adult services. Integrating care and support around their needs and ensuring that they have access to the services identified in their agreed care plan is vital (DH 2012).

Ideally, the young person and their family or carers should be involved in the transition process and should be provided with information about adult services, including their right to a social care assessment at age 18. Processes such as 'My Shared Pathway' and person-centred planning can help achieve this. My Shared Pathway is a tool used as part of a recovery approach to identify and achieve outcomes for service users in secure services. The young person should be involved in deciding how the transition should occur, that is, undertake shorter visits over a prolonged period before making the final transition or just transfer in one move. Social stories regarding the transition, pictures of the new placement and the staff, along with visits from the new staff, can all aid in preparing the young person for the transition and familiarise them with their new environment. This is particularly important if they are not having several visits. However, families and staff may have to work in the young person's best interest at times and withhold information regarding the transition until concrete plans are in place, in order to minimise the anxiety experienced through uncertainty. Guidance may also need to be given on the most suitable placement, using information gathered from assessments and informed by the young person's engagement in interventions.

Case example

So far this chapter has discussed the core features of ASD, as well as commonly associated factors that can be linked with high-risk behaviours, and the challenges of appropriately meeting the needs of these young people. To draw together the pertinent issues raised, a case study will be presented, based on a composite of young people with whom the authors have worked with in a clinical setting.

Billy was born two months prematurely after his father pushed his mother down the stairs. His father had a history of schizophrenia and his mother suffered from depression. When Billy was a baby he was not very demanding and would not seek out cuddles or attention from his mother, apart from when he needed to get his physical needs met. Billy's mother was quite neglectful as she spent lots of time in bed and only met the most basic needs for her child. Billy's father was detained in hospital under the Mental Health Act (1989) and his mother met a new partner. However, his mother and stepfather appeared to be much more interested in fighting with each other than giving any attention to Billy.

A health visitor noticed that Billy was not reaching his developmental milestones and, at 18 months, had not started talking or walking. His mother felt like she was a bad parent and this increased her depression. She also felt angry towards Billy for not 'being normal' and she did not want to give him any affection. By the time Billy was 3 years old he had started to display aggressive behaviours such as smashing his toys and biting people. His mother found it difficult to cope with these behaviours and would leave Billy in his room for hours on end. Sometimes he would be left in his own urine and faeces for long periods of time and nobody would respond to his cries. After a while, Billy would stop crying.

At age 4, Billy went to nursery. He had started talking a little, but none of the other children wanted to play with him. Billy would sit on his own and not attempt to play with the others. He would also be aggressive to children in his group if they came too close to him, or made too much noise. During the early school years Billy's difficulties at school continued, with increased peer victimisation and academic failure. At home, Billy was being physically abused by his mother's partners. His aggressive behaviours increased at school and at home he began setting small fires in his bedroom. The fires made Billy feel happy and excited and he liked the feeling of being able to put them out.

At age 10, Billy's behaviour continued to get worse. He could not communicate his feelings to anyone and would avoid people and busy loud places, At this point Billy was referred to Child and Adolescent Mental Health Service (CAMHS) by his teacher, but his mother failed to take him to his appointment. Billy could not understand others' behaviour and felt very confused about why he had to do certain things. Billy's aggression also got worse and, by the age of 12, he had to be schooled on an individual basis, as teachers struggled to contain him when he became frustrated or did not want to do something. Billy was learning that if he was aggressive he would be removed from an unpleasant situation, or people would stop asking him to do things. He would often be left on his own for 'time out', which he quite enjoyed. He was shunned by other children, who said Billy smelt. The school contacted social services, who had noticed that Billy was coming into school dirty and also had cigarette burns on his upper arms.

Age 13, Billy was starting to become aware that he was different to other people and he felt very left out, sad and angry that he did not have any friends. He had also noticed that he had strange feelings 'down below' and wanted to touch girls. When he tried to talk to girls they laughed at him and ran away, which made Billy very angry. One day he was walking home from school and saw two very young girls (aged around 7 to 8) playing in the park. Billy went over to the girls and tried to get involved in their game. They did not run away from him, but when Billy tried to touch one of the girls on the chest she kicked him. Billy became very angry, dragged the girl behind some park equipment and sexually assaulted her.

The police came to talk to Billy about what he had done, but Billy did not feel it was a big deal. When the police would not stop talking, Billy punched one of them in the face. Billy was arrested, but sent home. Billy had some input from YOS following a referral order and was sent to do some work on understanding relationships, but he offended again and then again, and began to assault teachers at school. Billy was eventually sent to a hospital because professionals said he was 'too high risk'. Due to professionals suspecting that Billy had ASD he was referred to an ASD-specific unit. Billy did not mind, he was glad to get away from home.

Once in hospital, Billy was assessed by the MDT. An ADOS and an ADI-R were completed based on interviews with his mother, local services and teachers at his school, which indicated Billy met the diagnostic criteria for ASD; he was subsequently given the diagnosis. This diagnosis would not have been easy to make as, although it was clear that Billy would avoid social situations, there could have been a number of reasons for this. For example, based on his past experiences it would be understandable Billy would want to avoid others as he did not trust them and would want to avoid future harm by them. However, from the information provided and the assessments completed it was clear that Billy had developmental issues that suggested his social avoidance was also due to additional factors associated with ASD, such as poor social communication and understanding of social situations. The information provided by the interviewees was used to inform the ADI-R, a functional analysis of aggression and fire-setting. Psychometrics were adapted by simplifying the language and providing visual cues for responses. These adaptations enabled Billy to provide a self-report in areas including fire-setting, anger, sexual knowledge, self-esteem and social skills. A cognitive assessment identified that Billy had a borderline ID with specific deficits in verbal comprehension and processing skills. These results highlighted the need for visual aids and time required for Billy to respond to information provided verbally. He was also referred for a speech and language assessment to explore his communication deficits further and provide interventions if required.

Staff observed that Billy was initially very challenging of the boundaries on the unit and he displayed frequent aggression towards staff. However, a few weeks after admission it was noted that the frequency and the severity of the aggression had reduced, as Billy became more familiar with the routines and expectations of the unit.

Formulation

Biologically, Billy was born prematurely, which could have put him at risk of developmental delay. In terms of genetic vulnerability there is a history of paternal mental illness, which increases the risk of Billy developing mental health problems. There may also have been temperamental factors at play, which meant Billy may have been more irritable and harder to console. These predisposing factors may have been exacerbated by features associated with

ASD, such as sensory sensitivities, difficulties understanding social situations, communication deficits and problem-solving difficulties. In terms of early experiences there were likely to be attachment difficulties considering that Billy's mother was a victim of domestic violence and had her own difficulties coping. These circumstances were likely to have led Billy to develop low self-esteem and a lack of confidence in his own abilities. Billy may have developed beliefs that others cannot meet his needs and others are dangerous. Aggression was potentially a learnt behaviour, or a re-enactment of the behaviours displayed towards him, which became an effective strategy for keeping people away and avoiding situations that were aversive, thus preventing further trauma from occurring.

As Billy got older, he was exposed to a number of precipitating factors, including academic failure, social rejection and further abuse. Aggression became entrenched as a way to express his frustration, communicate feelings and attempt to control the environment. Fire-setting may have served sensory needs in terms of enjoying looking at flames. Billy also liked the sense of control achieved from putting small fires out. Billy engaged in fire-setting when he was feeling out of control and was experiencing negative affect, which he found difficult to manage. With the lack of alternative coping strategies, fire-setting became the only means by which Billy experienced positive affect. As Billy hit puberty he experienced increased confusion around his own identity and sexual feelings. Lack of understanding of these feelings and the lack of opportunities to meet sexual needs in an appropriate way due to social rejection, meant that he sought other opportunities available. Billy found it easier to get on with younger children due to his immature developmental level and his assumption that younger children wanted to spend time with him and were less likely to reject him. However, the combination of high sexual arousal, impulsivity and poor empathy relating to the victim, meant that Billy went on to sexually assault a girl.

To summarise, maintaining factors include, but are not limited to: his mother's lack of supervision and parental involvement, poor role models and lack of support, high-risk behaviours serving their function, lack of consideration of consequences and impulsivity.

Intervention

In the intervention plan it was recommended that Billy attend a social and emotional skills group to support the development of emotional awareness and regulation skills and to improve his ability to interact with peers. These skills were reinforced by his attendance in a variety of sessions provided by other members of the MDT, including structured physical activity and development of adaptive living skills. The practitioner psychologist also worked with nursing staff to develop a shared understanding of the functions of Billy's behaviour, so that front-line staff could reinforce positive behaviour and appropriate coping skills. When Billy had completed the initial group work and developed some basic psychosocial skills, he began to attend individual sessions with the practitioner psychologist focusing on reducing the risk of his re-engagement in sexually harmful behaviour. Billy engaged well in the work and, 18 months after admission, was able to make a transition to a residential school. It was recommended that the school was ASD specific, as Billy had responded well to the structured environment of the ASD-specific unit. Due to local services remaining in regular contact with the unit throughout Billy's admission they were fully aware of Billy's needs and the progress he had made. They were therefore able to source an appropriate placement with a comprehensive transition plan, which included building up relationships, by staff from the school spending time with staff and Billy in the unit, and Billy spending increasing amounts of time at the school over a four-week period. A social story was developed to support Billy in his understanding around why he was moving, how it would happen, what was expected from him and what he could expect from others. It was hoped that this approach would lessen anxiety about the move by increasing familiarity and predictability. A formal staff handover regarding effective care plans and Billy's communication passport (a book all about Billy) would take place to ensure continuity of care and ensure that Billy has a positive experience of transition.

Conclusion

This chapter has provided an overview of some of the main issues to consider when working with young people with ASD who display high-risk behaviours. It is important to emphasise that a thorough multidisciplinary assessment needs to be completed to ensure that all areas of the young persons strengths and difficulties are considered. In summary, although it is promising that research in this area is increasing rapidly, there is still a long way to go in terms of transferring theory into practice within the UK. As the research literature develops and clinicians grow in their expertise, it is hoped that the gap between secure and community services can be bridged, to allow this complex group of young people to receive an appropriate service, reducing the likelihood of their unnecessarily involvement with the CJS.

References

Allen, D., Evans, C., Hider, A., Hawkins, S., Peckitt, H., and Morgan, H. (2008) 'Offending behaviour in adults with Asperger's syndrome', *Journal of Autism and Developmental Disorder*, 38: 748–758.
Anckarsater, H., Nillson, T., Saury, J., Rastam, M., and Gillberg, C. (2007) 'Autism spectrum disorders in institutionalized subjects', *Nordic Journal of Psychiatry*, 62: 160–167.

APA (American Psychiatric Association) (2013) *Diagnostic and Statistical Manual of Mental Disorders*. 5th edn. Arlington, VA: American Psychiatric Publishing.

Barnard, J., Prior, A., and Potter, D. (2000) 'Inclusion and autism: Is it working?' Available at: http://www.scottishautism.org/about-autism/autism-policy/inclusion-in-autism-is-it-working/. Accessed 9 September 2014.

Barnard, J., Harvey, V., Potter, D., and Prior, A. (2001) 'Ignored or ineligible? The reality for adults with autism spectrum disorders', *The National Autistic Society*. Available at: http://www. bowdiges.org.uk. Accessed 5 August 2014.

Baron-Cohen, S. (1998) 'Autism and "theory of mind": An introduction and review', *Communication*, Summer, 48, 3: 9–12.

Baron-Cohen, S. (2001) 'Theory of mind and autism: A review', *Special Issue of the International Review of Mental Retardation*, 23: 1–35.

Golan, O., Baron-Cohen, S., Wheelwright, S. & Hill, J.J. (2006) 'Systemizing empathy: Teaching adults with Asperger Syndrome and High Functioning Autism to recognise complex emotions using interactive multimedia', *Development and Psychopathology*, 18, 589–615.

Barry-Walsh, J.B., and Mullen, P.E. (2004) 'Forensic aspects of Asperger's syndrome', *Journal of Forensic Psychiatry and Psychology*, 15(1): 96–107.

Binnie, J. and Blainey, S. (2013) 'The use of cognitive behavioural therapy for adults with autism spectrum disorders: A review of the evidence', *Mental Health Review Journal*, 18: 93–104.

Bradley, E.A., Summers, J.A., Wood, H.L., and Bryson, S.E. (2004), 'Comparing rates of psychiatric and behavior disorders in adolescents and young adults with severe intellectual disability with and without autism', *Journal of Autism and Developmental Disorders*, 34: 151–161.

Brereton, A.V., Tonge, B.J., and Einfeld, S.L. (2006) 'Psychopathology in children and adolescents with autism compared to young people with intellectual disability', *Journal of Autism and Developmental Disorders*, 36: 863–870.

Brodie, I., Goldman, R., and Clapton, J. (2011) 'Mental health service transitions for young people: Research briefing 37', *Social Care Institute for Excellence*. Available at: www.scie.org.uk/publications/briefings/briefing37/

Buie, T., Campbell, D.B., Fuchs, G.J., Furuta, G.T., Levy, J., VandeWater, J., Whitaker, A.H., Atkins, D., Bauman, M.L., Beaudet, A.L., Carr, E.G., Gershon, M.D., Hyman, S.L., Jirapinyo, P., Jyonouchi, H., Kooros, K., Kushak, R., Levitt, P., Levy, S.E., Lewis, J.D., Murray, K.F., Natowicz, M.R., Sabra, A., Wershil, B.K., Weston, S.C., Zelter, L. & Winter, H. (2010) 'Evaluation, diagnosis, and treatment of gastrointestinal disorders in individuals with ASDs: A consensus report', *Pediatrics*, 125(Supplement 1): S1–S18.

Cashin, A. and Newman, C. (2009) 'Autism in the criminal justice detention system: A review of the literature', *Journal of Forensic Nursing*, 5: 70–75.

Chakrabarti, S. and Fombonne, E. (2005) 'Pervasive developmental disorders in preschool children: Confirmation of high prevalence', *American Journal of Psychiatry*, 162: 1133–1141.

Chalfant, A.M. (2011) *Managing Anxiety in People with Autism*. Bethesda, MD: Woodbine House.

Chalfant, A.M., Rapee, R., and Carroll, L. (2007) 'Treating anxiety disorders in children with high functioning autism spectrum disorders: A controlled trial', *Journal of Autism and Developmental Disorders*, 37: 1842–1857.

Croen, L.A., Grether, J.K., and Selvin, S. (2002) 'Descriptive epidemiology of autism in a California population: Who is at risk?' *Journal of Autism and Developmental Disorders*, 32: 217–224.

De Bruin, R.I., Ferdinand, R.F., Meester, S., de Nijs, P.F., and Verheij, F. (2006) 'High rates of psychiatric co-morbidity in PDD-NOS', *Journal of Autism and Developmental Disorders*, 37: 877–886.
De la Cuesta, G. (2010) 'A selective review of offending behaviour in individuals with autism spectrum disorders', *Journal of learning Disabilities and Offending Behaviour*, 1: 47–58.
Dadds, M.R., Whiting, C. and Hawes, D.J. (2006) 'Associations among cruelty to animals, family conflict and psychopathic traits in childhood', *Journal of Interpersonal Violence*, 21: 411–429.
DH (Department of Health) (1983). *Mental Health Act*. London: HSMO
DH (Department of Health) (2008) *Refocusing the Care Programme Approach: Policy and Positive Practice Guidance*. London: Department of Health.
DH (Department of Health) (2012) *Transforming Care: A National Response to Winterbourne View Hospital*. London: Department of Health.
Einfeld, S.L., Ellis, L.A., and Emerson, E. (2011) 'Comorbidity of intellectual disability and mental disorder in children and adolescents: A systematic review', *Journal of Intellectual and Developmental Disability*, 36: 137–143.
Fite, P., Stoppelbein, L., and Greening, L. (2009) 'Proactive and reactive aggression in a child psychiatric inpatient population: Relations to psychopathic characteristics', *Criminal Justice and Behavior*, 36, 481–493.
Geluk, C.A.M.L., Jansen, L.M.C., Vermeiran, R., Doreleijers, T.A.H., van Domburgh, L., de Bildt, A., Twisk, J.W.R., and Hartman, C.A. (2012) 'Autistic symptoms in childhood arrestees: Longitudinal association with delinquent behaviour', *Journal of Child Psychology and Psychiatry*, 53: 160–167.
Ghaziuddin, M., Tsai, L., and Ghaziuddin, N. (1991) 'Brief report: Violence in Asperger syndrome – a critique', *Journal of Autism and Developmental Disorders*, 21: 349–354.
Gunasekaran, S. (2012) 'Assessment and management of risk in autism', *Advances in Mental Health and Intellectual Disabilities*, 6: 314–320.
Harada, Y., Hayashida, A., Hikita, S., Imai, J., Sasayama, D., and Sari Masutani, S. (2009) 'Impact of behavioral/developmental disorders comorbid with conduct disorder', *Psychiatry and Clinical Neurosciences*, 63: 762–768.
Hare, D.J., Gould, J., Mills, R., and Wing, L. (1999) 'A preliminary study of individual with autistic spectrum disorders in three special hospitals in England', *The National Autistic Society*. Available at: www.aspires-relaationships.com/3hospitals.pdf. Accessed 29 December 2007.
Haskins, B.G. and Arturo Silva, J. (2006) 'Asperger's disorder and criminal behaviour: Forensic-psychiatric considerations', *Journal of the American Academy of Psychiatry and the Law*, 34: 374–384.
Howlin, P. (2000) 'Outcome in adult life for more able individuals with autism or Asperger's syndrome', *Autism*, 4: 63–83.
Joshi, G., Petty, C., Wozniak, J., Henin, A., Fried, R., Galdo, M., Kotarski, M., Walls, S., and Biederman, J. (2010) 'The heavy burden of psychiatric comorbidity in youth with autism spectrum disorders: A large comparative study of a psychiatrically referred population', *Journal of Autism and Developmental Disorders*, 40: 1361–1370.
Kanne, S.M. and Mazurek, M.O. (2011) 'Aggression in children and adolescents with ASD: Prevalence and risk factors', *Journal of Autism and Developmental Disorders*, 41: 926–937.
Kaplan, H.I. and Saddock, B.J. (1998) *Synopsis of Psychiatry: Behavioural Sciences/Clinical Psychiatry*, 8th edn. Maryland: Lippincott, Williams & Wilkins.
Långström, N., Martin, G., Ruchkin, V., Sjöstedt, G., and Fazel, S. (2008) 'Risk factors for violent offending in autistic spectrum disorder', *Journal of Interpersonal Violence*, 24: 8.

Laugeson, E.A. and Frankel, F. (2010) *Social Skills for Teenagers with Developmental and Autistic Spectrum Disorders: The PEERS Treatment Manual*. London: Routledge.

Laugeson, E.A., Frankel, F., Mogil, C., and Dillon, A.R. (2009) 'Parent-assisted social skills training to improve friendships in teens with autism spectrum disorders', *Journal of Autism and Developmental Disorders*, 39: 596–606.

Lavis, P and Hewson, L. (2011) 'How many times do we have to tell you? A briefing from the National Advisory Council about what young people think about mental health and mental health services', *Young Minds Magazine*, 109: 30–31.

Lecavalier, L. (2006) 'Behavioural and emotional problems in young people with pervasive developmental disorders: Relative prevalence, effects of subject characteristics, and empirical classifications', *Journal of Autism and Developmental Disorders*, 36: 1101–1114.

Leyfer, O.T., Folstein, S.E., Bacalman, S., Davis, N.O., Dinh, E., Morgan, J., Tager-Flusberg, H., and Lainhart, J.E. (2006) 'Comorbid psychiatric disorders in children with autism: Interview development and rates of disorders', *Journal of Autism and Developmental Disorders*, 36: 849–861.

Lord, C., Rutter, M., and Le Couteur, A. (1994) 'Autism Diagnostic Interview – Revised: A revised version of a diagnostic interview for caregivers of individuals with possible pervasive developmental disorders', *Journal of Autism and Developmental Disorders*, 24: 659–685.

Lord, C., Rutter, M., DiLavore, P.C., and Risi, S. (2008) *Autism Diagnostic Observation Schedule Manual*. Los Angeles: Western Psychological Services.

Loveland, K. and Tunali-Kotoski, B. (2005) 'The School-Aged Child with an Autism Spectrum Disorder', in F. Volkmar, R. Paul, A. Klin, and D. Cohen (eds.), *The Handbook of Autism and Pervasive Developmental Disorders*, 3rd edn. New York: Wiley, 247–287.

Mandell, D.S. (2008) 'Psychiatric hospitalization among children with autism spectrum disorders', *Journal of Autism and Developmental Disorders*, 38: 1059–1065.

Mandell, D.S., Walrath, C., Manteuffel, B., Sgro, G., and Pinto-Martin, J. (2005) 'Characteristic of children with autistic spectrum disorders served in comprehensive community-based mental health settings', *Journal of Autism and Developmental Disorders*, 35: 113–121.

Matson, J.L. and Nebel-Schwalm, M.S. (2005) 'Comorbid psychopathology with autism spectrum disorder in children: An overview', *Research in Developmental Disabilities*, 28: 341–352.

Mattila, M.L., Kielinen, M., Jussila, K., Linna, S.L., Bloigu, R., Ebeling, H., and Moilanen, I. (2007) 'An epidemiological and diagnostic study of Asperger syndrome according to four sets of diagnostic criteria', *Journal of the American Academy of Child and Adolescent Psychiatry*, 46: 636–646.

Mesibov, G.B., Shea, V., and Schopler, E. (2004) *The TEACCH Approach to Autism Spectrum Disorders*. New York: Springer.

Moran, H. (2010) 'Clinical observations of the differences between children on the autism spectrum and those with attachment problems: The Coventry Grid', *Good Autism Practice*, 11: 46–59.

Morgan, C.N., Roy, M., and Chance, P. (2003) 'Psychiatric comorbidity and medication use in autism: A community survey', *Psychiatric Bulletin*, 27: 378–381.

Mouridsen, S.E. (2012) 'Current status of research on autism spectrum disorders and offending', *Research in Autism Spectrum Disorders*, 6: 70–86.

Mouridsen, S.E., Rich, B., Isager, T., and Nedergaard, N.J. (2008) 'Pervasive developmental disorders and criminal behavior: A case control study', *International Journal of Offender Therapy and Comparative Criminology*, 53: 196–205.

Murphy, D. (2010) 'Understanding offenders with autism-spectrum disorders: What can forensic services do?' *Advances in Psychiatric Treatment*, 16: 44–46.

NAS (National Autistic Society) (2010) 'Socialeyes: Exploring the social world with people on the autism spectrum', *National Autistic Society*. Available at: http://www.autism.org.uk/spell. Accessed 20 June 2014.

NAS (National Autistic Society) (2011) 'Autism and Asperger syndrome: Some facts and statistics', *National Autistic Society*. Available at: http://www.autism.org.uk/about-autism/myths-facts-and-statistics/some-facts-and-statistics.aspx. Accessed 20 August 2014.

NAS (National Autistic Society) (2013) 'What is autism?' *National Autistic Society*. Available at: http://www.autism.org.uk/about-autism/autism-and-asperger-syndrome-an-introduction/what-is-autism.aspx. Accessed 27 October 2014.

Newman, S.S. and Ghaziuddin, M. (2008) 'Violent crime in Asperger syndrome: The role of psychiatric comorbidity', *Journal of Autism and Developmental Disorders*, 38: 1848–1852.

NICE (National Institute for Health and Clinical Excellence) (2011) *Autism: Recognition, Referral and Diagnosis of Children and Young People on the Autism Spectrum. Clinical Guidelines CG128.*

NICE (National Institute for Health and Clinical Excellence) (2012) *Autism: Recognition, Referral, Diagnosis and Management of Adults on the Autism Spectrum. Clinical Guidelines CG142.*

Palermo, M.T. (2004) 'Pervasive developmental disorders: Psychiatric co-morbidities, and the law', *International Journal of Offender Therapy and Comparative Criminology*, 48: 40–48.

Paterson, P. (2007) 'How well do young offenders with Aspergers syndrome cope in custody?' *British Journal of Learning Disability*, 36, 54–58.

Raggi, C., Xenitidis, K., Moisan, M., Deeley, Q., and Robertson, D. (2013) 'Adults with autism spectrum disorder and learning disability presenting with challenging behaviour: How tolerant should we be?' *Journal of Intellectual Disabilities and Offending Behaviour*, 4: 42–52.

Realmuto, G. and Ruble, L. (1999) 'Sexual behaviors in autism: Problems of definition and management', *Journal of Autism and Developmental Disorders*, 29: 121–127.

Ruble, L.A. and Dalrymple, N.J. (1993) 'Social/sexual awareness of persons with autism: A parental perspective', *Archives of Sexual Behaviour*, 22: 239–240.

Schieve, L.A., Gonzalez, V., Boulet, S.L., Visser, S.N., Rice, C.E., Van Vaarden Brau, K., and Boyle, C.A. (2012) 'Concurrent medical conditions and health care use and needs among children with learning and behavioural developmental disabilities, National Health Interview Survey, 2006–2010', *Research in Developmental Disabilities*, 33(2): 467–476.

Schwartz-Watts, D.M. (2005) 'Asperger's disorder and murder', *Journal of the American Academy of Psychiatry and the Law*, 33: 390–393.

Scragg, P. and Shah, A. (1994) 'Prevalence of Asperger's syndrome in a secure hospital', *British Journal of Psychiatry*, 165: 679–682.

Siminoff, E., Pickles, A., Charman, T., Chandler, S., Loucas, T., and Baird, G. (2008) 'Psychiatric disorders in children with autism spectrum disorders: Prevalence, comorbidity, and associated factors in a population-derived sample', *Journal of the American Academy of Child and Adolescent Psychiatry*, 47: 921–929.

Simpson, M. and Hogg, J. (2001) 'Patterns of offending among people with intellectual disability: A systematic review. Part I: Methodology and prevalence data', *Journal of Intellectual Disability Research*, 45: 384–396.

Siponmaa, L., Kristiansson, M., Jonson, C., Nydén, A., and Gillberg, C. (2001) 'Juvenile and young adult mentally disordered offenders: The role of child neuropsychiatric disorders', *Journal of the American Academy of Psychiatry and the Law*, 29: 420–426.

Smith, K.R.M. and Matson, J.L. (2010) 'Psychopathology: Differences among adults with intellectually disabled, comorbid autism spectrum disorders and epilepsy', *Research in Developmental Disabilities*, 31: 743–749.

Sopronoff, K., Attwood, T., and Hinton, S. (2005) 'A randomised controlled trial of a CBT intervention for anxiety in children with Asperger syndrome', *Journal of Child Psychology and Psychiatry*, 46: 1152–1160.

Staniforth, C. and Griffin, Y. (2013) *Characteristics of Young People with ASD in a Secure Psychiatric Hospital*. Unpublished study.

Sturmey, P. and Dalfern, S. (2014) 'The effects of DSM5 autism diagnostic criteria on number of individuals diagnosed with autism spectrum disorders: A systematic review', *Journal of Autism and Developmental Disorders*, 4: 249–252.

Sutton, L.R., Hughes, T.L., Huang, A., Lehman, C., Paserba, D., Talkington, V., Taormina, R., Wlaters, J.B., Fenclau, E. and Marshall, S. (2013) 'Identifying individuals with autism in a state facility for adolescents adjudicated as sexual offenders: A pilot study', *Focus on Autism and Other Developmental Disabilities*, 7: 175–183

Sverd, J. (2003) 'Psychiatric disorders in individuals with pervasive developmental disorder', *Journal of Psychiatric Practice*, 9: 111–127.

Sverd, J., Dubey, D.R., Schweitzer, R. and Ninan, R. (2003). 'Pervasive developmental disorders among children and adolescents attending psychiatric day treatment', *Psychiatric Services*, 54: 1519–1525.

Sverd, J., Sheth, R., Fuss, J., and Levine, J. (1995) 'Prevalence of pervasive developmental disorder in a sample of psychiatrically hospitalized children and adolescents', *Child Psychiatry and Human Development*, 25: 221–240.

Tiffin, P.A. and Le Couteur, A. (2005) 'Developmental Disorders', in S. Gowers (ed.), *Seminars in Child and Adolescent Psychiatry*. London: Gaskell, 124–144.

Treating Autism and Autism Treatment Trust (2013) 'Medical comorbidities in autism spectrum disorders: A primer for health care professionals and policy makers', *Treating Autism and Autism Treatment Trust*. Available at: www.autismtreatment.org.uk/wp-content/uploads/2013/07/Medical-Comorbidities-in-Autism-Spectrum-Disorders-2013.pdf. Accessed 30 September 2014.

Warren, Z., Veenstra-VanderWeele, J., Stone, W., Bruzek, J.L., Nahmias, A.S., Foss-Feig, J.H., Jerome, R.N., Krishnaswami, S., Sathe, N.A., Glasser, A.M., Surawicz, T., McPheeters, M.L. (2011) 'Therapies for children with autism spectrum disorders. Comparative effectiveness review no. 26'. Available at: http://www.effectivehealthcare.ahrq.gov/reports/final.cfm. Accessed 20 May 2014.

WHO (World Health Organization) (1992) *ICD-10 Classifications of Mental and Behavioural Disorder: Clinical Descriptions and Diagnostic Guidelines*. Geneva: World Health Organization.

WHO (World Health Organization) (2001) *Mental Health and Intellectual Disabilities: Addressing the Mental Health Needs of People with Intellectual Disabilities*, Report by the Mental Health Special Interest Group of the International Association for the Scientific Study of Intellectual Disabilities to the World Health Organization.

Williams, H., Chitsabesan, P., Davies, R., and Mounce, L. (2012) 'Nobody made the connection: The prevalence of neurodisability in young people who offend', *The Office of the Children's Commissioner*. Available at: http://www.childrenscommissioner.gov.uk/content/publications/content_633. Accessed 9 April 2015.

Wilson, C.E., Gillan, N., Spain, D., Robertson, D., Roberts, G., Murphy, C.M., Maltezos, S., Zinkstok, J., Johnston, K., Dardani, C., Ohlsen, C., Deeley, P.Q., Craig, M., Mendez, M.A., Happe, F. & Murphy, D.G. (2013) 'Comparison of ICD-10R, DSM-IV-TR and DSM-5 in an adult autism spectrum disorder diagnostic clinic', *Journal of Autism and Developmental Disorder*, 43, 2515–2525.

Wing, L. and Gould, J. (1979) 'Severe impairments of social interaction and associated abnormalities in children: Epidemiology and classification', *Journal of Autism and Childhood Schizophrenia*, 9: 11–29.

Wing, L., Leekam, S.R., Libby, S.J., Gould, J., and Larcombe, M. (2002) 'The Diagnostic Interview for Social and Communication Disorders: Background, inter-rater reliability and clinical use', *Journal of Child Psychology and Psychiatry*, 43(3): 307–325.

Winter, N., Holland, A.J., and Collins, S. (1997) 'Factors predisposing to suspected offending by adults with self-reported learning disabilities', *Psychological Medicine*, 27: 595–607.

Wolff, S. (1998) 'Schizoid Personality in Childhood', in E. Schopler, G.B. Mesibov, and L.J. Kunce (eds.), *Asperger Syndrome or High Functioning Autism?* New York: Plenum Press, 123–142.

Wong, S. (2000) 'Psychopathic Offenders', in S. Hodgins and R. Muller-Isberner (eds.), *Violence Crime and Mentally Disordered Offenders: Concepts and Methods for Effective Treatment and Prevention*. London: Wiley, 87–112.

Woodbury-Smith, M.R., Clare, I.C.H., Holland, A.J., and Kearns, A. (2006) 'High functioning autistic spectrum disorders, offending and other law breaking: Findings from a community sample', *Journal of Forensic Psychiatry and Psychology*, 17: 108–120.

Wozniak, J., Biederman, J., Faraone, S.V., Frazier, J., Kim, J., Millstein, R., Gershon, J., Thornell, A. Cha, K. & Snyder, J.B. (1997) 'Mania in children with pervasive development disorder-revisited', *Journal of the Academy of Child and Adolescent Psychiatry*, 36: 1552–1559.

14
Young People's Self-Disclosure in Secure Forensic Settings

Joel Harvey and Luke Endersby

Introduction

This chapter explores the act of self-disclosure for young people in forensic settings. Self-disclosure is a process whereby we verbalise personal thoughts, feelings, behaviours and autobiographical details, and let them become known to another. The general (non-forensic) adult psychotherapy literature has long understood the importance of self-disclosure for physical and psychological well-being (Jourard 1971; Besharat 2007; Forrest 2010). It could be argued that self-disclosure is equally important in forensic contexts, in order to improve the well-being of the young person and to ensure that information is obtained for an accurate assessment of risk to self and to others. However, it is also possible that there are specific costs to the young person when disclosing personal information about themselves in a secure forensic setting; these potential costs must also be considered when conceptualising the process of disclosure.

The extant literature on self-disclosure in the forensic psychology literature is relatively limited, and research that does exist focuses on adults (see Frost, Daniels and Hudson 2006; Ferguson, Ireland and Ireland 2013). Furthermore, whilst researchers have begun to examine the complexities of psychological therapeutic provision in prisons and other secure settings, there is little mention or consideration of the process of disclosure and what this *means* to the young person who is disclosing (Harvey and Smedley 2010).

Drawing on the clinical experience of the authors, this chapter sets out to consider the complexities of disclosure in secure forensic settings, and argues for the importance of explicit psychological thinking about the *process* of disclosure, alongside the content of the information disclosed. When thinking about disclosure, we are not only thinking about the disclosure of abuse, but of difficult thoughts, feelings, behaviours and past experiences more generally.

The role of the practitioner psychologist in forensic settings is to improve the well-being of the young people they are working with and to ensure the protection of the public from harm; self-disclosure is a key part of both tasks. Indeed, it is difficult to help someone, and to develop risk scenarios and risk management strategies, if the client is not expressing their internal thoughts and feelings.

However, the very dual nature of helping improve a client's well-being and managing risk makes self-disclosure complex in forensic settings. This dual focus can lead to ambiguity about the role of the practitioner psychologist, and this might impact upon self-disclosure from our clients. Indeed, the practitioner psychologist working in secure settings needs to reflect on the question: 'who is the client?' In other words, is it the 'young person', the 'prison', the 'public' or 'all of them'? An understanding of who the clients are, and the often multiple agendas that are at play, has implications as to how practitioner psychologists think about and respond to disclosure.

This chapter will begin by taking a brief look at the general psychotherapy literature which has taken a relational stance to client disclosure, viewing disclosure as a process that occurs in the context of interpersonal relationships. We will then consider studies that have examined self-disclosure among clients in forensic settings. This research has tended to take a more dispositional stance towards disclosure and has not conceptualised disclosure as a process occurring in the context of a relationship. Having examined the forensic literature, we will then put forward a contextual conceptual model of disclosure that takes into account individual and contextual factors.

A relational stance to disclosure

Self-disclosure is the process of sharing thoughts and feelings with another that would not previously have been known unless the client disclosed this material (Yalom 1970). That material can be autobiographical memories, thoughts (intentions, aspirations), fantasies, feelings and behaviours. It has been recognised that we come to understand our own emotional experiences through language (Kahn et al. 2008), and thus self-disclosure is critical in that process. It is through the process of articulating our thoughts and feelings that we bring about understanding. Learning how, if and when to self-disclose is a key developmental task of adolescence.

When we turn to the psychotherapy literature we read that self-disclosure is an integral part of all therapies and a feature of human relationships. It has been argued that self-disclosure can help people recover from psychological difficulties (Forrest 2010). Forrest (2010) argues that self-disclosure and openness in therapy are essential in order to ensure that an appropriate intervention is provided.

Farber, Berano and Capobianco (2004) carried out a detailed analysis of the phenomenology of the process and consequences of disclosing in therapy with adults in the general community. They found that: 'disclosure in therapy may be more comprehensively understood as an essentially interpersonal processing where the desire to reduce the fever of distress is weighed against the anticipation of shame and vulnerability in the presence of another' (Farber, Berano and Capobianco 2004: 344). It is assumed here that we make decisions regarding whether to disclosure or not (Forrest 2010). Indeed, 'human beings are continuously confronted with the moment-to-moment choice of revealing or not revealing who they are, expressing or not expressing their real feelings and thoughts' (Forrest 2010: 1). But how is this decision-making played out in the context of secure forensic settings for young people? Are there factors that may inhibit or facilitate self-disclosure during therapy taking place within prisons or secure hospitals? We would argue, from our experience as practitioner psychologists in clinical forensic practice, that there are factors which can facilitate or inhibit a young person's disclosure.

Importantly, a balance must be reached in relation to how much a young person discloses. It has been argued that there is a curvilinear relationship between self-disclosure and general mental health; as Jourard (1971) states, disclosing too much or disclosing too little is problematic. So, on the one hand, too little disclosure can impair the progress of therapy. However, on the other hand, the client can become uncontained by their own level of disclosure. Indeed, when carrying out therapy with young people we first need to consider their ability to self-regulate and not put young people in a position where they are retraumatised by disclosing their own experiences. The response of the practitioner psychologist to disclosure is of paramount importance in helping the young person manage it.

It has also been argued that genuine disclosure is a marker of trust. Whilst disclosing to another requires a pre-existing level of trust, disclosing to another is, at the same time, a means of developing further trust and thereby of forming relationships. Indeed, Yalom (1970) argues that being able to self-disclose is a prerequisite for forming meaningful relationships. So, whilst we need some trust at the outset in order to disclose, it is through disclosing that trust might be established further. Conversely, though, disclosing can also erode trust, depending on how the person to whom one discloses then responds. Disclosure is not always without its costs. These costs might be particularly high in forensic settings where trust levels are low, as criminologists have shown (Liebling 2004). Young people involved in the youth justice system (YJS) bring with them a range of psychological and social difficulties; a lack of trust, a wary approach or an active avoidance of people in positions of authority. Young people bring with them a model of relating to themselves and to others, and this might substantially impact upon whether or not they decide to disclose.

A dispositional stance to disclosure

Whilst, in the general adult psychotherapy literature, the concept of self-disclosure has been given due consideration, it has only been examined to a limited extent in the forensic literature. The research that has been carried out in forensic settings has tended to take a dispositional stance to disclosure and has viewed disclosure more as a dispositional strategy. Moreover, a body of research exists on how to elicit confessions in relation to an alleged crime at the interview stage (Faller et al. 2001; Gudjonsson 2006), and research has also been carried out on deception (Granhag et al. 2004). Indeed, we might consider deception here as *disingenuous disclosure*. However, less has been written about the function and outcome of *genuine* self-disclosure within the context of a therapeutic relationship in secure settings.

Frost, Daniels and Hudson (2006) carried out a study in New Zealand with clients who had committed child sexual offences, and looked at the *strategies* people use during disclosure. They argued that knowledge of these strategies could help practitioners understand how clients engage, what function their disclosure has and how one might increase the effectiveness of interventions. They put forward a 'disclosure management model', and suggest that people differ in relation to two factors. The first factor is their goals of disclosure, so what they want to attain through the disclosure encounter; the authors argue that clients may emphasise the attainment of *self-validation* through disclosure or they may emphasise validation *by others* through the disclosure encounter. The second factor is their communication strategy: being open or closed in their communication. From these two factors (each with two levels), the authors suggest four 'disclosure management strategies'.

Following this study, in the UK Ferguson, Ireland and Ireland (2013) developed an assessment tool to assess 'disclosure styles' and to explore the relationship between 'disclosure style', personality and self-esteem. The authors went on to conclude that 'willingness to disclose information about one's offending behaviour was a critical factor within motivation to engage' (Ferguson, Ireland and Ireland 2013: 106) and that the development of an assessment tool of disclosure styles can assist in understanding client engagement. They argue that the tool could be used to see what factors are associated with it and can also help identify barriers to disclosure.

These studies bring self-disclosure onto our radar when working with clients in forensic contexts. Within these two studies, there is an implicit assumption that there are particular internal 'styles' of disclosing. If we are able to identify these styles we can then use this information to help us, as practitioners, work with clients. However, it is notable that this conceptualisation of personal 'styles' for the person disclosing does not take into account the 'others' in the relationship, namely the therapist being disclosed to *and* the system in which the disclosure is taking place – a system, such as a prison or secure hospital, where there is an imbalance of power between staff and service users, where there are reduced levels of autonomy and 'rules' for self-presentation. Furthermore, 'style' of disclosure might also be related to the level of shame a person can tolerate. The relational process of disclosing to another can be potentially shaming and the practitioner must be mindful of this. Indeed, young people might be experiencing trauma-related symptoms and these might impact upon their willingness, or ability, to disclose.

A contextual conceptual model for understanding disclosure in forensic practice

We would like to put forward a conceptual model of disclosure that draws upon both the general psychotherapy literature and the forensic literature. As we have seen, the general psychotherapy literature takes a more relational perspective and sees disclosure unfolding in a therapeutic relationship. We would like to take some of the thinking from the general adult psychotherapy literature and consider it within the context of young people in secure forensic settings.

Our starting premise is that it is important to acknowledge the significance of disclosure as a relational process and as an *event* in its own right. When working as a practitioner psychologist in forensic settings, it is tempting to solely focus on the content of a disclosure rather than to take a broader perspective and to attend to it *also* as a relational process. We would argue that it is important to also acknowledge and understand the social and psychological significance of disclosure having taken place. For example, when a young person discloses that they have recently taken drugs in the prison, we might be drawn to finding out when he took them, what he used, how often he had taken them, how much he had taken, whether he was with someone else and whether he planned to continue to use. Whilst this information may be useful to develop a psychological formulation and manage potential risk, we must acknowledge and validate that a disclosure has taken place and recognise the process of disclosure as being significant in its own right. We are conceptualising disclosure as a relational process, and argue that we need to think about the young person, their development, the institutional context and the political sphere, and the interactions therein, when working in secure settings. We think that an analysis that focuses on individual factors alone is too limited, and that it is important to take a contextual approach to understanding therapy provision and self-disclosure.

Individual

There are a number of different individual-level factors that might impact upon a young person's self-disclosure. Young people bring with them a number of different experiences, strengths and difficulties. A young person might have a history of mental health difficulties and substance misuse (SM) problems (Lader, Singleton and Meltzer 2000; Kroll et al. 2002; Harrington and Bailey 2005). For example, if a young person is severely depressed and withdrawn, this will impact upon his ability to disclose his current concerns. He may lack motivation and energy, feel hopeless, and not see the point in disclosing his thoughts and feelings to a therapist. In another example, a person admitted to a secure unit might be actively psychotic, and experience paranoid delusions and command hallucinations. Here, disclosure to others might be an issue. Finally, a person might be uncontained and disinhibited in their presentation, and be keen to disclose, revealing aspects of themselves that perhaps they would have preferred to have kept private. In varied ways, then, mental health symptoms may thus decrease or increase a person's level of disclosure and what they disclose.

Furthermore, the young person might have had prior experiences of abusive or neglectful relationships with caregivers, difficulties trusting others and a reluctance to seek support from others (Harvey 2007, 2011). Young people have different internal working models of relating to themselves and others; they have different attachment styles (Adshead 2004; Rogers and Budd, Chapter 15, this volume). Depending upon their early life experiences, young people will have different expectations of relationships. Those who have been brought up in cumulative traumatic environments will not have had the opportunity to develop a secure base and to seek support from others. Why would such a client disclose to someone, if they have experienced such a punitive, abusive reaction by a caregiver? Having not been 'held in mind' by a significant other, disclosing to another might seem of limited value. To sum up, the young person's manner of disclosure might be affected by the difficulties and experiences they import with them into the prison. More generally, we also need to think about attachment and the stage a young person is at in their development. Adolescence is a period of developing autonomy, and to seek support and disclose to another might be seen as relinquishing control rather than gaining control over a difficult situation (Harvey 2007).

Contextual

We will now examine the context in which a young person may be disclosing. We must acknowledge that a young person does not self-disclose in a vacuum. To focus on disclosure styles or personality characteristics offers only a decontextualised conceptualisation of self-disclosure. We need to think about the relationship between the individual and their environment. Specifically considering secure settings, there are a range of factors that might impact upon disclosure.

Prisons, for example, are argued to be low trust environments where concerns over safety permeate (Liebling 2004). Moreover, they are at once highly structured and unpredictable environments. Staff and prisoners change, significant events occur, such as acts of violence and suicide, and prisoners often have to endure a number of transition points through their sentences. The same points apply to patients in secure hospital settings. These factors can all impact on self-disclosure.

The environment of the prison or the secure hospital brings with it conditions that require the young person to present as contained, or to 'manage their impression' in the presence of others; therefore, the level of disclosure, and the content of disclosure, within therapy requires careful thought (Harvey 2007, 2011). Young people who have received therapy need to leave the therapy room without showing visible vulnerability for their own safety. Equally, however, too little disclosure might hinder the outcome of the therapy. The question of whether or not it is safe to disclose and begin to process psychological difficulties with a practitioner psychologist needs to be carefully considered by the young person and the psychologist.

In secure settings we also need to consider: How supportive are staff on the wing or ward? How do staff use their authority? It could be argued that if the relationships between staff and young people are positive then this might create a more supportive milieu within the therapy room that would enable disclosure. However, in a harsh, control-oriented, unpredictable environment, such a context could impact upon therapy adversely. For instance, prison life might resonate with a negative and abusive internal working model of relationships. The prison can enact the role of the abusive parent, by being controlling, strict, restrictive and responsible, demanding and inhibiting. Due consideration needs to be given to these dynamics and the reciprocal roles that might be enacted.

The relationships between peers might also be important. It has been recognised that there is a culture of 'not grassing' on other peers, and this could prevent an individual from talking about concerns they may relate to bullying or the supply of drugs on the unit, for example (Ireland 2002; Crewe 2009). Moreover, peers might tell each other not to trust the team, and this could impact on the client's willingness to disclose. Furthermore, among the group self-disclosure might be perceived as a sign of weakness, and such a cultural belief could be significant when providing therapy in a prison or hospital. Young people communicate with one another and do not exist in a vacuum.

As well as the young person's own relationships, the relationships between the staff as a team could also have an important influence on client disclosure more generally. It is important to think about the culture of staff (Crawley and Crawley 2008). If there is a blame culture based on fear among staff, it could serve as a barrier to disclosing. If staff are practising in a manner that is defensive of their own profession, position or 'status', rather than working in a defensible manner with the client, then patients might become reluctant to engage at a therapeutic level and reveal their personal concerns.

Beyond these immediate relationships, we must also include wider systemic issues that impact upon practice in both secure and community settings. Over the years, risk assessments of future violence have become dominant within forensic practice (see Logan and Johnstone 2013; Chapter 5, this volume). The risk-led practice agenda may impact upon the process of disclosure. In contexts where risk to others is a central concern in respect of a particular individual, the client's disclosure has ramifications for decisions that affect his liberty. For example, if a client discloses sexual thoughts, then he could have his leave from a secure hospital into the community cancelled, he could endure increased monitoring, and thus he might come to feel that his autonomy has been reduced. Therefore, in addition to the very real intra-psychic influences on disclosure, such as shame or embarrassment, the individual has to make a pragmatic judgement about sharing information that may have profound, long-term material influence over their life and liberty. Whilst practitioner psychologists and other forensic practitioners with a duty of care to the public have a pressing reason to understand risk, we can understand why clients might have a pressing wish to hide their risk and 'protect' themselves, as they might see it. Indeed, clients might be thinking: 'what's at stake here if I talk? What's at stake if I don't?'

The importance of taking a relational–contextual approach

Having explored this conceptualisation of disclosure, we will now consider some clinical benefits of taking a contextual–relational approach to disclosure in our work with young people in forensic settings. Why is it important to take a relational–contextual approach to understanding disclosure? There might be a range of contextual factors at play, as we have outlined, but why do practitioner psychologists, and other professionals, need to attend to these? It is vitally important that practitioner psychologists are not facilitating trauma re-enactment.

Firstly, we would argue that, by acknowledging disclosure as a relational process and taking into account context, forensic practitioners can better understand disclosure as an important event in its own right. The process can then be better understood and managed, rather than being overshadowed by the content of the information. By placing an emphasis on disclosure as an important process itself, we can acknowledge to the young person, and to the team we are working with, that the young person has disclosed information against the odds. It is a milestone when the client has related to another and has placed some trust in them. Moreover, what is significant is that when disclosures are made within a therapeutic relationship in the general community the client might directly calculate the benefit of doing so in the context of the relationship 'at hand'. However, in a forensic context, patients or prisoners in this complex system make this assessment about relationships 'not at hand'. Information may be passed through different professionals and agencies beyond the therapist, and yet the young person has still disclosed.

Secondly, by thinking about context, we can think about the extent to which the young person felt *compelled* to disclose within the context of a power-laden environment, or whether it was because of the development of the therapeutic relationship. This needs careful thought and ensures that we, as therapists, hold in mind the power imbalance that exists. This is a general consideration with all aspects of providing therapy in prisons. It is ethically important.

Thirdly, taking a contextual approach might help us understand why some young people might disclose information that is not genuine. Of course, there may be individual reasons for this, but we should also consider the function of non-genuine disclosure within a contextual framework. What is the person attempting to achieve within a secure setting in particular? For example, a young person might think that if he tells you something it is a marker of progress and thus may begin to engage in an 'imaginary' way. This kind of participation in order to satisfy the demands of the system has been described by the criminologist Pat Carlen as 'imaginary penalty', where clients, and staff, may be going 'through the motions' of engagement in order to satisfy objectives without substance (Carlen 2008). Or the young person might decide to engage in non-genuine disclosure to get their needs met or to avoid receiving a sanction.

Fourthly, many of the young people in forensic services have been required to disclose so many times that, in the process, they might construct a narrative which is useful for professionals, or that professionals have constructed for them, but which no longer therefore feels like it is authentically their own. From a young age, they might have been assessed by various professionals from Child and Adolescent Mental Health Services (CAMHS), youth offending team (YOT) practitioners and social workers. The client has been in a system where the events and experiences that they disclose already 'belong' to the 'other', and perhaps have lost their personal relevance to the client. This might be one factor to consider when thinking about why some young people might be emotionally detached from what they are disclosing, or about the manner in which they are disclosing.

Fifthly, by acknowledging that disclosure might be difficult in forensic contexts, we can also ask young people about the likelihood that they would feel able to disclose if they *were* to have concerns. For example, in assessing the risk of self-harm we might ask if they would disclose thoughts of self-harm should they have these thoughts. Some young people might say that they would not and professionals would not find out if they had suicidal thoughts. This is important information for the practitioner to know in order to think about risk management and how to help the client develop trust. Having a conversation about *potential* disclosures can enable the young person and the practitioner psychologist to think together about what would help the young person feel safer. They can have a conversation *about* a conversation, and ask questions such as: 'What would make telling someone easier?' It is important that practitioners can appreciate *why* a person is not disclosing and then begin to engage the young person in a conversation about the event of disclosing or not. Explicitly recognising *barriers* to disclosure with young people, and appreciating the young person's dilemma, in whether to disclose or not, may be the start of some useful work. For example, this conversation might include understanding their experience of disclosing to other professionals in the past and what helped facilitate or inhibit this.

Sixthly, by placing disclosure in context, we can understand better the reasons for what we call 'non-compliance' and a 'lack of engagement'. By paying attention to attachment, coupled with an understanding of the forensic environment, forensic practitioners can establish the potential reasons why a person might not engage or self-disclose. That then provides a more nuanced appreciation of the young person's position, rather than seeing them as 'difficult' or 'deliberately obstructive'. Such an understanding is important, especially in relation to risk assessments, because it will enable practitioners to develop a better understanding of the conditions in which disclosure is more difficult for young people and conditions where it might be easier.

Seventh, a reluctance to disclose, or to engage at all, may also serve as an 'act of rebellion', as Goffman (1963) calls it, but that rebellion might be a 'normal' response to attempts to encroach on a client's individuality. It may be an attempt to represent their humanness. It could be argued that 'non-disclosure' or 'self-concealment' is an attempt to protect the self from being violated. Once information has been shared with a member of the team, these so-called 'facts' are then available to staff at any time of day. This construction of information comes, in part, from the client's disclosure, and also from their non-disclosures, because the lack of disclosure may be recorded too. However, non-disclosure can ultimately heighten a client's level of risk and prevent them from progressing through the system through being seen as 'non-compliant'.

Finally, if we take a relational and contextual approach towards disclosure, and place thinking about disclosure at the centre of our practice, we might think more about how to respond to disclosure when it occurs. By exploring context, we can see that a young person's sense of self can be fragile, given their previous life experiences and destabilising environment. Therefore, *how* this disclosure is handled is important. For example, when a young person who has been convicted of a sexual offence against a peer of his age discloses that he has sexual feelings towards a peer on the ward, we need to ensure that the fact he has disclosed this is recognised as significant and positive in itself, whilst also being clear about information sharing with the multidisciplinary team (MDT).

The response requires careful thought so as not to shut down any subsequent disclosures. Of course, the information needs to be shared and appropriate action taken, but given that the *event* of disclosure is significant in itself, it is important that thought is given to how information is then subsequently shared to others in the team or other agencies.

Summary

In summary, in this chapter we have argued for the contextual positioning of self-disclosure when working with young people in forensic practice. At this stage, these ideas are exploratory and we think it would be important for research to develop a greater understanding of the *experience* of self-disclosure by forensic clients. How do young people in a medium secure unit, for example, experience telling professionals personal information that they have kept secret for several years? How do they find that professionals respond to their disclosures, both in the here and now of the therapy, and in the period after disclosure? Given that some young people might feel compelled to disclose, whereas they might not have chosen to do so otherwise, do the potential benefits of disclosure for their well-being diminish or are they sustained? In other words, does the perceived openness or compulsion to disclosure mediate the relationship between disclosing and the outcome of disclosing? We would suggest that it is healthiest for people to come to experience disclosure on their own terms, without feeling pressurised, but this would require testing.

Disclosure is a complex arena and requires careful thought at the individual professional level, MDT level and institutional level. Self-disclosure requires attention as a process, in order to improve our practice when working with clients with complex histories held in complex systems.

References

Adshead, G. (2004) 'Three Degrees of Security: Attachment and Forensic Institutions', in G. Adshead and F. Pfäfflin (eds.), *A Matter of Security: The Application of Attachment Theory to Forensic Psychiatry and Psychotherapy*. London: Jessica Kingsley Publishers, 147–166.

Besharat, M.A. (2007) 'Measure of patient's response style to therapist and therapy: The development of the patient response style scale (PRSS)', *Acta Medica Iranica*, 45(5): 415–423.

Carlen, P. (ed.) (2008) *Imaginary Penalties*. Cullompton: Willan Publishing.

Crawley, E. and Crawley, P. (2008) 'Understanding Prison Officers: Culture, Cohesion and Conflict', in J. Bennett, B. Bowling, and A. Wahidin (eds.), *Understanding Prison Staff*. Cullompton: Willan Publishing, 134–152.

Crewe, B. (2009) *The Prisoner Society: Power, Adaptation and Social Life in an English Prison*. Oxford: Oxford University Press.

Granhag, P.A., Andersson, L.O., Strömwal, L.A., and Hartwig, M. (2004) 'Imprisoned knowledge: Criminals' beliefs about deception', *Legal and Criminological Psychology*, 9: 103–119.

Faller, K.C., Birdsall, W.C., Henry, J., Vandervort, F., and Silverschanz, P. (2001) 'What makes sex offenders confess? An exploratory study', *Journal of Child Sexual Abuse*, 10(4): 31–49.

Farber, B.A., Berano, K.C., and Capobianco, J.A. (2004) 'Clients' perceptions of the process and consequences of self-disclosure in psychotherapy', *Journal of Counseling Psychology*, 51(3): 340–346.

Ferguson, K., Ireland, C.A., and Ireland, J.L. (2013) 'Developing a self-report measure to assess disclosure strategies in adult male prisoners and its association with personality', *Journal of Forensic Practice*, 15(2): 97–108.

Forrest, G.G. (2010) *Self-Disclosure in Psychotherapy and Recovery*. Plymouth: Jason Aronson Inc. Publishers.

Frost, A., Daniels, K., and Hudson, S.M. (2006) 'Disclosure strategies among sex offenders: A model for understanding the engagement process in groupwork', *Journal of Sexual Aggression*, 12(3): 227–244.

Goffman, E. (1963) *Asylums: Essays on the Social Situation of Mental Patients and Other Inmates*. London: Penguin Press.

Gudjonsson, G.H. (2006) 'Sex offenders and confessions: How to overcome their resistance during questioning', *Journal of Clinical Forensic Medicine*, 13: 203–207.

Harrington, D. and Bailey, S. (2005) *Mental Health Needs and Effectiveness of Provision for Young Offenders in Custody and in the Community*. London: Youth Justice Board.

Harvey, J. (2007) *Young Men in Prison: Surviving and Adapting to Life Inside*. Cullompton: Willan Publishing.

Harvey, J. (2011) 'Young prisoners and their mental health: Reflections on providing therapy, Special Issue: Young Prisoners', *Prison Service Journal*, 197: 26–31.

Harvey, J. and Smedley K. (2010) 'Introduction', in J. Harvey and K. Smedley (eds.), *Psychological Therapy in Prisons and Other Secure Settings*. Abingdon: Willan Publishing, 1–25.

HMCIP (2007) *The Mental Health of Prisoners: A Thematic Review of the Care and Support of Prisoners with Mental Health Needs*. London: HM Inspectorate of Prisons.

Ireland, J. (2002) *Bullying among Prisoners: Evidence, Research and Intervention Strategies*. Hove: Bruner-Routledge.

Jourard, S.M. (1971) *Self-Disclosure: An Experimental Analysis of the Transparent Self*. New York: Wiley.

Kahn, J.H., Vogel, D.L., Schneider, W.J., Barr, L.K., and Herrell, K. (2008) 'The emotional content of client disclosures and session impact: An analogue study', *Psychotherapy Theory, Research, Practice, Training*, 45(4): 539–545.

Kroll, L., Rothwell, J., Bradley, D., Shah, P., Bailey, S., and Harrington, R.C. (2002) 'Mental health needs of boys in secure care for serious or persistent offending: A prospective longitudinal study', *Lancet*, 359: 1975–1979.

Lader, D., Singleton, N., and Meltzer, H. (2000) *Psychiatric Morbidity among Young Offenders in England and Wales*. London: Office of National Statistics.

Liebling, A. (2004) *Prisons and their Moral Performance: A Study of Values, Quality and Prison Life*. Oxford: Oxford University Press.

Logan, C. and Johnstone, L. (eds.) (2013) *Managing Clinical Risk: A Guide to Effective Practice*. London: Routledge.

Yalom, I.D. (1970) *The Theory and Practice of Group Psychotherapy*. New York: Basic Books.

15
Developing Safe and Strong Foundations: The DART Framework

Andrew Rogers and Miranda Budd

Introduction

This chapter aims to provide an overview of an emerging therapeutic approach for working with adolescents in secure settings who present with high vulnerability and high-risk behaviour towards both themselves and/or others. The approach has evolved over the past ten years through clinical experience and clinical practice within a variety of secure settings in the UK. The overarching framework is defined as the developmentally informed attachment, risk and trauma (DART) approach. The DART approach is unique because it brings together an understanding of complex presentations, and makes real and pragmatic links between theory and practice, pitching the interventions in a developmentally congruent way, while maintaining an awareness of the importance of understanding and managing risk. Rather than more traditional approaches in secure settings for young people, which are often drawn from adult practice that may have a particular focus on offending behaviour and risk, this approach understands high-risk behaviours as being driven by adaptive attachment strategies. The framework proposes that these are strategies that need to be understood within the broader developmental context, traumatic experience, and emotional and mental well-being of the young person and their system.

The DART approach is underpinned by an attachment and trauma 'meta-framework'. In addition to an evolutionary and developmental underpinning, the framework draws from the theoretical basis of attachment theory (e.g. Bowlby 1988), the Dynamic Maturational Model of Attachment (Crittenden 2005), trauma (e.g. Briere and Scott 2006), developmental trauma (Van der Kolk 2005), neuroscience (e.g. Perry 2008), mentalisation (Allen and Fonagy 2006) and trauma systems theory (e.g. Saxe, Ellis and Kaplow 2007), along with a multi-systemic formulation-driven approach to understanding and managing risk.

Current treatment models for young offenders

Currently, there are a limited number of treatment models for young offenders specifically within residential or secure settings. Much of the available research centres on the application of cognitive behavioural theory (CBT). Although there is not a plethora of information available, most studies in this domain either target recidivism and antisocial behaviour, or mental health problems (see Lipsey, Wilson and Cothern 2000 for a review). Koehler and colleagues (2013) completed a meta-analytic review to examine the effectiveness of young offender rehabilitation programmes in Europe. It was found that there were relatively sound effects for CBT, structured therapeutic communities and multimodal systems-oriented programmes, whereas pure punishment, deterrence and supervision-based interventions revealed either negligible or slightly negative outcomes. Redondo and colleagues (1999) completed a meta-analysis examining the effectiveness of different treatment techniques on criminal behaviour in young and adult offenders, and also found that behavioural and CBT techniques were most beneficial in reducing recidivism. Similarly, in 2005, Landenberger and Lipsey conducted a meta-analysis of 58 experimental and quasi-experimental studies of the effects of CBT on the recidivism of young and adult offenders, which confirmed prior positive findings. Koehler and colleagues' (2013) meta-analytic review also showed that the Risk-Need-Responsivity Model (RNR) is supported by robust empirical research (e.g. Andrews et al. 1990; Andrews, Bonta and Wormith 2006; Hanson et al. 2009; Andrews and Bonta 2010). According to RNR, treatment should correspond to the offenders' risk of reoffending, address their dynamic risk factors, and match their learning styles and capabilities.

There is also a growing evidence base for multi-systemic therapy (MST) for young offenders (e.g. Henggeler, Pickrel and Brondino 1999). MST is an empirically derived approach for the community-based treatment of young offenders. It is considered systemic, as it places emphasis on working with the youth's family, friends and school. More recently, Butler and colleagues (2011) assigned 108 families to either MST or 'treatment as usual' (TAU) delivered by youth offending teams (YOTs). The study found that although young people receiving both MST and YOT interventions showed improvement in terms of reduced offending, the MST model of service delivery significantly reduced the likelihood of non-violent offending during an 18-month follow-up period.

There are also more specific models of treatment for particular presentations. For example, the Good Lives Model – Comprehensive (GLM-C; Ward and Gannon 2006). The GLM-C is based on two types of theoretical resources: the original Good Lives Model of offender rehabilitation (GLM-O; Ward and Stewart 2003) and the integrated theory of sexual offending (ITSO; Ward and Beech 2005). GLM-C is multi-systemic, developmental and concerned with risk management. Understanding and formulating what need the sexually inappropriate behaviour is meeting is central to this approach.

Treatment models for working with challenging young people in residential settings

In recent years there has been a growth in methods to understand and work with young people who have experienced chaotic backgrounds and present with complex difficulties. There has been much work conducted in this area with children in the 'looked after' system (see Chapters 1 and 3, this volume, for further details on the looked after child (LAC) system). This includes work by Dan Hughes (2004), which, rather than focus on one-to-one therapy, places the relationship between the young person and their 'caregiver' at the centre of the intervention and as a primary facilitator of change. Hughes' work, drawing heavily on attachment theory, incorporates the use of 'playfulness, acceptance, curiosity and empathy' (PACE) in promoting the development of healthy attachments and relationships. Hughes (2004) emphasises the importance of actively facilitating the experience of safety that is necessary for a child to engage and explore unresolved difficult experiences. Co-regulation of affect and the co-construction of meaning are central to the treatment processes, just as they are central features in attachment security. Adopting a stance of acceptance and curiosity, empathy and/or playfulness, all the while committed to remaining emotionally engaged and available to the child, is a key aspect of the intervention.

In the UK, drawing on Hughes' work, Kim Golding (2006, 2007, 2012) has challenged traditional individual therapy interventions in isolation, and pioneered approaches to supporting foster carers to enhance caregiver sensitivity and provide 'therapeutic parenting' as the primary intervention for young people in the looked after system.

In the USA, Kinniburgh and colleagues (2005) have described a way of working with complex young people from an Attachment, Self-Regulation and Competency (ARC) framework. The ARC model attempts to provide a component-based framework for intervention. The goal of ARC is to address vulnerabilities created by exposure to overwhelming life circumstances that interfere with healthy development. It is grounded in theory about the effects of attachment disruption, trauma, and the impact on self-regulation and developmental competencies. This model emphasises the importance of understanding and intervening with the child as they are embedded within the system around them, with a philosophy that systemic change leads to effective and sustained outcomes.

Trauma systems therapy (Saxe, Ellis and Kaplow 2007) also places emphasis on the system around the young person. It is designed to address both a child's trauma-related symptoms and the perpetuating factors in the social environment. Trauma systems therapy is designed to build the capacity of others in the young person's environment to help the individual control his or her emotional and behavioural responses. It is now well recognised that post-traumatic stress disorder (PTSD) symptoms are highly reactive to ongoing stresses and threats within the social environment (e.g. Duncan et al. 2002; Saxe, Ellis and Kaplow 2007). Unfortunately, clinic-room-based interventions can be far removed from the social–environmental factors that drive young people's traumatic stress symptoms, and have been found to be less efficacious (Dulcan 2000). The notion of 'redefining therapy' with less emphasis on direct interventions with the individual and more aimed at the emotional and relational environment of the individual and their 'system' is highlighted by Rogers, McMahon and Law (2011). The other key theme highlighted by such treatment models and ideas, appears to be that the interventions are framed within the developmental context of the young person, irrespective of their chronological age.

A key feature of the DART approach, which draws on the emerging literature about early brain development, is that children and young people are not, and should not, be treated as 'mini-adults'. Young people are still in a period of enhanced dynamic development well into their twenties and their behaviour needs to be understood within this context. The following theoretical approaches to understanding behaviour are used to shape the DART framework.

Theoretical models informing DART

Attachment and trauma theory

Attachment theory underpins the DART framework. Attachment theory was first proposed by John Bowlby (1969/1982, 1973, 1980, 1988) and expanded with the work of Mary Ainsworth (Ainsworth et al. 1978) and Mary Main (Main and Solomon 1986). It is a theory of child development. It focuses on how children develop within relationships, and the impact that this has for later social and emotional development.

Disruption to the early attachment process through parental inconsistency, neglect and abuse has a direct impact on the development of a child's brain, attachment style and emotional regulation systems (e.g. Schore 2001). When children grow up in a neglectful, inconsistent or abusive environment, they will develop alternative attachment strategies that maximise their chances of receiving care from their caregiver or, in the most extreme cases, maximise their chances of survival. The developing brain wires itself, in an adaptive way, to manage these experiences. Individuals who have had a less than ideal early experience of care, including a lack of exposure to the process of co-regulation by a caregiver, are less likely to have developed the structures and connections in the brain which keep the thinking brain regulating the emotional brain in the face of danger or trauma (Schore 2001).

Mary Ainsworth expanded the concepts of attachment theory (Bretherton 1992) when she identified three attachment styles that a child may have with their primary caregiver. These are secure, insecure-avoidant and insecure-ambivalent. Secure attachments develop when children experience sensitive, consistent and responsive care. The child uses the parent as a secure base from which to explore and develop. A secure attachment will have a positive impact upon the child's development, increase resiliency and the likelihood of a psychologically healthy internal working model that enables the child to believe they are loveable, effective in relationships, and that others are caring, available and protective. In adolescence, securely attached individuals will be young people who are confident in their developing independence and relationships with peers and family members.

Insecure-ambivalent patterns of attachment may develop from inconsistent and insensitive patterns of parenting. The parent may find it difficult to attune to the child and therefore be unpredictable in their responses. The child may therefore become preoccupied with their caregivers' availability, as they are uncertain about its consistency. Children may be unable to effectively use their parent as a secure base from which to explore, and instead maximise their attachment-seeking behaviour to ensure that they do receive care from an inconsistent parent. These children may be resistant to being soothed, display a highly distressed response to relatively minor events and show dependency. Their internal working model will reflect this: beliefs about self are uncertain in terms of their worth to others, and beliefs about others are unreliable and untrustworthy. An individual with an insecure-ambivalent attachment pattern may develop enmeshed and entangled relationships with others, and display coercive behaviour, alternating between aggressive and helpless behaviour. As adolescents, there may be an increase in risky behaviour in order to maintain attention and care from others.

An avoidant-attachment pattern of relating to others suggests that the child's experience was of parents who were rejecting, consistently unavailable, intrusive and possibly hostile. In order to adapt to such a care environment and maintain proximity with their caregiver, the child learns to minimise their attachment behaviour. Therefore, they inhibit emotional expression, become undemanding, withdrawn and self-sufficient. Ainsworth's procedure, known as the 'strange situation', demonstrated clearly how an avoidant-attachment style can be observed through the separation and reunion behaviour between child and primary caregiver (Ainsworth et al. 1978). Children with an insecure-avoidant pattern of interaction consistently showed little or no distress on departure, little or no visible response to return and treated a stranger similarly to the caregiver. The internal working model is that of seeing the self as unlovable, of little worth, and the model of others as not available or intrusive and consistently unresponsive. Additionally, they may predict that others will be rejecting and hostile.

Further research by Mary Main and colleagues then identified a fourth attachment pattern, which they called disorganised/disoriented attachment (Main and Solomon 1986). If parents display insensitive, frightening or frightened behaviour, a disorganised attachment pattern of interaction will be evident. The child will seek protection and comfort, but the source of this comfort is the same person who is frightening, so the child will experience confusion. The child's behaviour will therefore be disorganised, as they are unable to organise their behaviour at times of stress in order to receive emotional support and safety.

In clinical practice, working with adolescents who display high-risk behaviour, it seems that young people do not necessarily present with a distinct and dominant attachment style at all times. They may, however, activate their different attachment strategies depending on the people they are relating to at that time. For example, a male young offender may display avoidant-attachment strategies with a powerful and relatively 'avoidant' or rejecting adult caregiver, but may display much more ambivalent strategies with a very empathic caregiver. At times, this can seem 'disorganised', but when taking into account the relational system the young person is in, it can be understood as activating multiple strategies at different times and with different caregivers.

Research on attachment styles in young offenders is extremely limited. There is slightly more information available relating to sex offenders; however, this is an area that needs further attention. Muris and colleagues (2004) explored the relationships between self-reported attachment style, parental rearing behaviours, and anger and hostility in adolescents. Results found that those who defined themselves as avoidant or ambivalently attached displayed higher levels of anger and hostility than adolescents who classified themselves as securely attached. Parental rearing practices that displayed low levels of emotions and warmth and high levels of rejection, control and inconsistency, were accompanied by high levels of anger and hostility. The study concludes that attachment style and parental rearing are involved in the development of anger and hostility in youths. Other studies have had similar findings. For instance, Kolvin and colleagues (1988) found that poor-quality 'mothering' was related to the number of convictions during adolescence and adulthood. In a series of meta-analyses of a large number of concurrent and longitudinal studies, Loeber and Stouthamer-Loeber (1986) found the best predictors of juvenile antisocial behaviour were parental child-rearing practices. Timmerman and Emmelkamp (2006) explored the relationships between attachment styles and diagnoses of Cluster B personality disorders in adult prisoners and forensic inpatients. The results showed that a criminal status, as well as forensic inpatient identity, were negatively associated with a secure attachment style, meaning that prisoners and forensic service users show more insecure attachment styles than controls from the general population. These findings are consistent with van Ijzendoorn and colleagues (1997) who also reported that the adult offender population generally has disproportionately more insecure attachment styles.

Ireland and Power (2004) explored whether offenders who bully others and/or are victimised themselves can be distinguished by their attachment styles and the level of emotional loneliness that they report. It was found that young offenders were more likely than adult offenders to report behaviours indicative of 'bullying others' and of 'being bullied'. Significant differences were restricted to avoidant attachment; 'bully/victim' reported higher avoidant scores than the other bully categories, with 'pure bullied' and those not involved reporting lower avoidant scores.

More work in this area has been undertaken with adults who commit sexual offences. Marshall (1989) developed an etiological model stressing the importance of insecure attachment and intimacy deficits in both the onset and maintenance of sex offending. Ward and colleagues (1996) examined attachment styles of sex offenders, and the results indicated that the majority of sex offenders were insecurely attached. However, the study found this attachment style to also be present in other groups of offenders, so hypothesised that it may be a general vulnerability factor, rather than specific to sex offences. Ward also suggested that the study provided evidence that child molesters were more likely to have a preoccupied or fearful attachment style than were rapists, and be less dismissive. Rapists were indiscriminable in some respects from violent non-sex offenders (i.e. both tended to be dismissive (avoidant)) and non-violent non-sex offenders were comparatively the most securely attached. Smallbone and Dadds (1998) had similar results. They found adult sex offenders to report significantly less secure maternal, paternal and adult attachment in comparison to individuals charged with property theft. They also postulated that certain combinations of childhood attachment experiences may relate more specifically to different kinds of sexual offending. Marsa and colleagues (2004) compared 29 child sex offenders, 30 violent offenders, 30 non-violent offenders and 30 community controls. A secure adult attachment style was four times less common in the child sex offender group than in any of the other three groups. Ninety-three per cent of sex offenders had an insecure adult attachment style.

As attachment processes are thought to be the foundation for emotional regulation, patterns of care seeking and relationships, and recognising and responding to emotions in ourselves and others, it is argued that they should also be considered as part of the foundation for resilience to traumatic life events. Insecure attachments can be viewed as risk factors that increase the likelihood of psychopathology (Kobak et al. 2006). Young people with disrupted or maladaptive attachment patterns, who then experience trauma, are therefore likely to experience a multitude of difficulties.

It has long been known that fragmented memories of traumatic events seem to dominate the lives of traumatised individuals. These memories may return as physical sensations, flashbacks, nightmares and even behavioural re-enactments. Children are particularly vulnerable to behavioural repetition (Horowitz and Becker 1971) and, as adults, those who have been traumatised are more likely to behave in an antisocial or self-destructive manner (Bloom 1999). A major causal factor for violence is believed to be re-enactment of victimisation (Van der Kolk 1989), although it is very important to acknowledge that not all those who have experienced victimisation will engage in this.

Traumatised children have great difficulty with self-regulatory functions (Cicchetti and Tucker 1994; Van der Kolk and Fisler 1994; Perry et al. 1995; Van der Kolk, Pelcovitz and Roth 1996; Putnam 1997; Perry and Pollard 1998; Schore 2001). Children who experience traumatic stress can have tremendous difficulty in controlling their emotions, behaviour and attention when faced with environmental threats, and in reconstituting themselves to terminate their extreme responses (Charney et al. 1993; Van der Kolk 1994; Perry et al. 1995; Perry and Pollard 1998; De Bellis 2001; Schore 2001). It is suggested, therefore, that those that have early attachment experiences that mean that their ability to regulate emotion and behaviour is already less well developed, may be more vulnerable in terms of finding themselves in situations that could be traumatic (through high-risk behaviour) and less likely to manage the emotional consequences of these.

While in the course of development, most children have the chance to invest their energies in growing various competencies, complexly traumatised children must focus on survival. It is suggested that these children need a flexible model of intervention, embedded in a developmental and social context that can address a continuum of trauma exposures, including ongoing exposure.

Understanding why young people behave in the way they do can reduce feelings of frustration, guilt and blame (Golding 2007), enhance 'carer sensitivity' and ultimately make it more likely that the young person will experience positive relational experiences. This, in turn, helps staff to accept the young person and the difficulties they display, and provides a greater sense of empathy for how hard relationships are for the young person. Thus, feeling understood and experiencing empathy is the starting point from which young people trust and learn new ways of relating to people.

Neurodevelopmental theory

If a child experiences high levels of, and repeated trauma, the brain can become hard-wired to danger, and they are more likely develop extremely sensitive brain systems to recognise and interpret potential threat (Sunderland 2006). In any given situation therefore, not only will the child be more likely to interpret an event or situation as threatening, they are more likely to react in a survival way (fight or flight), and be less able to regulate their behavioural and emotional response to that situation. This places a young person at a disadvantage early on, disrupting the typical developmental pathways and developing a trajectory to managing future threats and challenges in an arguably adaptive, but dysregulated manner. Such young people tend to present with poor emotional regulation skills, 'anger management' difficulties, utilise illicit substances as a method of self-medication, have poor understanding of boundaries, negative or hostile attribution bias, and associate with antisocial peers, who have similar difficulties. This is highly relevant to secure settings, where many people appear to have a history of early attachment disruption, neglect and trauma (Crighton and Towl 2008).

While it may be argued that early adversity is likely to place a young person at increased risk of future difficulties, recent advances in the understanding of brain development and brain 'reorganisation', particularly during key periods, such as infancy and adolescence, and lasting well into our twenties, highlight the real potential for influencing a more adaptive developmental trajectory that can impact at a biological, as well as psychological, level. The importance of adolescence as a critical period in which we can effect change is only strengthened by this. Bowlby himself argued that our attachment patterns are open to change throughout our lives (Bowlby 1988). The DART framework strongly advocates that *every* interaction with a young person, including those with domestic and maintenance staff, management, professionals and caregivers has the opportunity to be therapeutic (effecting change), by promoting positive attachment experiences and developing self-regulation strategies. Similarly, every interaction has the potential to reinforce previous maladaptive strategies, and reinforce a less adaptive developmental trajectory, including mistimed or misplaced individual therapy. Experience has demonstrated that the care systems that young people find themselves in often recreate the chaotic early parenting experiences that they are trying to address. It is suggested that, in this way, developmental trajectories towards diagnoses of personality disorder in adulthood are reinforced by the very systems that are trying to reduce psychopathology and high-risk presentations.

Risk

The concept of care-eliciting behaviour is proposed as an essential part of the phenomenon of attachment. From an attachment perspective, high-risk behaviour almost always generates high levels of emotion in others, which activates their attachment systems and results in care-enhancing or care-reduction behaviours. In this context, high-risk behaviour may therefore be best viewed and understood as adaptive 'attachment behaviour'. Attachment theory (and the concept of evolution) emphasises that a child must adapt to their early care-giving environment in order to maximise their chances of survival. It is therefore perhaps not surprising that children in chaotic, disruptive and neglectful care environments may adopt 'survival' behaviour early in life that may later, in different environments, be considered as challenging, risky or perplexing. For example, a high level of arousal activated through the body's fight or flight response may be adaptive and help a young person maintain their safety in an early care environment where domestic violence occurs. However, this response to stressful situations in the future may not be helpful. Similarly, patterns of initially challenging behaviour in young children, aimed at eliciting care and attention from parents and functionally successful in achieving this aim when younger, may become increasingly challenging, difficult to manage, and viewed as violent and aggressive as that child physically develops.

Lyons-Ruth (1996) reviewed attachment-related studies of early aggression to show that aggressive behaviour towards peers is related to disorganised or controlling patterns of attachment behaviour towards parents. The study also reports that disorganised attachment behaviours, in turn, predict aggression in school-age children, even when other family factors are controlled for. Another study (Cooper, Shaver and Collins 1998) explored the relationship between attachment styles, emotional regulation and adjustment in adolescence, and found that adolescents with anxious-ambivalent attachment styles had the highest levels of problematic and risky behaviours. An insecure attachment pattern has also been cited as a significant predictive risk factor for deliberate self-harm (Gratz, Conrad and Roemer 2010). There is already considerable evidence that adolescents who report weak attachment to their parents are more likely to be involved in early sexual activity, and to have large numbers of sexual partners (e.g. Smith 1997). These findings support the broader preposition that inadequate (but adaptive for the context) parent–child attachment is a risk factor for adjustment problems in adolescence, including high risk behaviour, such as substance abuse (Rice 1990).

Seeking to understand high-risk behaviour within an attachment framework means working towards identifying the need behind the behaviour. Both in forensic settings, where the system may be set up to be risk adverse, and care settings, where 'over-caring' may be present, such responses may actually serve to maintain the risk that both facilities are aiming to reduce. For example, placing individuals with insecure attachment patterns on one-to-one or intensive observations after deliberate acts of self-harm, while managing risk in the short term, may have the longer-term effect of maintaining the self-harm if the need is to elicit care and time from others. Alternatively, reducing the interaction with young people who are violent and rejecting of support (by ignoring them or isolating them in segregation or seclusion), may reinforce their model that others are hostile and rejecting and that they have to cope independently.

The DART framework proposes that risk behaviours be initially viewed and understood as adaptive attachment strategies, primarily aimed at survival, either through keeping people at a distance or by being care eliciting. These strategies have been developed early and, while appearing to be 'high risk', have (if you are working with the young person) to date achieved their aim (of survival). The authors hypothesise that the vast majority of high-risk (attachment) behaviours displayed by young people within the secure estate (but arguably anywhere) fall into eight broad categories (Table 15.1).

Clearly, many of these behaviours also indicate increased risk of vulnerability, including vulnerability from the negative and abusive actions of others. As such, those young people who display high-risk behaviours are almost universally vulnerable at the same time (although, particularly in the context of risk to others, this is often underacknowledged).

It is likely that the different risk behaviours will be displayed within different attachment patterns and styles, and rarely will a clinician observe all of the above behaviours being displayed by one young person at any one time. It is also likely that trauma will impact upon each young person in a different manner, as each individual varies in their experience of being parented, their attachment style, attachment behaviours, resiliency and effective coping strategies. However, there are key similarities, and the key feature of all of these behaviours is that they generate very high anxiety in the 'parent' or 'parenting system', leading to the activation of attachment patterns in the caregiving system and, all too often, a response driven primarily by this

Table 15.1 High-risk attachment behaviours

Risk to self	Risk to others
1. Self-harm (inc. alcohol/substance misuse)	4. Violence
2. Food-based difficulties (inc. restricting food/overeating)	5. 'Disgust' behaviours (inc. spitting, smearing, urinating, poor self-care)
3. Absconding (increasing vulnerability and increased risk from others)	6. Fire-setting
	7. Sexually harmful behaviour
	8. Frequent and unsubstantiated complaints

anxiety. As levels of anxiety climb, our ability to regulate our own emotions and our capacity to mentalise – providing attuned, co-regulated and objective responses – is reduced. As is our ability to make informed risk decisions. Put simply, the more anxious we get, the more stupid we get! As a result, our interactions with those young people displaying high-risk behaviour are often driven by emotion, rather than by objective and regulated appraisal of emotion and thought, and result in mirroring patterns of interaction that have their basis in the historical experiences of the young person. In effect, in our experience, the systems around the young people often come to reflect their early experiences of parenting, either ambivalent, avoidant and rejecting or chaotic and disorganised.

An attachment-informed framework

The DART framework has evolved through years of clinical practice within a variety of secure and residential settings. It is the combination of developmental, attachment and trauma theory applied to real-life settings where young people display and engage in high-risk behaviour. The DART approach provides a framework for those involved in the direct care of the young person to form a pragmatic, developmentally and contextually appropriate understanding of a complex presentation. This understanding, supported by psychologically informed formulation, then helps to inform and prioritise the most appropriate interventions. Although young people in secure settings are developmentally 'adolescent' in terms of their chronological age, it is posed that they may well have missed, or not yet completed, numerous pivotal tasks relating to their cognitive, emotional, moral and social development. It is also likely that the young person has had a disrupted (but adaptive at the time) attachment experience. All of which can mean the individual is vulnerable in traumatic and difficult situations and unable to cope with these well.

Within the context of such approaches, the DART framework does not necessarily propose anything particularly radical, certainly in terms of underlying theory. However, from clinical experience within various community and secure settings with youth who display high-risk behaviour, it is the operationalising of these theoretical underpinnings into practice that can be problematic, particularly in the face of sometimes extreme emotional and physical risks to self and others. The DART approach therefore proposes a framework that may help to bridge those theory-to-practice links, whilst paying considered attention to the risk the young person may pose. Understanding this risk, within an attachment and trauma framework, is suggested as essential to addressing the underlying need that drives the risk behaviour and thus reducing risk in the longer term.

Aims and principles of the DART framework

The DART model is underpinned by ten principles and has eight main aims. These principles and aims will guide the delivery of the model within any setting that it is applied. These are listed as follows:

Principles

Children are born dysregulated and learn adaptive strategies to manage both their emotions and behaviour through experience

This principle is shaped by attachment theory and suggests that children respond to their early care environment and adapt with attachment-seeking behaviours, in order to receive the care they require whilst growing and developing (Bowlby 1969/1982, 1973, 1980, 1988; Ainsworth et al. 1978; Main and Solomon 1986; Crittenden 2005). This principle is used to guide understanding and the formulation of the young person.

Attachment experience and trauma can impact upon brain development

The links between neurodevelopment, attachment and trauma were explored in the introduction to this chapter. There is growing evidence to suggest that early maltreatment affects brain development (e.g. Glaser 2000; De Bellis 2001; De Bellis et al. 2002; De Bellis et al. 2010). Studies comparing these children with those with no evidence of having been exposed to similar maltreatment demonstrate compelling differences in neuroanatomy and cognitive function, which suggest that the impact of maltreatment has the potential to cause significant impairment of brain structure and function (De Bellis et al. 1999). This knowledge will support an understanding of the young person, increase empathy and, therefore, the likelihood that those working with the young person will be able to build effective, attuned therapeutic relationships.

All young people should be understood within the context of their developmental experiences, trauma and adaptive strategies

This principle emphasises the importance of understanding the young person within the context of their life experiences. Dan Hughes (2004) highlights the importance of the relationship between the young person and the person or people who are caring for them, with this relationship being central to any intervention. Parenting with 'PACE', adopting a stance of *playfulness, acceptance, curiosity* and *empathy*, is a key aspect of the intervention.

Staff working directly with these young people are the primary facilitators of change and, as such, act as 'therapeutic parents'

Dan Hughes (2004) places much emphasis upon the relationship between young person and carer(s), as do many other clinicians and researchers.

Golding (2006, 2007, 2012), Kinniburgh and colleagues (2005) and Rogers and colleagues (2011) all challenge the effectiveness of individual therapy interventions in isolation, highlighting the role of the caregiving adults within the young person's system. Saxe, Ellis and Kaplow (2007) developed trauma systems therapy in order to build the capacity of others in the young person's environment to support the child.

The emotional well-being of staff is an essential ingredient to successful outcomes

This principle draws on the notion that the caregiver is better able to co-regulate distress in the young person if the caregiver themselves is regulated and calm. A distressed, highly anxious or highly aroused caregiver is likely to have a reduced capacity to effectively manage and soothe distress in the young person and teach the young person effective coping strategies. Golding (2008) emphasises the importance of the emotional well-being of the therapeutic parent, suggesting the need for rest and relaxation as an essential part of the parenting approach.

Secure settings themselves can sometimes be traumatised systems, and so the DART framework highlights the importance of staff support, through co-working and clinical supervision, to enhance understanding, minimise the risk of vicarious traumatisation and reduce feelings of hopelessness within staff.

Safety is paramount

Safety is central to the effective implementation of the DART approach. It is recognised that high-risk behaviour is likely to occur within secure settings and should not be ignored or downplayed.

Understanding the risk the young person poses to themselves and others is vital, as is involving the young person in their own assessment of risk as much as possible. Maintaining the young person's safety is important for their physical and psychological health and development. Maintaining the safety of those working with the young person is key for staff members' health and that of the young person. High-risk behaviour generates high levels of emotion in others. If staff members do not feel safe, it is likely that they will struggle to regulate their own emotions and then co-regulate the young person. Therefore, it will be difficult to implement the foundations of the DART framework, which is to provide a safe and secure base to enable the young person to feel physically and psychologically safe and then develop in other areas.

This principle is met through the completion of appropriate and robust risk assessment and management plans based on a structured professional judgement (SPJ) approach and underpinned by psychologically informed formulation. Where possible, the young person should be involved in the risk management process. In secure settings, risk management may include the provision of low stimulus and special observation measures.

There are hidden needs behind risk behaviours

Understanding high-risk behaviour and promoting safety means identifying hidden need(s). This knowledge can reduce the likelihood that previous unhelpful patterns of interactions are repeated and strengthened, as the cycle is interrupted and the young person is given the opportunity and supported to learn new ways of responding.

Primary interventions are underpinned by a consistent and attuned therapeutic parenting approach that is developmentally appropriate. Additional interventions should only occur when they are informed by a clear psychological formulation that integrates multiple theoretical perspectives

This principle strengthens the importance of a systemic intervention being the primary intervention, with the 'therapeutic parent' being at the centre. The DART house (see Figure 15.1) emphasises the foundations that need to be in place prior to more focused one-to-one work taking place, such as trauma-focused individual work. The DART house (adapted from Golding 2013), fits with the Pyramid of Need (Golding 2013), which takes into consideration what factors the young person needs, at what time. Should a young person require one-to-one therapy, the intervention should be driven by a comprehensive formulation of need, that draws from the available evidence, but also fits with what the young person needs and what they are able to engage with, rather than (all too often) being driven by the therapist's specific area of interest, therapeutic modality or simply what is available. Therefore, a range of different psychological therapeutic approaches may be required at different times, and it is argued that any assessment of therapeutic need should be overseen by those experienced and trained in a broad range of psychological knowledge and theory (not single models or single therapeutic modalities) and assessed only after balancing the potential risks and benefits of any such intervention. Clearly, this should also take into account the wishes and needs of the young people themselves.

The intervention starts as soon as the young person arrives: Every single interaction has the potential to promote positive and adaptive development

Given the emphasis of effective interventions occurring within the context of relationships, this approach means each interaction can be viewed as an opportunity for change. Each interaction can help a young person to learn a new model of being with others, promote a positive attachment experience and develop self-regulation strategies.

Continuity of care/placement stability is one of the most influential mediators of long-term negative outcomes

Placement moves can reduce the opportunity for a young person to experience a sense of belonging (Golding 2008). Instability reduces the opportunities for

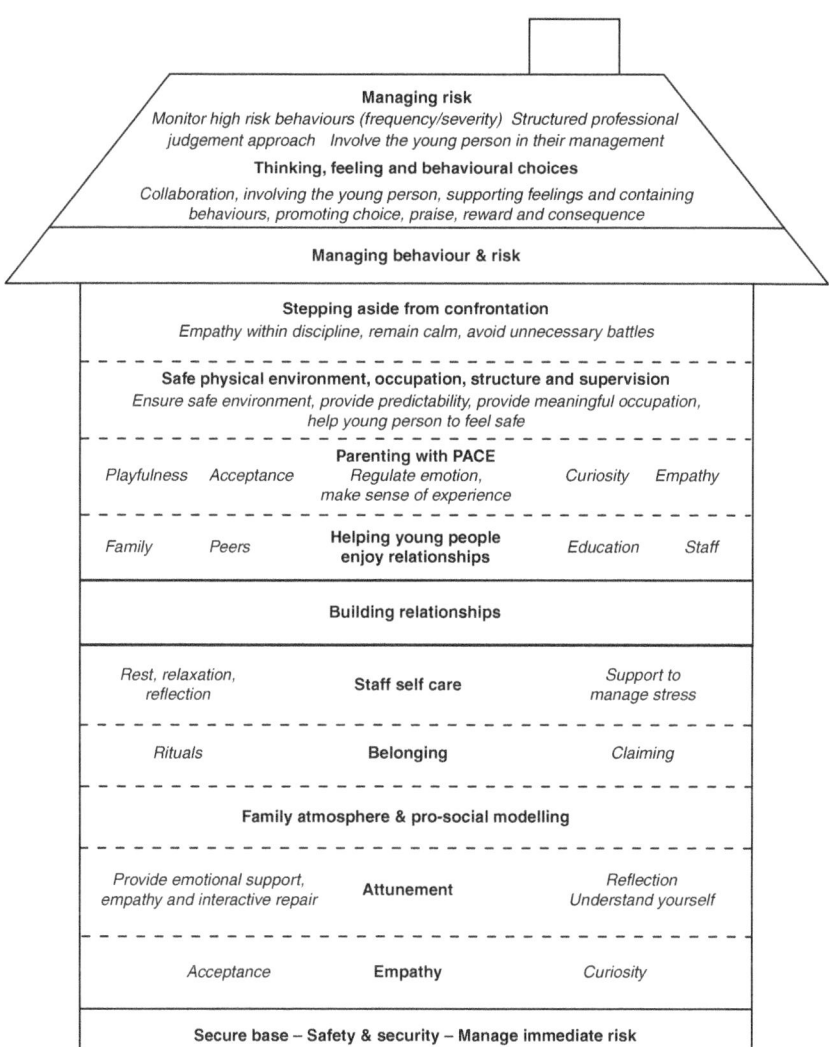

Figure 15.1 The DART house of parenting (adapted from Golding, 2013 – with permission)

the young person to feel settled, experience a reduction in anxiety and develop from a secure base. Opportunities to form meaningful attachments with others are also reduced. Placement moves can reinforce previously developed models and thinking patterns in relation to being 'unlovable' and 'out of control', which, in turn, can negatively affect their behaviour and well-being. Children who experience numerous changes in placements may be at particularly high risk of these deleterious effects (Newton, Litrownik and Landsverk 2000).

Aims

Reduce the severity and frequency of high-risk behaviours and promote safety

Safety is promoted through the implementation of the DART house as an intervention with the system around the young person. The DART framework is a whole systems approach, not an approach that focuses on individual therapy as a primary facilitator of change.

Clear risk assessment using a SPJ approach and robust risk management plans are essential and shared with all involved in supporting the young person. Wherever possible, any risks should be discussed openly with the young person, and the risk assessment and management plan should be developed in conjunction with the young person. The management plans should be underpinned by a psychological formulation, which addresses the hidden need that is being expressed and met through the risk behaviour. Potential high-risk scenarios identified within the risk assessment should be highlighted and safety plans should be developed alongside the young person, to be implemented should the scenarios arise. Risk behaviours should be monitored in terms of at least their frequency and severity, and feedback provided on a regular basis to the wider system. Regular reviews of presenting risk behaviour and clear communication is essential.

To raise caregiver sensitivity through understanding complex presentations

Increasing understanding and sensitivity starts with training for all staff working with the young person in a developmental attachment and trauma approach. Training is then followed with regular psychological consultation, supporting carers and staff to maintain perspective, be 'therapeutic parents' and parent with 'PACE'. Consultation should involve the dynamic development of a shared formulation, to support understanding and raise caregiver empathy and sensitivity.

Facilitate emotional regulation

Staff members have a pivotal role in helping young people regulate their emotions and, in that sense, they co-regulate the emotions young people experience. For example, noticing if the young person is becoming aroused (e.g. anxious or angry) out of context, or at a more exaggerated level than is appropriate for the situation, labelling this with the adolescent, coaching and supporting them to regulate their arousal level, and providing attuned care and concern. This can work best if the young person and staff member have previously developed a 'safety plan' which details triggers, how the young person feels, what this will look like to others and what helps. This safety plan can then be referred to, as the situation has already been discussed and both the young person and staff member will have an idea about how best to respond.

Emotional regulation skills can also be taught 'in vivo' through coaching, modelling, or during therapeutic sessions (that involve the caregivers), where psychoeducation can be provided, and 'safe place' visualisation exercises (Golding 2008) and relaxation techniques can be practised. Such strategies can also be taught within a group setting, such as a relaxation group or mindfulness group. Both interventions aim to develop the young person's emotional coping and increase emotional awareness and emotional regulation skills.

Facilitate self-regulation of behaviour

The implementation of behavioural strategies, such as reward programmes and clear consistent consequences for unacceptable/unsafe behaviour will help a young person to regulate their own behaviour. While working with a young person, allowing a careful balance between responsibility and clear expectations is paramount. Interventions such as these are best delivered within the context of relationships, such as by key workers, but having clear expectations for all staff to follow is key.

Promote prosocial relationships with staff and peers

Staff members will have a pivotal role in prosocial modelling and acceptable ways of dealing with difficult situations. The importance of readdressing and talking about difficult situations that occur (e.g. an argument or unacceptable behaviour) once the 'emotional temperature' has reduced is emphasised. This will allow repair and reattunement once a disruption has occurred, allowing the young person to learn new ways of interacting with others. The aim is to ensure the young person understands that it is the behaviour that is not acceptable, not the young person themselves, and that relationships can repair after conflict.

Reduce placement moves

This is implemented through having a shared understanding of the young person's behaviour and a shared management plan for managing challenging behaviour. It will be important to get 'buy-in' to this early on. Clinical experience suggests that once a difficult situation has arisen, there can frequently be a tendency for different support teams within a system to react differently, often in reactive and unhelpful ways, with little reflection or thinking through.

To address the needs of young people who are 'at risk' of developing more chronic and enduring mental health problems

It may be argued that early attachments are one of the foundations for emotional resilience and well-being. It is within the context of early relationships that young people develop their 'internal working model', so this experience can mean they either develop positive beliefs about themselves and the world around them, or unhelpful ones, which may lead to later problems with self-esteem. As attachment styles are heavily implicated in a young person's ability to regulate their emotions, including distress, and employ healthy coping strategies, it makes sense that an intervention with attachment and trauma theory at the centre will increase resilience in young people.

Pathway approach based on supporting and building adaptive development

Attachment theory states that a child needs a secure base from which to develop. If a child has not consistently experienced a secure base, this can impact upon how much they have then explored their environment and developed in other areas. It is therefore hypothesised that if the foundations of the DART framework are created with the secure setting, the young person will then have the opportunity to continue their development in a more positive trajectory.

Developing the framework in a secure setting

The DART framework has been developed to inform work with young people placed within a secure setting, as all young people in these settings, regardless of their offence history, will have experienced some form of attachment relationships. In the UK, these secure settings include: young offender institutes (YOIs), secure training centres (STCs), secure children's homes (SCHs) and secure hospital settings. The approach is designed for young people up to the age of 21, but arguably such a developmentally informed approach could be relevant well into adulthood. The index offence or arrest history would not include or exclude a young person from the DART approach.

The application of the framework to different forensic settings might vary as a function of the size of the institution. In a smaller secure hospital setting, for example, the DART framework may be helpful when adopted as a therapeutic model to underpin the way the whole unit works. In a larger setting, such as a YOI, whilst it may be helpful to consider it as a model to underpin the way the whole YOI functions, it is likely that the DART framework could be rolled out within a smaller complex needs unit, rather than across the whole YOI.

The challenge, of course, is applying the DART framework in practice within a secure setting. A key emphasis of the approach is to be pragmatic and realistic in meeting the needs of the young people, given the resources available. As such, the DART approach tries to put the theoretical perspectives and underpinning framework into practice within the secure establishment. To date, this has been piloted within the secure estate using small, dedicated units, staffed by prison staff, who are supported in their care delivery by multidisciplinary Forensic Child and Adolescent Mental Health Services (FCAMHS). Rather than an arguably traditional 'in-reach' mental health approach (e.g. in some ways a separate 'expert' team, reaching in), the F-CAMHS team preferred to use the term 'embedded' (e.g. actively involved with the prison staff in modelling and influencing the delivery of care). A whole systems approach is essential in bringing those in the system around the young person to a shared understanding, using the DART framework as a reference point.

The DART approach puts the day-to-day staff (prison officers) at the centre of treatment, recognising that they have a pivotal role in developing the environmental and relational conditions that can promote safety (relational security) and change for the young people. Staff are supported in this through informal and formal psychological consultation, coaching and 'modelling', always highlighting 'attachment-informed' ways of interacting (e.g. attunement, co-regulation, interactive repair and parenting with PACE).

As with promising community interventions for high-risk youth, the framework recognises that a 'multi-systemic' approach is needed, with a creative and flexible integration of psychological approaches, addressing environmental and system factors as well as working directly with the individual. The approach attempts to maintain a care environment attuned to the young person's developmental needs and underpinned by a clear psychological formulation. There is priority emphasis given to effective risk management, safety and supporting staff, to regulate their own emotions and provide secure, 'therapeutic' parenting. This may or may not be supplemented by specific individual therapy as guided by the formulation. A particular importance is placed on assessing the appropriate timing and modality of intervention. The inadvertent pressure from the system to provide individual interventions too early in the process, before the environmental conditions are in place to ensure the greatest potential for that intervention to be successful, are resisted. For example, to offer interventions that explore traumatic experiences before having developed appropriate emotional regulation skills and a supportive social network, are likely to be unsuccessful, and may even be harmful and retraumatising. Wherever possible, family members and members of external organisations (such as YOTs) should be invited to at least one therapeutic session and all review meetings. The aim would be to share the formulation (understanding) of the young person's difficulties in order to increase understanding and empathy with the difficulties the young person has, and increase understanding about effective management of risk (including addressing the underlying needs of the young person).

It is proposed that the DART framework firstly helps staff members increase their understanding of complex, challenging and high-risk behaviour in young people (raising caregiver sensitivity) and, secondly, it then makes clear links to developmentally appropriate interventions to manage risk and promote adaptive development. With understanding comes the opportunity for change. Without this, there is a risk that the system around the young person will repeat early, inconsistent and unhelpful environments that will only serve to reinforce maladaptive patterns of interactions and behaviours. This, of course, is not good for the young person, but it also means that services may be left with ineffectual ways of managing challenging and high-risk behaviour, and it is argued may even increase the risk of those behaviours in the longer term.

With the cornerstone of the DART framework lying within an integrated whole systems approach to meeting the needs of the young person, the key to successful delivery is a coherent framework for understanding young people and their behaviour. This understanding is initially developed through a comprehensive and developmentally sensitive staff training programme, and a genuine multi-agency commitment to the framework. Training is not enough, however, and continuous support is provided through psychologically informed consultation to help manage the anxiety in the system, maintain the therapeutic and reflective culture of the unit, and enhance objective decision-making. Psychological consultation has been shown to increase the confidence of staff and effect changes in perceptions of young people through theoretical understanding (Evans et al., 2011).

The DART approach is summarised within a 'house' framework (adapted for work with high-risk adolescents from pioneering work by Kim Golding, 2008 and 2013), with different parts and aspects of delivery explained from the foundations up.

Linking theory to practice: The DART house

An adapted version of the house of parenting (Golding 2013) is used to underpin the DART framework in terms of delivery of care. The house model of parenting is based upon knowledge of child development, formation of secure attachment relationships in infancy, and how this can be adapted to help older children to also achieve a more secure attachment. The house of parenting draws on the work of a number of clinicians who have explored ways of helping children with attachment difficulties, for example Mary Dozier (2005), Vera Fahlberg (2002), and, most notably, the work of Dan Hughes (2004) and Kim Golding (2013).

The secure base

The ground floor of the house emphasises the importance of providing a secure base, a safe environment, both physically and psychologically (see Figure 15.1). Figure 15.1 operationalises some of the key points and strategies in providing a secure base. Safety and security is considered early on in the DART approach, due to the high level of risk that may well be present in secure settings (see Figure 15.2). It is recognised that many other parenting approaches promote positive engagement and interactions before dealing with negative behaviour

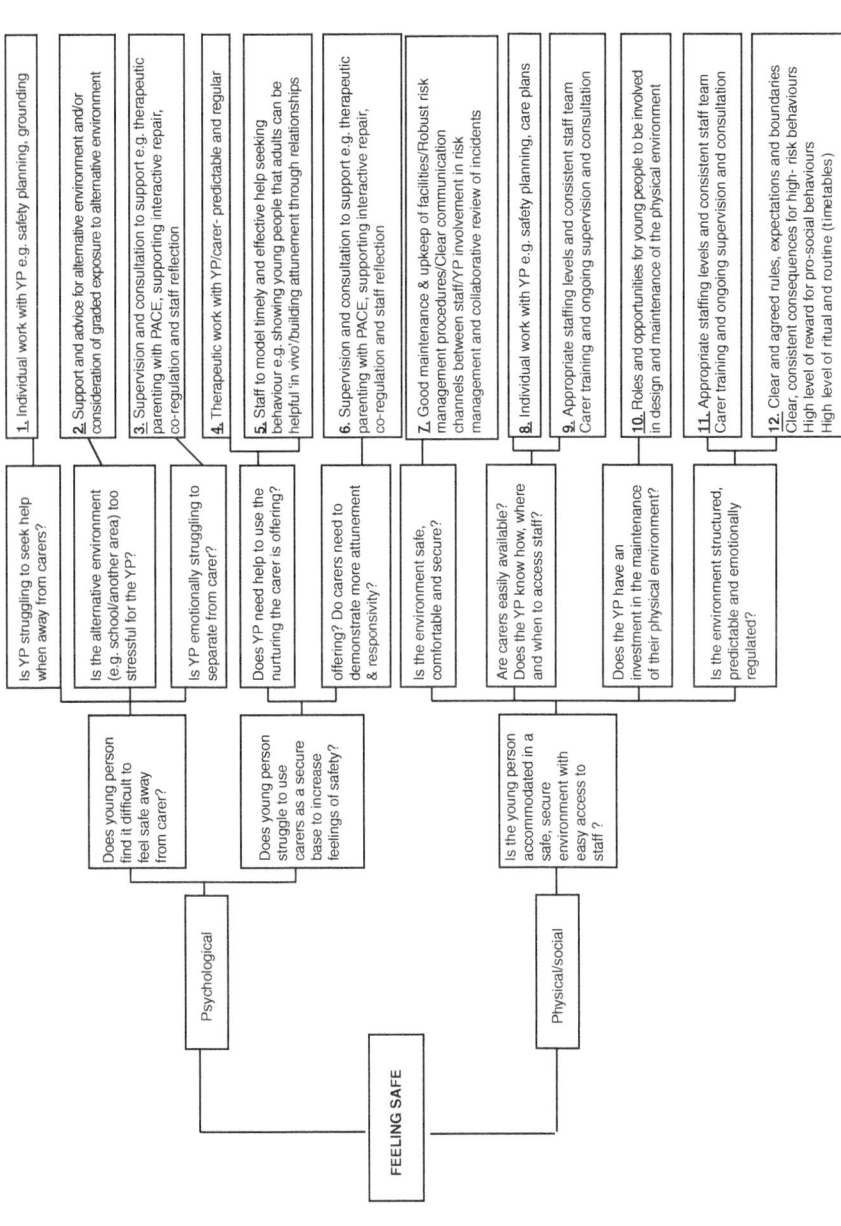

Figure 15.2 Feeling safe (adapted from 'Pyramid of Need', Kim Golding (2007) – personal correspondence – with permission)

(e.g. Webster-Stratton 2006; Golding 2006). Whilst the DART framework does not disagree with this, the secure base recognises that, when working with a dysregulated adolescent, it may first be necessary to have clear strategies to manage immediate violent or self-harm behaviour when this arises. Maintaining safety and providing containment for both the young person and staff will help staff to remain calm when working with high levels of arousal. Involving young people in their own risk management is a key element in the DART approach.

As part of creating a secure base, staff members need to work from a secure and regulated position in order to regulate and inform the emotional tone of the environment (see Figure 15.2, boxes 3, 5, 6, 9, 11 and 12). In order to provide optimal care, the staff member needs to self-regulate and feel safe themselves. A secure base is at the heart of attachment theory and also provides the foundation of the house. Young people need to feel safe and secure. From this secure base, the individual can begin to build up confidence and explore the world around them. Within such an environment, young people can develop emotionally and cognitively. In particular, they will develop the capacities for emotional regulation and reflective function. The physical and psychological changes which occur as a result of a child being exposed to dangerous or threatening situations can be countered by the creation of a safe, protective environment (Bloom 1999).

Emphasis is also placed upon avoiding dialectically opposed 'extremes' in terms of care delivery. For example, there is a risk of overemphasising the need for care and/or over-caring for a young person in distress, and therefore neglecting the need for exerting some control in terms of providing safety (risk management). All too often systems become driven by either a 'care' narrative or a 'control' narrative, rather than a recognition that a balance of the two is required to promote positive developmental trajectories. This care–control dynamic is a fine balance to achieve in practice, particularly with high-risk behaviour. It is proposed that either extreme is not developmentally appropriate and is potentially harmful to promoting positive development. Too much an emphasis on over-care is likely to lead to the young person becoming over-reliant on others for co-regulation and not developing the self-regulation skills necessary to independently manage distress or manage their behaviour. High-risk behaviour can often therefore be reinforced, as the behaviour is used in increasing severity as an attempt to retain co-regulation and avoid rejection. Similarly, too much emphasis on control may also lead to overdependence on external 'controls', such as locked doors, and/or an experience of learned helplessness, powerlessness and invalidation, leading to desperate and high-risk attempts to take power and control back. The DART model promotes regular reappraisal of the care–control dynamic, including in discussion with the young person.

Staff members are charged as 'therapeutic parents', and an important part of their role is to recreate multiple experiences of a typical relational pattern of attunement, co-regulation and interactive repair (see Figure 15.2, boxes 1, 3, 4, 5, 6, 8, 11 and 12, and Figure 15.3). It is suggested that these multiple experiences help develop attachment security by providing a relational experience that the young person needs, but may have missed out on. Interactive repair is a key process within the staff–young person relationship. This refers to the repairing of a therapeutic relationship after breakdown (e.g. when a young person has become aggressive towards a member of staff following a boundary having been put in place). Once immediate risk has been managed, and a level of emotional regulation achieved, staff and the young people are encouraged to review the incident, highlighting where misunderstandings may have occurred, where safety was compromised and implementing any sanctions required (see Figure 15.2, boxes 7, 11 and 12). If staff have made a mistake or, on reflection, recognise they have overreacted, they are encouraged to model an appropriate apology. Discussions also take place on how to avoid similar incidents in the future. This is often a very challenging process, but one that is key in delivering the message that it is the behaviour that is not accepted, not the person.

Comfort and co-regulation

This section of the house places emphasis on 'therapeutic parents' remaining calm and 'regulated'. To maintain such an atmosphere, 'therapeutic parents' will need to avoid being drawn into the emotional state being experienced by the young person (see Figure 15.3). In our experience, in order for the 'therapeutic parents' to remain calm, team support is vital. This includes safe spaces for staff and team meetings, supported by management, during which frustrations can be aired and support between the team members be given. Supervision and consultation from a psychological perspective is also important during this time. Providing consultation and advice, using the DART framework, offers an understanding of the challenging behaviour that a young person may present with. This consultation may take place in the more formal time slot of the weekly meeting, or during informal discussions in the staff office.

Building relationships

This section of the house model relates to the building of relationships (see Figure 15.4). Dan Hughes (2006) suggests a certain attitude (PACE) that 'therapeutic parents' can adopt, which will help them to maintain a level of emotional engagement. If staff can remain curious (C) about why the young person is behaving as they are, they will be less likely to become dysregulated themselves. Dysregulation and feelings of frustration are problematic, as these can then lead to punitive or inconsistent care. Curiosity leads to understanding, which helps the 'therapeutic parent' to accept (A) the young person and

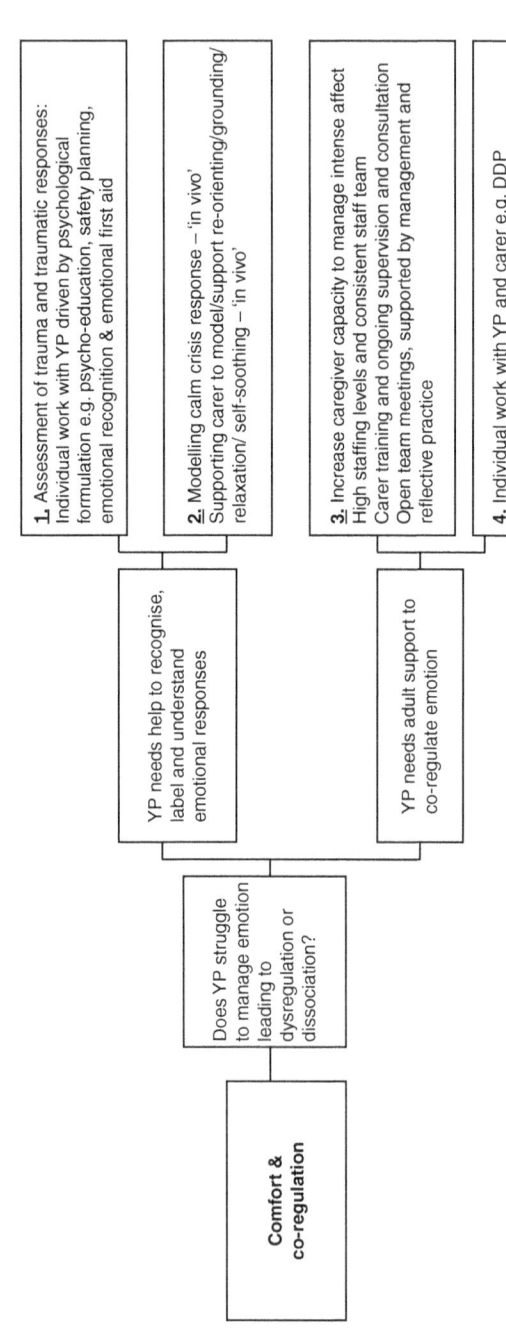

Figure 15.3 Comfort and co-regulation (adapted from 'Pyramid of Need', Kim Golding (2007) – personal correspondence – with permission)

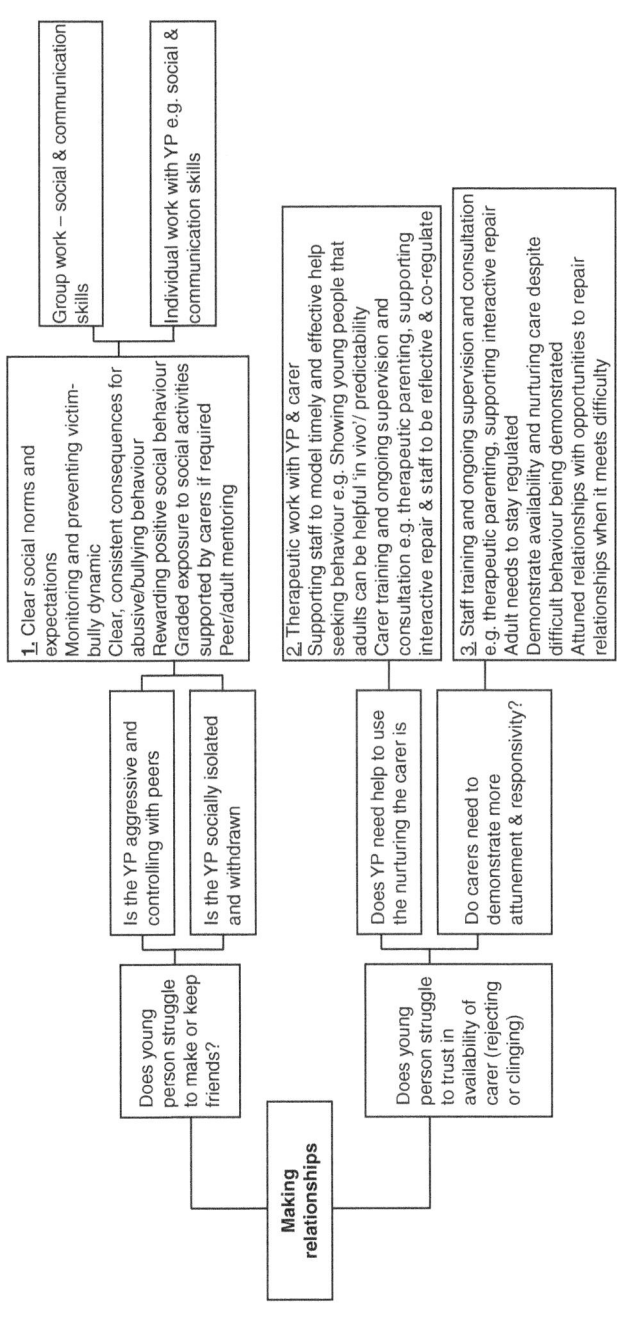

Figure 15.4 Making relationships (adapted from 'Pyramid of Need', Kim Golding (2007) – personal correspondence – with permission)

the reasons for their behaviour. This, in turn, will help the 'therapeutic parent' to provide the young person with empathy (E) and support alongside the discipline they need. At times, a playful (P) stance promoting a sense of fun can also diffuse a situation and help the young person to behave in a more acceptable way.

Positive relationships are seen as a vital source from which a young person can elicit care and comfort when needed (see Figure 15.4, boxes 2 and 3).

Managing behaviour and risk

The roof of the house represents the management of high-risk behaviour (see Figure 15.5). Effective parenting is supported by good behaviour management, which is underpinned by a balanced SPJ approach to risk assessment and management, and proportionate reward and/or consequence. Behaviour management is a key part of the DART approach, recognising the need for a balance between effective and attuned care and safety, security and effective

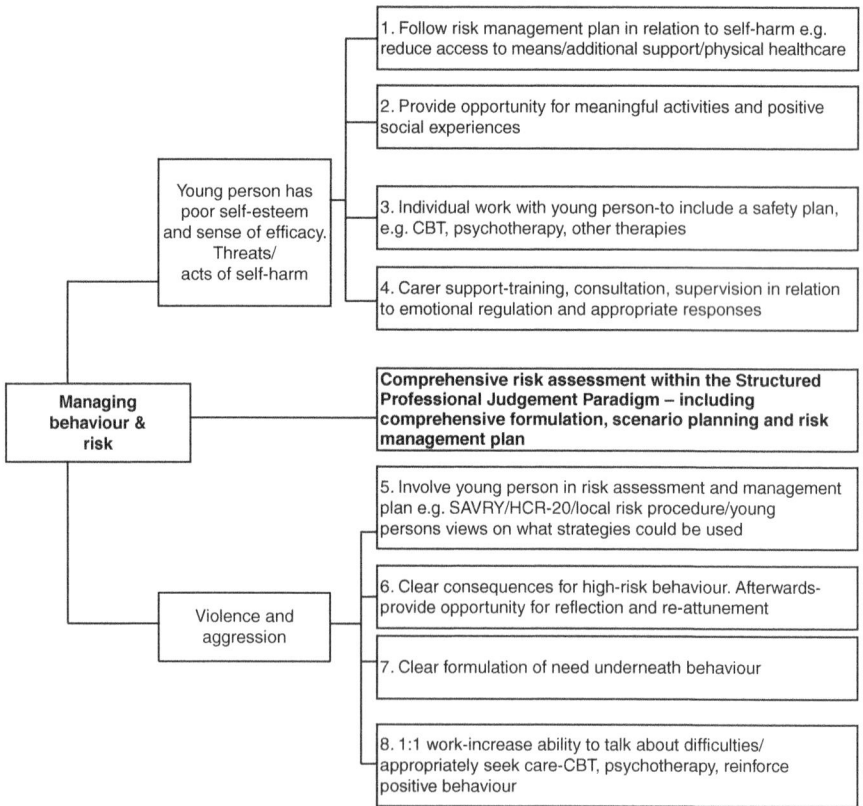

Figure 15.5 Managing behaviour and risk (adapted from 'Pyramid of Need', Kim Golding (2007) – personal correspondence – with permission)

boundaries, and consequences. Where possible, the young people are involved collaboratively in the management of their own behaviour. Young people need boundaries to feel safe and the feeling of safety links back into the ground floor of the house.

Findings from a pilot implementation

Our understanding in relation to effective interventions for high-risk youth in secure settings is growing, but there is much work still to be done. Proposed interventions with this population are limited and the DART framework is in its infancy. However, evaluation of this approach has begun. In 2011, Ryan and Mitchell evaluated the effectiveness of a complex needs provision within a YOI in the UK, where the DART framework underpinned practice. The complex need provision housed up to ten young people and aimed to provide individualised care to this small group, who could not be supported on the typical residential units within the YOI due to the high-risk behaviour they displayed.

Upon admission and discharge to the provision, demographic information and data from four measures was collected between February 2008 and July 2009. The measures included the Health of the Nation Outcome Scales for Children and Adolescents (HoNOSCA) and Health of the Nation Outcome Scales (HoNOS) Secure. The Social and Behavioural Engagement Rating Scale (SABER; Ryan and Mitchell 2011), which examines seven areas of daily functioning, was developed for the study. Finally, data from the incentives and earned privileges (IEP) scheme operated by the YOI was used. The IEP scheme encourages individuals to earn rewards for good behaviour, and young person can have an IEP status of basic, standard or enhanced.

The average age of the young men admitted to the complex needs unit was 16.6 years. Thirty-seven per cent had been, or were currently on a Care Order, and 66 per cent had been in local authority care at some point. In total, 14 individuals (34 per cent) had previously been in custody and 72 per cent had convictions for violence, sexual offences or arson. Compared with national statistics, the young offenders admitted had elevated needs in multiple areas. When supported within the general accommodation (main wings) within the YOI, they presented high risks to themselves and/or others, had difficulty engaging with the regime and needed a high level of support from other agencies, particularly mental health services. On average, young people spent 68 days on the unit.

Results indicated that the HoNOSCA scores at admission to the unit showed a high incidence of severe problems with behaviour, emotional regulation relationships and social engagement. In most domains, there were reductions in the mean scores and in the number of young people with 'severe' problems on discharge.

HoNOS Secure scores upon admission highlighted the need for a highly structured and high-staffed secure environment; risk to others and vulnerability were both high. Significant reductions were observed in scores for risk to others and need for both physical and staff security. Mean scores at discharge were lower in all domains except vulnerability from others. SABER scores at admission were generally high in all domains except self-care; high scores at discharge were reduced in all domains, and mean scores were significantly lower in all domains except social behaviour. Significant improvements were also shown through the young person's IEP status, that is, a reduction in challenging behaviour meant a reduced need for sanctions and therefore a higher IEP status and more access to privileges. The study also reported a marked reduction in unmet emotional needs and high-risk behaviours, and an improvement in peer relationships and engagement with the YOI regime. However, although one-third of young people were successfully transitioned back to main location, results did suggest that supporting transition more effectively was an area that needed further work.

Ryan and Mitchell (2011) did not formally evaluate relationships with staff, although they do note that both mental health workers and custodial staff reported an improvement over time. The authors align this with the attachment and trauma theory which underpins the DART framework, which would anticipate improvements in behaviour and social engagement as self-regulation improves through experiencing safety, stable and supportive relationships. Currently, evaluation of this approach within the YOI has been taken forward, and assessments that attempt to measure attachment and quality of relationships have been included. Initial results are promising, with significant results being found for improvement in relationships and a move towards interactional styles being described as 'secure'. At present, this data is in the process of being prepared for publication.

Summary

This chapter aimed to summarise a framework for working with young people in secure settings who present with complexity, high vulnerability and high-risk behaviour towards themselves and others. The DART framework is still very early in its development, but draws on current theory and practice. It seeks to bring together an understanding of complex presentations within secure settings, making real links between theory and practice, and places an emphasis on understanding and effectively managing risk. It is posed that a wider systems approach to understanding, managing and working with adolescents who present with high-risk behaviours should be underpinned by a psychologically informed, multi-systemic formulation that includes understanding high-risk behaviours in terms of the young person's early attachment experiences and experiences of trauma.

There are clearly areas for future research and the need to evaluate the application of this framework in different secure settings is essential, as no doubt there will be a variation in barriers to effective delivery, and there will be aspects of the framework which require additional thought and adjustment.

Future evaluation of the application of the framework with males and females will be important. The majority of studies have examined interventions with male young offenders and this undoubtedly reflects the fact that most young offenders are male. However, more studies are now required for both genders. There is evidence to suggest that there are gender differences in attachment-seeking behaviour within attachment styles (Wekerle and Wolfe 1998). Of course, future research would also benefit from the inclusion of service-user feedback.

References

Ainsworth, M., Blehar, M., Waters, E., and Wall, S. (1978) *Patterns of Attachment: A Psychological Study of the Strange Situation*. Hillsdale, NJ: Lawrence Erlbaum.

Allen, J. and Fonagy, P. (2006) *Handbook of Mentalization-Based Treatment*. England: John Wiley & Sons.

Andrews, D. and Bonta, J. (2010) *The Psychology of Criminal Conduct*, 5th edn. Newark: LexisNexis.

Andrews, D.A., Bonta, J., and Wormith, S. (2006) 'The recent past and near future of risk and/or needs assessment', *Crime and Delinquency*, 52(1): 7–27.

Andrews, D., Zinger, I., Hoge, R., Bonta, J., Gendreau, P., and Cullen, F. (1990) 'Does correctional treatment work? A clinically relevant and psychologically informed meta-analysis', *Criminology*, 28(3): 369–404.

Bloom, S.L. (1999) 'Trauma theory abbreviated', *The Sanctuary Model*. Available at: http://www.sanctuaryweb.com/bloom.php. Accessed 12 December 2014.

Bowlby, J. (1969/1982) *Attachment and Loss*, vol. 1: *Attachment*, 2nd edn. New York: Basic Books.

Bowlby, J. (1973) *Attachment and Loss*, vol. 2: *Separation: Anxiety and Anger*. New York: Basic Books.

Bowlby, J. (1980) *Attachment and Loss*, vol. 3: *Loss: Sadness and Depression*. New York: Basic Books.

Bowlby, J. (1988) *A Secure Base: Clinical Applications of Attachment Theory*. New York: Basic Books.

Bretherton, I. (1992) 'The origins of attachment theory: John Bowlby and Mary Ainsworth', *Developmental Psychology*, 28(5): 759.

Briere, B. and Scott, C. (2006) *Principles of Trauma Therapy: A Guide to Symptoms, Evaluation and Treatment*. London: Sage.

Butler, S., Baruch, G., Hickey, N., and Fonagy, P. (2011) 'A randomized controlled trial of multisystemic therapy and a statutory therapeutic intervention for young offenders', *Journal of the American Academy of Child and Adolescent Psychiatry*, 50(12): 1220–1235.

Charney, D., Deutch, A., Krystal, J., Southwick, S., and Davis, M. (1993) 'Psychobiologic mechanisms of posttraumatic stress disorder', *Archives of General Psychiatry*, 50: 295–305.

Cicchetti, D. and Tucker, D. (1994) 'Development and self-regulatory structures of the mind', *Developmental Psychopathology*, 6: 533–550.

Cooper, M., Shaver, P., and Collins, N. (1998) 'Attachment styles, emotion regulation and adjustment in adolescence', *Journal of Personality and Social Psychology*, 74: 1380–1397.

Crighton, D.A. and Towl, G.J. (2008) *Psychology in Prisons*, 2nd edn. Oxford: Wiley-Blackwell.

Crittenden, P.M. (2005) 'Attachment theory, psychopathology and psychotherapy: The dynamic-maturational approach', *Psicoterapia*, 30: 171–182.

De Bellis, M. (2001) 'Developmental traumatology: The psychobiological development of maltreated children and its implications for research, treatment, and policy', *Developmental Psychopathology*, 13: 539–564.

De Bellis, M.D., Hooper, S.R., Woolley, D.P., and Shenk, C.E. (2010) 'Demographic, maltreatment, and neurobiological correlates of PTSD symptoms in children and adolescents', *Journal of Pediatric Psychology*, 35(5): 570–577.

De Bellis, M.D., Keshavan, M.S., Shifflett, H., Iyengar, S., Beers, S.R., Hall, J., Moritz, G. (2002) 'Brain structures in pediatric maltreatment-related posttraumatic stress disorder: A sociodemographically matched study', *Biological Psychiatry*, 52: 1066–1078.

De Bellis, M.D., Baum, A.S., Birmaher, B., Keshavan, M.S., Eccard, C.H., Boring, A.M., Jenkins, F.J., and Ryan, N.D. (1999) 'Developmental traumatology part I: Biological stress systems', *Biological Psychiatry*, 45: 1259–1270.

Dozier, M. (2005) 'Challenges in foster care', *Attachment and Human Development*, 7: 27–30.

Dulcan, M. (2000) 'Does community mental health treatment of children and adolescents help?' *Journal American Academy of Child and Adolescent Psychiatry*, 39: 153–154.

Duncan, S.C., Strycker, L.A., Duncan, T.E., and Okut, H. (2002) 'A multilevel contextual model of family conflict and deviance', *Journal of Psychopathology and Behavioural Assessment*, 24: 169–175.

Evans, K., Law, H., Turner, R.E., Rogers, A and Cohen, K. (2011). 'A pilot study evaluating care staff's perceptions of their experience of psychological consultation within a mental health setting', *Child Care in Practice*, 17(2).

Fahlberg, V. (2002) *Child's Journey through Placement*. 2nd edn. London: Jessica Kingsley Publishers.

Glaser, D. (2000) 'Child abuse and neglect and the brain: A review', *Journal of Child Psychology and Psychiatry*, 41(1): 97–116.

Golding, K. (2006) *Thinking Psychologically about Children Who Are Looked after and Adopted: Space for Reflection*. Chichester: John Wiley & Sons.

Golding, K. (2007) *Nurturing Attachments: Supporting Children Who Are Fostered or Adopted*. London: Jessica Kingsley Publishers.

Golding, K. (2012) *Creating Loving Attachments: Parenting with PACE to Nurture Confidence and Security in the Troubled Child*. London: Jessica Kingsley Publishers.

Golding, K. (2013) *Nurturing Attachments Training Resource: Running Parenting Groups for Adoptive Parents and Foster or Kinship*. London: Jessica Kingsley Publishers.

Gratz, K., Conrad, S., and Roemer, L. (2010) 'Risk factors for deliberate self-harm among college students', *American Journal of Orthopsychiatry*, 72: 128–140.

Hanson, R.K., Bourgon, G., Helmus, L., and Hodgson, S. (2009) 'The principles of effective correctional treatment also apply to sexual offenders: A meta-analysis', *Criminal Justice and Behavior*, 36(9): 865–891.

Henggeler, S., Pickrel, S., and Brondino, M. (1999) 'Multisystemic treatment of substance-abusing and dependent delinquents: Outcomes, treatment fidelity and transportability', *Mental Health Services Research*, 1: 171–184.

Horowitz, M. and Becker, S. (1971) 'The compulsion to repeat trauma: Experimental study of intrusive thinking after stress', *Journal of Nervous and Mental Disease*, 153: 32–40.

Hughes, D. (2004) 'An attachment-based treatment of maltreated children and young people', *Attachment and Human Development*, 6: 263–278.

Hughes, D. (2006) *Building the Bonds of Attachment: Awakening Love in Deeply Troubled Children*, 2nd edn. Jason Aronson. Lanham, Maryland.

Ireland, J.L. and Power, C.L. (2004) 'Attachment, emotional loneliness, and bullying behaviour: A study of adult and young offenders', *Aggressive Behaviour*, 30(4): 298–312.

Kinniburgh, K., Blaustein, M., and Spinazzola, J. (2005) 'Attachment, self-regulation and competency', *Psychiatric Annals*, 35: 424–430.

Kobak, K., Cassidy, J., Lyons-Ruth, K., and Ziv, Y. (2006) 'Attachment, Stress and Psychopathology: A Developmental Pathways Model', in D. Cicchetti and D.J. Cohen (eds.), *Developmental Psychopathology*, vol. 1: *Theory and Method*, 2nd edn. London: John Wiley & Sons, 333–369.

Koehler, J.A., Losel, F., Akoensi, T.D., and Humphreys, D.K. (2013) 'A systemic review and meta-analysis on the effects of young offender treatment programs in Europe', *Journal of Experimental Criminology*, 9(1): 19–43.

Kolvin, I., Miller, F.J., Fleeting, M., and Kolvin, P.A. (1988) 'Social and parenting factors affecting criminal-offence rates. Findings from the Newcastle thousand family study (1947–1980)', *The British Journal of Psychiatry*, 152: 80–90.

Landenberger, N.A. and Lipsey, M.W. (2005) 'The positive effects of cognitive-behavioural programs for offenders: A meta-analysis of factors associated with effective treatment', *Journal of Experimental Criminology*, 1(4): 451–476.

Lipsey, M., Wilson, D., and Cothern, L. (2000) *Effective Intervention for Serious Juvenile Offenders*. Washington, DC: Office of Juvenile Justice and Delinquency Prevention.

Loeber, R. and Stouthamer-Loeber, M. (1986) 'Family factors as correlates and predictors of juvenile conduct problems and delinquency', in M.H. Tonry and N. Morris (eds.), *Crime and Justice: An Annual Review of Research Vol. 7*. Chicago: University of Chicago Press, 29–149.

Lyons-Ruth, K. (1996) 'Attachment relationships among children with aggressive behaviour problems: The role of disorganised early attachment patterns', *Journal of Consulting and Clinical Psychology*, 64: 64–74.

Main, M. and Solomon, J. (1986) 'Discovery of an Insecure-Disorganized Attachment Pattern', in T.B. Brazelton and M.W. Yogman (eds.), *Affective Development in Infancy*. Norwood, NJ: Ablex, 95–124.

Marsa, F., O'Reilly, G., Carr, A., Murphy, P., O'Sullivan, M., Cotter, A., and Hevey, D. (2004) 'Attachment styles and psychological profiles of child sex offenders in Ireland', *Journal of Interpersonal Violence*, 19(2): 228–251.

Marshall, M.L. (1989) 'Intimacy, loneliness and sexual offenders', *Behaviour Research and Therapy*, 27(5): 491–504.

Muris, P., Meesters, C., Morren, M., and Moorma, L. (2004) 'Anger and hostility in adolescents: Relationships with self-reported attachment style and perceived parental rearing styles', *Journal of Psychosomatic Research*, 57(3): 257–264.

Newton, R.R., Litrownik, L.J., and Landsverk, J.A. (2000) 'Children and youth in foster care: Disentangling the relationship between problem behaviours and number of placements', *Child Abuse and Neglect*, 24(10): 1363–1374.

Perry, B.D. (2008) 'Child maltreatment: The role of abuse and neglect in developmental psychopathology', in T.P. Beauchaine and S.P. Hinshaw (eds.), *Textbook of Child and Adolescent Psychopathology*. New York: Wiley, 93–128.

Perry, B. and Pollard, R. (1998) 'Homeostasis, stress, trauma, and adaptation: A neurodevelopmental view of childhood trauma', *Child Adolescent Psychiatry Clinics North America*, 7: 33–51.

Perry, B., Blakley, T., Baker, W., and Vigilante, D. (1995) 'Childhood trauma, the neurobiology of adaptation, and "use-dependent" development of the brain: How "states" become "traits"', *Journal of Infant Mental Health*, 16: 271–291.

Putnam, F. (1997) *Dissociation in Children and Adolescents: A Developmental Perspective*. New York: Guildford Press.

Redondo, S., Sanchez-Meca, J., and Garrido, V. (1999) 'The influence of treatment programmes on the recidivism of juvenile and adult offenders: A European meta-analytic review', *Psychology, Crime and Law*, 5(3): 251–278.

Rice, K. (1990) 'Attachment in adolescence: A narrative and meta-analytic review', *Journal of Youth and Adolescence*, 19: 511–538.

Rogers, A., McMahon, J., and Law, D. (2011) 'Expanding therapy: Challenging the dominant discourse of individual therapy when working with vulnerable children and young people. A discussion paper', *Clinical Psychology Forum*, 222: 9–14.

Ryan, T and Mitchell, P. (2011) 'A collaborative approach to meeting the needs of adolescent offenders with complex needs in custodial settings: An 18-month cohort study', *Journal of Forensic Psychiatry & Psychology*, 22(3): 437–454.

Saxe, G.N., Ellis, B.H., and Kaplow, J.B. (2007) *Collaborative Treatment of Traumatized Children and Teens: The Trauma Systems Therapy Approach*. New York: Guilford Press.

Schore, A. (2001) 'The effects of early relational trauma on right brain development, affect regulation, and infant mental health', *Journal of Infant Mental Health*, 22: 201–269.

Smallbone, S.W. and Dadds, M.R. (1998) 'Childhood attachment and adult attachment in incarcerated adult male sex offenders', *Journal of Interpersonal Violence*, 13(5): 555–573.

Smith, C. (1997) 'Factors associated with early sexual activity among urban adolescents', *Journal of the National Association of Social Workers*, 42: 334–346.

Sunderland, M. (2006) *The Science of Parenting*. London: Dorling Kindersley.

Timmerman, I.G.H. and Emmelkamp, P.M.G. (2006) 'The relationships between attachment styles and Cluster B personality disorders in prisoners and forensic inpatients', *International Journal of Law and Psychiatry*, 29: 48–56.

Van der Kolk, B. (1989) 'The compulsion to repeat the trauma: Re-enactment, revictimization and masochism', *Psychiatric Clinics of North America*, 1292: 389–411.

Van der Kolk, B. (1994) 'The body keeps the score: Memory and the evolving psychobiology of posttraumatic stress', *Harvard Review of Psychiatry*, 1: 253–265.

Van der Kolk, B. (2005) 'Developmental trauma disorder: Toward a rational diagnosis for children with complex trauma histories', *Psychiatric Annals*, 35: 401–408.

Van der Kolk, B. and Fisler, R. (1994) 'Childhood abuse and neglect and loss of self-regulation', *Bull Menninger Clinics*, 58: 145–168.

Van der Kolk, B., Pelcovitz, D., and Roth, S. (1996) 'Dissociation, somatization, and affect dysregulation: The complexity of adaptation of trauma', *American Journal of Psychiatry*, 153: 83–93.

Van Ijzendoorn, M.H., Feldbrugge, J.T.T.M., Derks, F.C.H, de Ruieter, C., Verhagen, M.F.M., Philipse, M.W.G., van der Staak, C.P.F., Riksen-Walraven, J.M.A. (1997) 'Attachment representations of personality-disordered criminal offenders', *American Journal of Orthopsychiatry*, 67(3): 449–459.

Ward, T. and Beech, A. (2005) 'An integrated theory of sexual offending', *Aggression and Violent Behaviour*, 11(1): 44–63.

Ward, T. and Gannon, T.A. (2006) 'Rehabilitation, etiology and self-regulation: The comprehensive Good Lives Model of treatment for sexual offenders', *Aggression & Violent Behaviour*, 11: 77–94.

Ward, T. and Stewart, C.A. (2003) 'The treatment of sex offenders: Risk management and good lives', *Professional Psychology: Research and Practice*, 34(4): 353–360.

Ward, T., Hudson, S.M., and Marshall, L.M. (1996) 'Attachment style in sex offenders: A preliminary study', *Journal of Sex Research*, 33(1): 17–26.

Webster-Stratton, C. (2006) *The Incredible Years*. London: Longden.

Wekerle, C. and Wolfe, D.A. (1998) 'The role of child maltreatment and attachment style in adolescent relationship violence', *Development and Psychopathology*, 3: 571–586.

Index

Note: Locator's followed by 'b' refer to boxes.

acceptance and commitment therapy (ACT), 245–6
actuarial risk assessment (ARA), 100–1, 105
Adaptive Behaviour Assessment System: Version 2 (ABAS-II), 292
Adolescent Mentalisation-based Integrative Therapy (AMBIT), 273
adolescents
  antisocial behaviour, 123, 125, 138
  with autism spectrum disorder (ASD), 318–23, 326–7, 330–2, 334
  DART approach, 356, 360–1, 365, 367, 372, 374, 376, 378, 383–4
  evidence-based psychotherapies, 32, 54–5, 57, 133
  with intellectual difficulties (ID), 289–90, 293, 295–9, 301, 303, 306
  mental health service, 47–8, 67, 69–70
  MTFC schemes, 134
  multimodal interventions, 124
  psychologically informed approaches, 3, 7, 17–18
  risk assessment, 97–8, 100, 103–4, 106, 113
  in secure settings, 72
  self-harm, 229–32, 238, 244
  sexually harmful behaviour, 168–74, 176–7
  social isolation, 123
  substance misuse (SM), 130, 254, 257, 260–4, 266, 269, 273
  Violent behaviour, 144, 162
  Well-being, 161
  see also fire-setting
Adult mental health services (AMHS), 20, 24, 37, and 331–2
Agency for Healthcare and Research Quality (AHRQ), 331
Alcohol Use Disorders Identification Test (AUDIT), 263
American Psychiatric Association (APA), 206, 287, 318

Antisocial behaviour co-coordinators (Abs), 288
Antisocial behaviour orders (Asbos), 287–8
Assessment of Risk and Manageability of Individuals with Developmental and Intellectual Limitations who Offend (ARMADILO), 296
Assessment, Care in Custody and Teamwork (ACCT), 238
Assessment, Intervention and Moving-On project (AIM)
  AIM-2 assessment (case study), 186–7
  ASSET, 104
  ERASOR protocol, 177
  Intervention packages, 179–80
  J-SOAP-II protocol, 177
  Services in Manchester, 102–3
  Youth offending service (YOS), 178
Attachment, Self-Regulation and Competency (ARC) framework, 358
Attachment theory, 108, 172, 356, 358–60, 365, 368, 374, 378
Attention deficit hyperactivity disorder (ADHD)
  Antisocial acts, 123
  ASD and, 320–1, 332
  Diagnostic labels, 46
  Fire-setting (case study), 209, 219
  ID and, 289, 306, 308
  MST case vignette, 53
  Pharmacological interventions, 124, 129
  Prevalence rate, 68–9
  Self-harm behaviour, 232
  SM difficulties, 267
Autism Diagnostic Observation Schedule: Version 2 (ADOS-2), 327
autism spectrum disorder (ASD)
  assessment
    psychosocial functions, 327–8
    risk factors, 328–9
  case study, 333–7
  co-morbidity, 319–20

definition, 317–18
difficulties associated with, 316–17
formulation, 327–9
impact on diagnosis, 320–1
intervention
   co-morbid mental health problems, 330
   cognitive behavioural therapy (CBT), 330–1
   environment, 331
   psychosocial, 329–30
   systemic, 331
offending and, 323–6
prevalence, 318–19
reasons for referral, 321–3
transition, 331–3

Beck Youth Inventories: Version 2, 293, 306
behavioural difficulties, 123, 125, 274, 321
behavioural problems, 4, 56, 78, 124, 126–8, 138, 306
black and minority ethnic (BME) communities, 69
Bradley Report, 304

Cannabis Youth Treatment Trial (CYT), 272
Care Programme Approach (CPA), 332
case study
   AIM-2 assessment, 186–7
   attention deficit hyperactivity disorder (ADHD), 53, 209, 219
   autism spectrum disorder (ASD), 333–7
   child and adolescent mental health services (CAMHS), 53, 209–10, 279–80, 306, 308, 334
   fire-setting, 209–11, 215
   forensic child and adolescent mental health services (FCAMHS), 49–51
   high-risk behaviour, 333–6
   intellectual disabilities (ID), 306–10
   multi-systemic therapy (MST), 53–4, 130–3
   offending behaviour, 307
   problem sexual behaviour (PSB), 49–50, 189–90
   psychological assessment, 8–10
   secure settings, 77b, 79b, 80b–1b, 84b, 85b

self-harm, 238–48
sexually harmful behaviour, 185–93
structured professional judgment (SPJ), 110–11
substance misuse (SM), 275–80
whole systems approach, 130–3
youth violence risk assessment, 110–17
child abuse and neglect, 52
child and adolescent mental health services (CAMHS)
   case vignette, 53, 209–10, 279–80, 306, 308, 334
   child protection principles, 268
   comprehensive approach, 73, 100
   Lola-Rose's experience, 20, 23–4, 37–9
   multi-systemic factors, 264
   non-genuine disclosure, 352
   presenting concerns, 6
   referral pathways, 58
   risk assessment checklist, 101
   services and settings, 1
   systemic intervention, 244
   therapeutic approach, 49
   Tier 3 functions, 48
   traditional, 60, 197
   treatment models, 273
   UK context, 254–5, 260, 272
Child and Adolescent Self-Harm in Europe (CASE), 228–9
children
   with ASD, 318–19, 321–3, 325–7, 330–2, 334, 336
   communication strategies, 147
   competencies of a practitioner psychologist, 13
   DART approach, 358–60, 363, 365, 368, 371, 374, 376, 383
   evidence-based psychotherapies, 32, 54
   fire-setting behaviour, 205–6, 208, 213, 216, 218–19
   health needs, 45
   with intellectual disabilities, 288–92, 294, 296, 300, 305, 308
   MTFC, 55
   parenting skills, 153

children – *continued*
  predisposing factors (formulation), 106, 109
  psychological therapies, 260, 276
  risk assessment protocols, violence, 102–4
  in secure setting, 64–6, 68–73, 75–6, 81, 87, 89
  self-harming behaviour, 226, 228–9, 231, 238–9
  sexual activity, 167
  sexual offences against, 97, 169–71
  sexually harmful behaviour, 174–7, 185, 194
  systemic intervention, 59
  violence risk assessment, 97–8, 101–4, 106, 109–10, 113–14, 116
  violent behaviour, 98, 101
  welfare concerns, 146
  whole systems approach, 123–5, 129–30, 133–4, 137
  see also looked after child (LAC); secure children's homes (SCHs)
children and young people's increasing access to psychological therapies (CYP IAPT), 260
Children's Acts 1989 and 2004, 45, 65–6, 176, 305
cognitive analytic therapy (CAT), 82–3
cognitive behaviour therapy (CBT)
  for ASD, 330–1
  DART approach, 382
  in FAIV intervention, 158
  Fit for aggression plan, 54
  FSE (Fire Safety Education), 218
  for intellectual difficulties (ID), 300, 302
  harmful sexual behaviour, 183
  in prison and secure settings, 82
  offending behaviour programmes, 11
  for self harm, 244–5
  for substance misuse, 270–1
  young offender rehabilitation programmes, 357
community forensic services
  forensic child and adolescent mental health services (FCAMHS), 47–51
  multisystemic therapy (MST), 51–4
  youth offending teams, 46–7

Comprehensive health assessment tool (CHAT), 263
Consolidated Framework for Implementation Research (CFIR), 136–7
criminal justice system (CJS)
  AIM interventions, 179
  antisocial behaviours, 123
  ASD, 316, 337
  children's right protection, 176
  intellectual difficulties (ID), 289–90, 296, 310
  prison setting, 84
  psychologically informed planned environments (PIPEs) services, 78
  secure children's homes (SCHs), 67
  substance misuse (SM), 257, 270–1, 273, 276
  traditional services, 57
  young offenders (in England and Wales), 66
  young people's support, 44–6

Department of Health (DH), 45, 56, 72–3, 124, 175
detention and training orders (DTOs), 66
developmentally informed attachment, risk and trauma (DART) framework
 aims
  caregiver sensitivity, 372
  emotional regulation, 372–3
  healthy coping strategies, 373–4
  pathway approach, 374
  placement moves reduction, 373
  prosocial relationships with staff and peers, 373
  safety promotion, 372
  self-regulation of behaviour, 373
 attachment-informed framework (real life settings), 367
 challenges, secure setting, 374–6
 house model of parenting
  behaviour and risk management, 382–3
  comfort and co-regulation, 379–82
  secure-base, 376–9
 pilot implementation, 383–4

principles
  brain development (attachment and trauma experience), 368
  care/placement stability, 370–1
  emotional well-being of staff, 369
  hidden needs, identification, 370
  positive and adaptive development, 370
  safety, 369
  staff as 'therapeutic parents,' 368–9
  systemic intervention, 370
  understanding of life experience, 368
theoretical models
  attachment and trauma theory, 359–63
  high-risk behaviour, 364–7
  neurodevelopmental theory, 363–4
therapeutic approach, 356
treatment models
  residential settings, 358–9
  young offenders, 357–8
Diagnostic and Statistical Manual of Mental Disorders (DSM-5 or ICD-10 diagnosis), 8, 287, 292, 318
Diagnostic Interview for Children and Adolescents – Revised (DICA-R), 69
dialectical behaviour therapy (DBT), 82, 243–4, 246, 271
disorganised/disoriented attachment, 361
Division of Clinical Psychology (DCP), 3, 10

Early Assessment Risk List for Boys (EARL-20B), 103
Early Assessment Risk List for Girls (EARL-20G), 103
Estimate of Risk of Adolescent Sexual Offence Recidivism Version 2.0 (ERASOR), 103, 177, 296

FACE – Child and Adolescent Risk Assessment Suite (FACE-CARAS), 104
Facing Up to Offending: The Use of Restorative Justice in the Criminal Justice System (Criminal Justice Joint Inspection), 184
family group conferencing (FGC), 56
family intervention projects (FIPS), 56
fire deviant behaviour, 205
fire play, 204–6, 210–12, 214, 221

Fire safety education (FSE), 217–19
fire-setting
  arson offences, 204–5, 208
  behaviour assessment, 204
  case example, 209–11
  definition, 205
  formulation
    developmental method, 214
    dynamic behavioural model, 213
    Jake's case study, 215
    key aims, 215
  intervention
    areas of, 219–21
    cognitive approaches, 218–19
    fire safety education, 217–18
  motivating factors, 208–9
    behavioural context, 212
    community factors, 212
    developmental context, 212
    family factors, 212
    fire-related factors, 212
    social context, 212
  non-pathological group, 208
  pathological group, 208
  prevalence studies, 205–7
  psychosocial characteristics, 207–8
  reasons, 208–9
  risk prediction and management, 216–17
  terminologies, 204–5
  by young women, 209
Fire setting Risk Interview, 213
forensic child and adolescent mental health services (FCAMHS)
  case vignette, 49–51
  definition, 47
  psychological work, 49
  range of services, 48
forensic mental health services (Lola-Rose's experience)
  access, 30–1
  author's reflection, 40–1
  background, 22–5
  engagement, 30–1
  ethical considerations, 22
  family outcomes, 33–5
  holistic approaches, 37–9
  motivation, 30–1

forensic mental health services
  (Lola-Rose's experience) – *continued*
  psychologist's reflections, 25–6, 28–30,
    32, 35–6, 39
  reflection on methods, 33–5
  relationships with professionals, 26–8
  youth justice manager's reflections, 26,
    30, 32–3, 36–7, 39–40
forensic services
  autism spectrum disorder (ASD),
    316–337
  DART framework, 356–385
  fire-setting, 204–221
  forensic mental health settings, 20–41
  intellectual disabilities (ID), 286–310
  needs of young people, 3–5
  overview, 5–7
  practitioner psychologists' role, 2, 7–8,
    49, 73, 295, 345
  psychological practice in community
    settings, 44–60
  psychologically informed approaches,
    1–18
  secure settings, 64–90
  self–disclosure, 344–354
  self–harming behaviour, 226–248
  sexually harmful behaviour, 167–197
  substance misuse (SM), 253–280
  violence among young people, 143–163
  whole systems approaches, 123–138
  youth violence risk assessment, 96–117
four Ps model (youth violence risk
  assessment), 106, 108
Framework for the Assessment and
  Intervention with Violence (FAIV)
  adaptations and changes, 157
  assessment of violence risk, 151–2
  assessment-interfering behaviours,
    153–4
  child welfare, 146
  client-related variables, 145–6
  clinical concerns, 148
  collaboration, 156
  definition, violence, 144, 146
  developmental considerations, 147–8
  formulation, 154–7
  individual or problem focus, 155
  individual's insight and understanding,
    146–7

informants, 153
intervention, 157–8
potential victims (violence risk), 152–3
practice guidelines, 143–6, 160
quality of therapeutic relationship,
  148–9
risk assessment technique, 153
risk management or risk reduction, 159
social-ecological model, 150, 161
stability, 149
systemic approaches, 158–9
theoretical approaches, 162
theoretical orientation, 154–5
therapeutic process, common factors,
  160
therapeutic relationship, 149
treatment-interfering behaviours,
  159–60, 160
violence risk assessment, 151–2
Functional Assessment of Self-Mutilation
  (FASM), 237
functional family therapy (FFT)
  antisocial behaviour, 55–6, 125
  evidence-based intervention, 15, 127–8,
    158
FCAMHSs, 44

Good Lives Model (GLM), 161, 179, 181,
  196, 219, 301, 357–8

Health and Care Professions Council
  (HCPC), 7, 13
Health of the Nation Outcome Scales
  (HoNOS) Secure, 383–4
Health of the Nation Outcome Scales for
  Children and Adolescents
  (HoNOSCA), 383
high-risk behaviour
  ASD patients, 16, 316–18, 322–4, 328–9,
    331, 337
  attachment perspective, 364–5
  care delivery, 378
  case vignette (Bill), 333–6
  clinical formulation, 80, 356, 361
  DART model, 17, 366–7, 369–70, 372,
    375–6
  harm reduction, 275
  NICE guidelines, 332
  of intellectual disability (ID) patients,
    286, 290, 293, 299, 301, 303, 310

paranoid psychosis, 102
psychologically informed services, 1–3
secure settings, 67, 76, 356, 383
SM difficulties, 264
SPJ approach, 382
statutory services, 6
of traumatized children, 363
whole systems approach, 14
YOI regime, 384
Historical Clinical Risk-20, V2 (HCR-20 V2), 101

Impact of Events Scale (IES), 294–5
incentives and earned privileges (IEP) scheme, 383–4
integrated theory of sexual offending (ITSO), 357
intellectual disabilities (ID)
  assessment
    criminal justice process, 296–7
    criteria, 292–3
    psychological formulation, 298–9
    psychosocial functioning, 293–5
    risk factors, 295–6
  case study, 306–10
  co-morbidity, 289
  definition, 286–7
  ethical consideration, 304–6
  intervention
    adaptation, 301–2
    environmental factors, 302–4
    individual and group work, 299–301
  prevalence, 287–9
  reasons for referral, 289–91
International Classification of Diseases (Version 10, ICD-10), 287, 289, 318
Internet-Assessment Intervention and Moving-On (I-AIM), 103

juvenile enhanced thinking skills (JETS), 81
Juvenile Sex Offender Assessment Protocol (J-SOAP-II), 103, 177

Key Elements of Effective Practice (KEEP), 259–60

Local Safeguarding Children's Board (LSCB), 176

looked after child (LAC), 14, 44, 55–7, 231, 358

Millon Adolescent Clinical Inventory (MACI), 70, 170
modular approach to therapy for children (MATCH), 133
motivational enhancement therapy (MET), 271
Multidimensional Treatment Foster Care (MTFC), 15, 44, 55–7, 59, 125, 127, 133–4, 158
multidisciplinary team (MDT), 16, 65, 74, 110, 227, 237, 248, 305, 307, 326, 335–6, 353–4
Multiplex Empirically Guided Inventory of Ecological Aggregates for Assessing Sexually Abusive Adolescents and Children (MEGA), 103, 177–8
multisystemic therapy (MST)
  benefits, 59–60
  case vignette, 53–4, 130–3
  challenges, 57–9
  –child abuse and neglect (MST-CAN), 52
  community-based treatment, 357
  contingency management programmes, 272
  evidence-based intervention, 137
  family intervention, 51–2
  home-based model, 271–2
  intervention, 51–2, 270
  looked after children, 55–7
  other evidence-based interventions, 54–5
  –problem sexual behaviour (MST-PSB), 52–3, 179, 182–4, 185, 187, 189, 196
  referral behaviour formulation, 53
  secure setting, 87
  –substance abuse (MST-SA), 53
  standard, 52
  systemic or individually-focused approaches, 158
  whole system approach, 125, 127–30
Multisystemic Therapy – child abuse and neglect (MST-CAN), 52
Multisystemic Therapy – problem sexual behaviour (MST-PSB), 52–3

Multisystemic Therapy – substance abuse (MST-SA), 53

National Autistic Society (NAS), 317, 327
National Children's Home, 168
National Health Service (NHS), 20, 44, 67, 73, 89, 196
National Institute for Health and Care Excellence (NICE) guidelines
  Alcohol Use Disorders Identification Test (AUDIT), 263
  antisocial behaviour, 123, 125
  ASD, 321, 327, 330
  Care Programme Approach (CPA), 332
  conduct disorder, 219
  contingency management programmes, 272
  high-risk behaviours, 300
  intellectual difficulties (ID), 305
  multimodal interventions, 52
  self harm, 228–9, 235, 243
  substance misuse (SM), 260, 271
National Treatment Agency (NTA), 254, 256–8, 261–2, 264, 269–70
neurodevelopmental theory, 363–4
nonsuicidal self-injury (NSSI), 228, 237, 243

Obsessive Compulsive Disorder (OCD), 320, 322
Offender Health Research Network (OHRN), 263
offending behaviour
  actuarial risk assessment (ARA) approach, 100
  adolescence, 148, 169
  ASD patients, 316, 324–5
  case vignette (Johnny), 307
  childhood trauma, 46
  DART approach, 356
  drug use, 132
  Good Lives Model, 219
  group-based programmes, 81
  ID patients, 286
  juvenile sexual offenders, 171
  mental health assessment, 278
  multisystemic therapy (MST), 51
  personality disorder traits, 170
  psychologically informed approaches, 2–3, 11, 13

risk assessment, 111, 114–16
secure settings, 89
SM treatment, 259, 262–3
Office for Standards in Education, Children's Services and Skills (OFSTED), 56, 58, 66
Office of Juvenile Justice and Delinquency Prevention (OJJDP), 125
Onset and the Asset (tool), 46

playfulness, acceptance, curiosity and empathy (PACE), 358, 368, 371–2, 375, 379
post-traumatic stress disorder (PTSD), 46, 69, 87, 279, 359
practitioner psychologists
  competencies, 13
  consultation, 12
  forensic services, 7–8
  formulation, 10–11
  intervention, 11–12
  psychological assessment, 8–10
  training, 12–13
practitioner skills
  adapting, 160
  clinical optimism, 161
  clinical supervision, 162
  evaluating, 160
  experiencing setbacks, 161
  intervention approach, 161–2
  monitoring, 160
  systemic variables, 161
  working hypothesis, 161
problem sexual behaviour (PSB)
  case study, 49–50, 189–90
  emerging models, 196
  multisystemic therapy, 52–3, 129–30, 179, 182, 185, 187
Programme for the Education and Enrichment of Relational Skills (PEERS), 330
Promoting Action on Research Implementation in Health Services (PARiHS), 136
Psychiatric Intensive Care Unit (PICU), 238, 246, 248
psychodynamic theory, 7
psychological assessment, case vignette, 8–10

psychological theory, 10, 76–7, 101, 179, 234, 269, 274
psychological thinking, 1–2, 8, 17, 344
psychologically informed environments (PIEs), 14, 78
psychologically informed planned environments (PIPEs), 78
psychological theory, 10, 76–7, 101, 179, 234, 269, 274
  and knowledge, 7, 10, 17, 49, 154, 370
psychological therapy, 82–3

randomised controlled trial (RCT), 32, 55, 126, 128–30, 137–8, 330
restorative justice approaches (sexual abuse)
  in Australia, 185
  in New Zealand, 184
  in UK, 184
Risk-Need- Responsivity Model (RNR), 357
Risk for Sexual Violence Protocol (RSVP), 101, 111–12
Royal College of Psychiatrists (RCP), 101

Screening Questionnaire Interview for Adolescents (SQIfA), 263
Secure Accommodation Network, 69–70
secure children's homes (SCHs)
  ASD patients, 323
  challenges, 89
  DART framework, 374
  health needs, 69–70
  health services, 73–4
  positive impact (young people), 72
  relational security, 85
  reoffending rates, 72
  secure settings, 65–70, 72–4, 85, 88–9
  staffing ratios, 88
  young people in, 70
secure settings
  case example, 77b, 79b, 80b–1b, 84b, 85b
  challenges, 83–5
  clinical outcomes, young people, 72
  creating dependency, 85–6
  front-line staff support, 86–7
  mental health services, 72–3
  outside world connection, 87–8
  overview, 64–5

psychological assessment and formulation, 79–81
psychosocial impact, 71
psychologically informed practice, 77–9
  challenges, 88–9
  role of psychology, 73–7
  secure children's homes (SCHs), 66–7
  secure mental health hospitals, 67–8
  Single modality interventions, 81–2
  young offender institutions (YOIs), 65–6
  young people's characteristics, 68–71
self-disclosure
  conceptual model, 348
  contextual-level factors, 349–51
  dispositional stance, 347–8
  individual-level factors, 348–9
  relational stance, 345–6
  relational–contextual approach, 351–4
  role of the practitioner psychologist, 344–5
self-harm
  assessment
    areas of, 235–6
    case study, 238–48
    client's response, 237–8
    intervention plan, 233–5
    use of tools, 236–7
  definition, 227–9
  disclosure context, 227
  practitioner psychologist's role, 226–7
  prevalence, 229–31
  psychological formulation, 233–5
  risk factors, 231–3
  social media and, 233
Sexually Harmful Adolescent Risk Protocol (SHARP), 104
sexually harmful behaviour
  adolescent perpetrators, 168–9
  assessment
    actuarial risk assessments (ARAs), 177
    AIM2 (Aim Project 2012), 178
    ERASOR, 177
    J-SOAP-II, 177
    MEGA, 177–8
  case study, 185–93
  challenges, practitioners, 193–5
  characteristics, 169–75
  definition, 168
  intervention

sexually harmful behaviour – *continued*
  AIM model, 179–81
  Good Lives Model (GLM), 181–2
  multi-systemic therapy – problem sexual behaviour (MST-PSB), 182–4
  restorative justice approaches, 184–5
  policies and legislation, 175–6
  risk factors, 169–75
  terminologies, 168
  underreporting, 167
Social and Behavioural Engagement Rating Scale (SABER), 383–4
Social Care Institute of Excellence (SCIE), 123
social learning theory, 55, 108, 133, 173
social psychology, 9, 13, 135
specific, measurable, attainable, relevant and time-bound (SMART) format, 274
Stalking Assessment Manual (SAM), 101
Strength and Difficulties Questionnaire (SDQ), 293
Structure, Positive, Empathy, Low Arousal, Links (SPELL) framework, 331
Structured Assessment of Violence Risk in Youth (SAVRY) tool, 70, 79, 103, 111–12, 151, 296, 307, 382
structured professional judgement (SPJ)
  Actuarial Risk Assessment (ARA) approach, 100
  case study, 110–11
  DART Framework, 372, 382
  fire-setting, 216
  formulation, 105–9
  key steps, 101–5
  limitation, 114
  risk assessment process, 14, 96, 295, 328, 369
substance misuse (SM)
  assessment
    comprehensive model, 266–8
    confidentiality, 268
    level and impact of use, 262–4
    motivation level, 265–6
    New Zealand, 261–2
    risk and safeguarding concerns, 264–5
  case study, 275–80
  criminality factors, 253

formulation, 269–70
intervention
  adolescent mentalisation-based integrative therapy (AMBIT), 273
  cognitive behaviour therapy (CBT), 270–1
  contingency management programmes (including MST-CM), 272
  dialectical behaviour therapy (DBT), 271
  multi-systemic therapy (MST), 271–2
  systemic/family-based interventions, 272–3
the UK context
  legal status, 258
  national policies, 258–61
  practice guidelines, 258–61
  prevalence, 256–7
  sentencing, 258
  service types, 253–6
treatment models
  development of formulation, 273–4
  goal focused, 274
  guiding principles, 273
  integrated therapeutic models, 274–5
  systemic involvement, 274
  youth justice system (YJS, in UK), 253–4, 256, 272–3
suicide, 23–4, 26, 31, 68, 71, 228–31, 237, 241–2, 244, 271, 350
Suicide Attempt Self-Injury Interview (SASII), 237
systemic theory, 14

theory of mind, 113–14, 298, 324–6, 328–9
trauma systems theory, 356
trauma theory, 359, 367, 374, 384

UN Convention on the Rights of the Child, 45, 176

violence among young people
  definition (violence), 144
  official crime statistics (USA and UK), 143
  risk factors, 149–51
  social-ecological model, 149–51

whole systems approach
  conduct problems, review of intervention, 123–5
  evidence-based interventions, implementation, 134–6
    challenges, 137
    feedback-informed services, 137–8
  evidence-based multi-systemic therapy, 125–7
  functional family therapy (FFT), 127–8
  multidimensional treatment foster care (MTFC), 133–4
  multisystemic therapy (MST), 128–30
    case example, 130–3
Winterbourne View Report, 305

young offender institutions (YOIs), 1, 64–6, 69, 72–3, 85, 88–9, 292, 323, 374
young people's needs
  with autism spectrum disorder (ASD), 331
  evidence-based intervention, 158
  with intellectual difficulties (ID), 298
  with mental health problems, 373–4
  psychologically informed system, 3–5, 76
  secure system 67–9
  youth justice system, 45–8
youth justice system (YJS), 2, 44–5, 68, 153, 253, 346
youth offending services (YOSs), 1, 14, 160, 256, 263, 322
youth violence risk assessment
  approaches
    actuarial risk assessment (ARA), 100–2, 104–5
    risk assessment checklist, 101
    unstructured clinical judgment (UCJ), 99–100
    structured professional judgment (SPJ), 96, 100–6, 110–11, 114

formulation models, 107–9
  case study, 110–17
  developmentally informed, 109
  systems informed, 109
  trauma informed, 109–10
  vulnerability informed, 110
homicide, international statistics, 96
protocols
  Assessment, Intervention and Moving-on Project (AIM) protocol, 102–4
  Asset protocol, 102, 104
  Early Assessment Risk List for Boys (EARL-20B), protocol, 103
  Early Assessment Risk List for Girls (EARL-20G), 103
  Estimate of Risk of Adolescent Sexual Offence Recidivism Version 2.0 (ERASOR), 103
  FACE – Child and Adolescent Risk Assessment Suite (FACE-CARAS), 104
  Internet-Assessment Intervention and Moving-on (I-AIM) protocol, 103
  Juvenile Sex Offender Assessment Protocol (J-SOAP-II), 103–4
  Multiplex Empirically Guided Inventory of Ecological Aggregates for Assessing Sexually Abusive Adolescents and Children (MEGA), 103
  Sexually Harmful Adolescent Risk Protocol (SHARP), 104
  Short-Term Assessment of Risk and Treatability: Adolescent Version (START: AV), 103
  Structured Assessment of Violence Risk in Youth (SAVRY), 103
relevant factors, 98–9
state intervention, 97–8
types of offences, 97

Printed and bound in Great Britain by
CPI Group (UK) Ltd, Croydon, CR0 4YY